ADOLESCENT PSYCHIATRY

DEVELOPMENTAL AND CLINICAL STUDIES

VOLUME VII

Annals of the American Society for Adolescent Psychiatry

ADOLESCENT PSYCHIATRY

DEVELOPMENTAL AND CLINICAL STUDIES

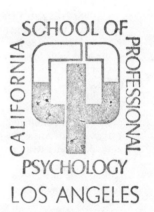

SCHOOL OF

CALIFORNIA PROFESSIONAL

PSYCHOLOGY

LOS ANGELES

VOLUME VII

Edited by
**SHERMAN C. FEINSTEIN
PETER L. GIOVACCHINI**

The University of Chicago Press
Chicago and London

The University of Chicago Press, Chicago 60637
The University of Chicago Press, Ltd., London

International Standard Book Number: 0-226-24052-5
Library of Congress Catalog Card Number: 70-147017

CONTENTS

PERSPECTIVES ON THE EFFECTS OF SOCIAL AND CULTURAL CHANGE
SIDNEY L. WERKMAN, Special Editor

PART III. PSYCHOPATHOLOGY AND ADOLESCENCE

PART IV. THERAPEUTIC APPROACHES IN ADOLESCENT PSYCHIATRY

PERSPECTIVES ON PSYCHOPHARMACOLOGY AND THE ADOLESCENT
ARTHUR D. SOROSKY, Special Editor

PART V. LEGAL AND PSYCHIATRIC PERSPECTIVES ON DELINQUENCY AND ACTING OUT
RICHARD C. MAROHN, Special Editor

PREFACE

The United Nations General Assembly declared 1979 the International Year of the Child to focus on the concerns for children and adolescents throughout the world and to celebrate the twentieth anniversary of the United Nations Declaration of the Rights of the Child. The American Society for Adolescent Psychiatry recognizes the rights and needs of young people and through its official publication, *Adolescent Psychiatry*, emphasizes the subtle interrelationships between current world political tides and the developmental and clinical studies with which we are occupied.

The papers in this seventh volume of the Annals of the American Society for Adolescent Psychiatry reflect the tumultuous occurrences of the recent past. It is amazing how many of these events are directly or indirectly related to adolescence. For example, we have seen the spread and felt the impact of various religious movements. The formation of such groups and the blind devotion that characterizes cults become subjects that have to be understood. Many of us suspect that the forces that are intrinsic to the adolescent processes are somehow involved in the reactions of masses to charismatic and in some instances dangerous and destructive leaders.

Obviously, the significance of these questions transcends a particular group; we have seen how such phenomena involve nations and threaten our civilization. Alongside an interest in what have been regarded as fringe movements has been a comparable preoccupation with the impact of geographical displacement, during and following the Vietnamese War, on adolescents and their families. Possibly, this represents an intuitive awareness of parallel constellations intrinsic to the microcosmic cult and macrocosmic tyranny. Here is an instance in which our clinical understanding can extend to global issues.

As clinicians, we have to continue directing our attention to our patients, and the papers dealing with both diagnostic and technical problems reflect such a focus. In the clinical area, this volume represents a natural continuation of previous volumes. Quite early in the history of this publication, clinical articles tended to deal with patients suffering from structural problems. This, undoubtedly, is related to the subject itself, the adolescent patient whose character structure is in a state of flux. Still, more is involved than the loose personality structure of adolescence in determining the types of patients that so many authors write about. Those adolescents, and adults as well, who find their way to psychiatrists' offices, increasingly reveal the manifestations of early developmental defects. We continue publishing papers concentrating on primitive fixations as seen, for example, in borderline patients in general and in this issue, delinquency, in particular. The emphasis is on serious psychopathology.

Perhaps we have created a full circle. The types of psychopathology we encounter may be typical of personalities that are especially susceptible to the omnipotent promises of religious and political leaders. There may be a reciprocal relationship between emotional illness and the formation of institutions that are congruent with the defensive adaptations of a large segment of the clinical population. It is unlikely that the basic structural problems of adolescence have substantially changed throughout the years. Some psychoanalysts have reevaluated Freud's early cases and were able to formulate them in terms of ego defects similar to those we often discover in our adolescent patients. If anything has changed, it is the manifestations of psychopathology. This would lead to the construction of new adaptive techniques which affect our culture and in turn our culture contributes to the further elaboration of coping mechanisms.

Thus, psychopathology and cataclysmic world conditions are, in some way, related. This is a subject which is much beyond our expertise as psychiatrists who treat adolescent patients. Still, our insights about the adolescent process will broaden our understanding and tolerance in many areas that are meaningful for numerous humanistic purposes.

SHERMAN C. FEINSTEIN
PETER L. GIOVACCHINI

PART I

ADOLESCENCE: GENERAL CONSIDERATIONS

EDITORS' INTRODUCTION

The chapters in this section always cover a large spectrum. This year we note a continuum from such global factors as modifications of a conceptual system, the psychoanalytic model, to focal issues such as the setting up of mental health consultation programs in high schools. There is no discernible point of convergence among these chapters. However, whether the topic is theoretical, clinical, or administrative, we note that the problems being discussed are meaningful to all of the frames of reference emphasized by the various authors. This again points to the fact that working in isolation, that is, parochially limiting oneself to just one viewpoint, has disadvantages. Our perspective is not constricted by blinders as we absorb ideas and experiences that, at first, seem to have no relevance to our interests. The creative mind constantly discovers relevance.

Peter Blos in a seminal essay outlines a theory of adolescence and clarifies his findings, which diverge from the usual psychoanalytical model. He discusses recapitulation theory and examines impeded ego development during latency owing to narcissistic fixations, completion of the Oedipus complex during adolescence rather than latency, and resolution of the negative Oedipus complex. He considers preoedipal vicissitudes and their impact on adolescence, the second individuation process, and its relevancy for an understanding of adolescent individuation with its regression in the service of development normative for adolescence. To be taken into consideration by clinicians are several suggestions about resistances and analytic treatment in adolescents.

Hilde Bruch defines the therapeutic task as helping the anorectic in

searching for autonomy and self-directed identity by evoking awareness of impulses, feelings, and needs. Therapeutic focus must be on
failure in self-expression, on the defective tools and concepts for organizing and expressing needs, and on the bewilderment in dealing
with others. A basic attitude of deep mistrust must be approached. The
anorectic thinks of herself as isolated on an island in a river, excluded
from joining the mainstream of life.

Saul V. Levine discusses the psychosocial needs of adolescents. He
writes that two factors are necessary: a belief system, and a sense of
belonging. The extent to which an external belief system and a sense of
belonging to a participating community exist in any social system will
by and large determine the success or failure of the program, the future
direction of the young person, and acceptance by the dominant society.

James S. Gordon reviews the historical impact of running away on
American society and the ambivalence with which it has been regarded. From being viewed as a social, economic, and moral offender,
the runaway began to be seen as a psychiatric casualty of adolescence,
a predictor of delinquency and psychopathology. In recent years this
pathological definition has given way to the view of running away as
part of a process of personal growth and social struggle, stimulated by
broken families, poverty, or cultural dislocation. Most adolescent
runaways feel pushed out or thrown away by their parents and society.
Gordon describes the development of the runaway house movement to
its current status as a community-based, multidisciplinary counseling
center where young people have the opportunity to redefine the meaning of running away from a stigmatized act into a catalyst for change in
the individual, the family, and the community.

Robert L. Arnstein traces the development of the concept of identity
crisis and examines the problems of transition to adulthood. He is
convinced that such transition requires emancipation from the family,
choice of a career or work, and the consolidation of a personal identity.
Containing both conscious and unconscious elements, late adolescence
allows a degree of conscious experimentation which allows partial
identifications with an eventual opportunity for a final choice. Arnstein
also believes societal influences can be a factor in the choice and
discusses several current trends.

Henry O. Kandler reviews the development of school consultation
as a dynamic system of interaction between mental health specialists
and the educational system involving individual evaluation and treat-

ment of students, psychoanalytically oriented supervision of school staff, and consultation based on expert knowledge and education. The consultant must understand the social structure, the methods of administration, and the power sources in order to be effective.

1   MODIFICATIONS IN THE CLASSICAL PSYCHOANALYTICAL MODEL OF ADOLESCENCE

PETER BLOS

The decades I have spent in clinical research of adolescence have resulted in the harvest of many findings: they encompass a body of knowledge—theoretical and practical—which I shall outline here in a systematic and comprehensive form. In doing so, I intend to clarify especially those of my findings which diverge from the familiar or widely accepted view of the adolescent process. My psychoanalytic investigations have always issued from clinical observations which presented me with intriguing problems of theory and technique due to their particularly perplexing nature. Whatever my clinical observations were at that time, they continued to sustain my attentiveness to comparative considerations along similar lines in other cases. An investigative approach of this nature leads either to a verification, to a revision, or to a rejection of whatever the theoretical inference might have been. In some instances, clinical observations have led to theoretical constructs and finally to propositions which, tested over time, have become part of my psychoanalytic thinking about adolescence. I am fully aware that much of what I shall lay before you in this presentation remains controversial and debatable for many of my colleagues. This fact is no deterrent to me but, rather, an incentive to report my findings, because I consider controversy a desirable and productive enterprise as long as it is rooted in the unique methodology of psychoanalytic observation.

Before I proceed, a word of caution is in order. I fear I might possibly convey the impression of not appreciating sufficiently the vast psychoanalytic research that has so immensely enriched our knowledge of the adolescent process. It is in many instances quite beyond my faculty to sort out authorship and origins and accord credit to the many suggestive and seminal ideas which, as by a quantum leap, coalesce in a new theorem. I owe more to what I have read and heard over time than I can possibly acknowledge by searching my memory most diligently. I have therefore omitted references altogether. In a chapter of this kind, in which I summarize my own thoughts, I must leave much of the referential associations to the reader. What gives me the courage to present an exclusively theoretical paper derives from my conviction that therapeutic advances in the field of psychological, emotional, and developmental disturbances have been always predicated on vigorous and often daring theory building. The history of psychoanalysis offers the most convincing evidence of this fact.

My presentation has one other shortcoming which I will announce before you discover it yourself with a sense of disappointment. This so-called shortcoming lies in the nature of my subject. Due to the broad theoretical scope which forms the framework of this essay, I had to forgo the customary inclusion of illustrative case material. This can be found in the various papers the essence of which I reformulate here in order to weave them into the fabric of the current theory of adolescence. I suggest that you review in your mind's eye your own cases alongside my exposition.

The issue I shall discuss first concerns the psychoanalytic recapitulation theory of adolescence. According to this view, the revival of infantile sexuality and of the vicissitudes of early object relations is initiated by the biological event of puberty. In accordance with the classical recapitulation theory, the revival and renewed resolution or transformation of the Oedipus complex represents one, if not *the*, essential aspect of the adolescent process. It is beyond doubt that oedipal issues emerge at adolescence with regularity. However, we must acknowledge the fact that a decisive expansion of the ego has accrued from middle childhood, that is, latency, which has altered, qualitatively and quantitatively, the reexperience of the oedipal conflict on the adolescent level. The resourcefulness of the adolescent ego is able to cope with the revival of infantile object relations in consonance with bodily maturation, thus bringing the state of infantile dependencies to a close. This achievement usually, if not always, contains rectifications or resolutions of conflicts or immaturities which were carried forward from the infantile period to the adolescent level. In this sense we speak of adolescence as a "second chance." This normative developmental advance is forfeited whenever the child fails to acquire the appropriate ego differentiation or ego supremacy during the latency period.

What I have foremost in mind when I speak of an impeded ego development during latency refers to drive fixations on the level of infantile narcissism. Consequently, oedipal passions remain weak, their conflict resolution incomplete, and the superego never gains the autonomous sway over infantile self-idealization that is preconditional for the entry into the latency period. Looking at this constellation from the side of the ego, one would refer to the fact that no clear or stable line of demarcation between fantasy and reality has become part of the latency ego structure, thus stunting the ego's capacity to assess self and object critically. "I am what I do" becomes facilely replaced by "I am what I wish to be" or "I am what others think I am." Under these conditions it is only natural that the voice of the self-observing ego remains weak, contradictory, or silent. The repercussion of this state on reality testing, especially in the world of object relations, never fails to alert the clinical observer to a developmental anomaly. However, one cannot ignore the fact that, regardless of drive fixation and ego immaturity, some latency children are capable of the most remarkable cognitive and creative achievements, the defensive nature of which does not reveal itself until adolescence.

What follows from such a developmental lag is an abortive adolescence or a failure in the autonomous mastery of internal, disequilibrating tensions and in the capacity to use selectively the social surround in terms of sublimatory and identificatory adaptations. Under these circumstances, the social field fails to acquire an age-relevant presence on which to articulate the emerging needs for new object relations beyond the family matrix. Consequently, new object relations within the peer group show the characteristics of simple object substitutions rather than those of elaborated replacements. In other words, adolescent development takes its normative course only if the latency ego has progressed along age-adequate developmental lines. Considering adolescent therapy, it follows that latency ego deficits often demand our attention above all else, even though sexual and dependency conflicts occupy the forefront of the behavioral and mental stage. While such conflicts are real enough, they have to be scrutinized as to their defensive aims which push these conflictual, typically adolescent themes into the forefront of the patient's awareness.

I shall now pursue another strand of the recapitulation theory of adolescence. I refer to the implication that the resolution of the Oedipus complex has brought about the closure of the phallic phase, thereby structuring the superego and ushering in the latency period. With the advent of adolescence, the conflicts of the phallic phase are resuscitated due to the biological condition of physical maturation and the human-specific incest taboo. From my work with adolescents— male and female—I have gained the impression that the decline of the Oedipus complex at the end of the phallic phase represents a suspension of a conflictual constellation rather than a definitive resolution. Because we can ascertain its continuation on the adolescent level, the resolution of the Oedipus complex is completed—not just repeated— during adolescence. It should be made explicit at this point that I refer to both the positive and the negative components when speaking of the Oedipus complex in general.

My attention was directed to the above considerations by clinical observations, namely, by the fact that the negative Oedipus complex presents a most difficult therapeutic problem in the treatment of the adolescent. I had not observed a similar severity, marked by stubborn repression and denial, in the analysis of most children. The love for the parent of the opposite sex is always intensified during adolescence. However, a distinction, even if obvious, needs to be made at this point. The term "oedipal love" implicitly refers to the sexual component of infantile object relations, in contrast to feelings of affection, admiration, and loyalty which never cease to flow—ambivalently and reciprocally—between the child and both parents. My clinical observations concerning the negative Oedipus complex lead me to the conclusion that oedipal love, directed toward both mother and father, does not burden the young child with intrinsic contradictions or mutual exclusiveness, as is the case in adolescence when the polarities of masculinity and femininity reign supreme. Their coexistence cannot be tolerated by the sexually maturing individual. In other words, the state of bisexuality is tolerated in the prelatency child without the catastrophic disharmony at puberty. It is the positive Oedipus complex which falls under repression or finds its resolution through identification and the regulatory influence of the superego at the termination of the phallic phase. It remains the task of adolescent oedipal resolution to transmute the negative Oedipus complex, the sexual love for the parent of the same sex.

Clinically, this aspect of the oedipal constellation appears at adolescence in a paradoxical disguise that is in evidence whenever a drive fixation on the negative oedipal position is interwoven with symptom formation or characterological defenses. Such pathological development is often not recognizable on first sight, especially when the adolescent pushes heterosexual behavior and fantasies into the center of his therapy sessions or of his life in general. The urgency of and the preoccupation with sexual affects and desires during adolescence are familiar to us. In fact, their attendant conflicts, anxieties, and defenses play a large part in our interpretative work. It has been my experience that, alongside the adolescent effort to reach a heterosexual identity, we have also to reckon with an intrinsically defensive element that aims at keeping the conflict of the negative oedipal love in repression. I have called this adolescent maneuver the oedipal defense.

If you contemplate for a moment your therapeutic work with the male adolescent (of middle and late adolescence), I think you will agree with me when I say that it is, relatively speaking, less laborious to deal with the defenses against sexual and erotic fantasies and feelings in relation to mother or sister than to father or brother. The affects directed toward the female remain in the realm of a gender-appropriate position and are ego syntonic. In contrast, the uncovering of the negative oedipal fixation leads inescapably into the realm of homosexuality, latent or manifest, and into the center of sexual identity problems. Should these remain unaltered by the adolescent process we might speak of a secondary adolescent fixation. In that case, the adolescent choice of defense will determine the adult character consolidation, and, due to the unaltered infantile libidinal position, this fixation engenders adult love life with disharmonious affects and moods. The dread, horror, and ego-dystonic nature of homosexuality or perversion is often voiced quite directly by the adolescent girl or boy and constitutes in many cases the first productive approach to the problem of sexual identity.

It might now be stated: since the resolution of the negative Oedipus complex is the task of adolescence, the coming to terms with the homosexual component of pubertal sexuality is an implicit developmental task of adolescence. In fact, we might say that sexual identity formation is predicated on the completion of this process. Our adolescent patients display always the twofold oedipal strivings because the incompatibility of their heterogenous objects and aims brings the maturing individual up against an either-or of decisive finality.

I would like to remind you of a common adolescent complaint, namely, the sense of vocational indecision or noncommitment, or floundering or academic failure in college. These problems are frequently adjuncts of a symptom complex we are called on to unravel. On first sight, defeats of this nature look like oedipal inhibitions, especially whenever a boy sets out to follow in the vocational footsteps of his father or, generally, when the young person feels called upon to fulfill the ambitions which one or both parents harbor for their offspring. The oedipal factor plays, no doubt, a decisive role. But in juxtaposition to it—as we see in so many cases of gifted boys—operates the infantile trend of renouncing oedipal competition and envy in exchange for the regressive contentment derived from standing in the glow of shining grandeur that radiates from the imago of the oedipal father. In this way, the small boy once experienced the pleasures—pervasive but hardly acknowledged—of the submissive passive position. In this connection we must remember that every boy had once—fleetingly or more lastingly—identified with the role of the envied and admired procreative woman, the mother. I have observed how these trends in the small boy become pathologically aggravated when the father, disillusioned in his conjugal life, shifts his need for emotional fulfillment from his wife to his son.

Whenever I hear a father say in the consultation that precedes treatment, "The only one I love in this world is my son," I feel alerted to the central complex of the patient. Having followed such cases in treatment, I was repeatedly impressed by the emergence of the Janus-faced oedipal passions and of the alternating conflicts they inexorably contain. Should the conflicts which are attached to the incest taboo and bisexuality remain beyond resolution, the adolescent patient protects himself by a stubborn denial of any self-limitation, that grave affront to narcissism. We see here, once again, how ego maturation takes its cue from drive maturation. How intrinsically social facilitations are part of this process should be self-evident. However, it needs emphasizing in this context that the use the individual is able to make of such facilitations remains predicated on drive and ego maturation or, in other words, on the unimpeded forward movement of the adolescent process.

We have reached the point in this presentation where it behooves us to contemplate some inherent puzzlements which issue from the foregoing propositions. Let me give you an account of the questions which I had asked myself. Psychoanalytic theory has shown us in great clarity the course which the positive oedipal attachment follows from early childhood through adolescence to adulthood. All along this course, there remains one unaltered characteristic, namely, its implicit gender appropriateness; the object remains one of the opposite sex. We have come to consider gender polarity along the shift from infantile to adult sexuality as a developmental axiom. Some amendments, however, become plausible and exigent when we follow the developmental course of the negative oedipal constituent. Its sex-inappropriate nature is bound to reach an impasse at puberty when sexual maturation can no longer accommodate infantile negative oedipal strivings. Obviously, there is no displacement of these object-directed drive components available within the sexual identity whose definitive structure is acquired during adolescence. One might relegate the transformation of the drive component under consideration entirely to neutralized—that is, desexualized—emotional attitudes, to character traits, and to sublimatory endeavors. This would be the logic by which the classical psychoanalytic theory explicates the resolution of the negative Oedipus complex; the implicit dynamics of these transformations are by now taken as self-evident in the light of clinical experience.

The schema just outlined has only partially been borne out in my analytic work with adolescents. I have found it necessary to postulate an intermediate step in the process. Freud's (1914) ideas concerning narcissism and ego ideal are here brought to bear on the adolescent process. If you permit me, I shall present a condensed version of the proposition which my clinical observations have suggested and confirmed over the years. The negative oedipal attachment is a narcissistic object tie ("I love what I wish to be"). At adolescence, the libido invested in this tie becomes desexualized and, thus, initiates the narcissistic structure of the adult ego ideal. From an adaptational or psychosocial point of view one might speak of this process as the socialization of oedipal narcissism. At the adolescent junction I speak of, the infantile ego ideal of self-aggrandizement, as an always attainable gratification and self-esteem regulator, becomes transformed into the adult ego ideal, which constitutes a drive toward perfection. The infantile belief in the realizability of perfection becomes replaced during late adolescence by the drive toward its approximation. Thus, it becomes a journey without arrival. Its intention and direction are ego syntonic and always unequivocal; by implication, there is no place for doubt or thought. Whatever the edict that emanates from the adult ego ideal, it is self-evident to the rational mind as well as to the emotional being. Should this not be the case, we very likely deal with superego issues which so often resemble those of the ego ideal. This dubious accountability is one more reason for outlining differentiating criteria which lie beyond the well-known reactions of guilt or shame as indicative of superego or ego ideal neglect.

The above thoughts are derived from clinical observations which demonstrated to me that the resolution of the negative oedipal conflict in adolescent analysis effects a personality change of a particular nature; we recognize these changes in an emerging self-determination, in a projection of the self into a realistic adult life, and, last but not least, in the tolerance of self-limitations. The intrinsic precondition for this developmental advance to adulthood lies in the deidealization of self and object or, in more general terms, in the acceptance of life's existential imperfections. These budding characteristics, which stood in such marked contrast to the patient's preanalytic life, became to me trustworthy indicators of the adult ego ideal in *statu nascendi*. I credited the decline and paling influence of the infantile ego ideal or, conversely, the emergence and structuralization of the adult ego ideal to the analytic work which had brought about the resolution of the negative Oedipus complex. The dynamics of this structural innovation of adolescence lead me to say that the adult ego ideal is the heir to the negative Oedipus complex.

An adolescent issue of overriding importance centers on the alternation of regressive and progressive movements which last over a considerable time of adolescent growth. We are accustomed to recognize in regressive phenomena a normative adolescent characteristic. A shift in emphasis, however, has been noticeable ever since infant research has so vastly extended our knowledge of the preoedipal child. The reflection of earliest structure formation in the adolescent process has become an integral aspect of adolescent psychology. The vicissitudes of preoedipal object relations and the varied traumatizations of normal childhood are, to a great extent, offset as to their noxious potential by subsequent ego development and structural stabilizations. However, they never can be discounted in their effect on the oedipal stage, its formation, conflict, and resolution. There is no doubt that preoedipal components have increasingly attracted our attention in the treatment of the adolescent child.

Viewing this development from the vantage point of adolescence, I

13

have referred to it as the second individuation process. One crucial developmental advance to be accomplished at adolescence deals with the self-divestiture of infantile dependencies. They are, at this advanced stage, of an internalized nature and referred to as object representations or imagoes. Should they be persistently externalized or projected onto the outer world during adolescence, the disengagement from infantile dependency objects is thwarted or precluded. This kind of adolescent pathology is well known to us. In the first—the infantile—stage of individuation the young child gains relative independence from the physical presence of the mother through internalization. Once the small child has acquired a representational imagery of its surround, physical and emotional, his maturational potential, motoric, sensory, and cognitive, dashes forward into an outburst of new faculties and masteries.

I have paid explicit attention to the individuation process of infancy because of its relevancy for an understanding of adolescent individuation. The first step in infancy accomplishes a relative independence from external objects, while the second—namely, the adolescent step of individuation—aims at the independence from internalized infantile objects. Only when this last process is completed can childhood be transcended and adulthood attained. This internal change comes about through the normative adolescent regression which is nondefensive; due to this fact I have called it regression in the service of development. At no other developmental stage, except, perhaps, at Mahler, Pine, and Bergman's (1975) rapprochement subphase (pp. 76–108), is regression an obligatory condition of growth. It is by way of nondefensive regression that the adolescent comes in contact with lingering infantile dependencies, anxieties, and needs. These are now revisited with an ego equipment infinitely more resourceful, stable, and versatile than the one which the small child had at its disposal.

The ego of this advanced stage is, as a rule, sufficiently reality bound to forestall a regressive engulfment within the undifferentiated stage, namely, in a stage of ego loss or psychosis. It is a well-known fact that the adolescent process and psychotic illness are related by a developmental risk which, in my opinion, lies in the individual's capacity to keep the nondefensive regression of this age within bounds—that is, staying this side of the undifferentiated stage. It is only through a delimited regression that infantile object dependencies can be overcome. It remains a constant query for the therapist to differentiate between what in the clinical picture is defensive regression, causing developmental arrest and symptom formation, and what is regression in the service of development, which we have come to identify as a prerequisite for progressive development to take its course and sustain its momentum. I know that the chaotic and inconsistent behavior of the adolescent often defies our wish for clear-cut differentiations, but I also know that relevant clues are forthcoming if the clinician's patience and attentiveness do not grow weary.

These deliberations of preoedipality in relation to adolescent psychic restructuring permit me to say that the preoedipal stage of object relations rivals the oedipal stage in their respective contributions to adolescent personality formation. However, there are good reasons to designate the oedipal stage as the *primum inter pares*, because—at that particular juncture—a forward step in psychic organization has been reached which reflects an entirely new—namely triadic—complexity of conflictual object relations. Their resolution is memorialized in the definitive structure of the superego. Within this developmental context we speak of the phase-specific infantile neurosis which is self-liquidating in the normal course of development. Whenever neurotic psychopathology prevails in childhood or adolescence, we can be certain that preoedipal traumatic remnants have been carried forward and have worked their way into oedipal formations.

As a common example I mention the "abandonment malaise" of the adolescent who tells us in endless variations of his conviction that "nothing will ever work out in his or her love relationship," or that he or she "will never accomplish anything the world needs, admires, and loves." Encouraging beginnings always fall apart.

The roots of such dysphoric moods are of preoedipal origin, even though we usually encounter them amalgamated with oedipal anxiety, guilt, and inhibitions. Excessive indulgences, such as the overeating of the adolescent girl or drug use in both sexes, point to preoedipal fixations, even though a pseudo-oedipal stance is often forcefully and frantically displayed. From clinical work we have learned that the persistent, irrepressible psychic irritants of a preoedipal nature make their appearance in treatment, demanding therapeutic interventions able to reach the primitive emotions and infantile needs which appear in all kinds of sophisticated disguises. In practice, the treatment strategy veers constantly between preoedipal and oedipal realms, while the therapist attempts to relate both to the adolescent's present life situation or the other way round. The respective vehicles of these efforts are—in ascending levels of abstraction—advice, judgment, explanation, interpretation, and reconstruction. Preoedipal components in adolescent therapy often lie concealed behind the patient's guarded, critical, and suspicious attitude or behind his unshakably trusting expectancy of the good life which the therapist will deliver. A precious sense of security and safety derives from being part of an idealized object, the preoedipal mother, reified in the person of the therapist. Parenthetically I might mention that fathers as idealized maternal imagoes appear more frequently in contemporary adolescent patients than in those of the past, because many more parents now share the caretakership of their small children. Be this as it may, the revival of the idealized parent imago in the person of the therapist demands a most delicate work of actuating object deidealization. What, at best, is the outcome of this process we refer to as trust, the bedrock of the therapeutic alliance.

The adolescent patient needs to be exposed—gradually and repeatedly—to a disillusionment in self and object. Over time, this leads to a tolerance of imperfection, first in the object and finally extending to the self. How difficult and painful the process of deidealization of object and self is for the adolescent never ceases to impress me. Indeed, I feel inclined to say that the process of deidealization of object and self represents the single most distressful and tormenting aspect of growing up—if any such generalization can be made. The magnitude of this step at adolescence is comparable to the Copernican revolution which deprived man of his place in the center of the universe, a truly sobering, existential awareness. Having made this cosmic analogy, I might mention in passing that not until adolescence does a true sense for the tragic emerge as implicit in the acceptance of the human condition. In contrast, the young child tends to fix blame and experiences feelings of sadness, fright, anger, or abandonment. Mourning follows a different pathway before and after the second individuation and the deidealization of self and object, both of which are completed during adolescence. For the work of mourning to take its course, the attainment of what I shall call mature ambivalence is essential; otherwise, a split in the ego of the postadolescent personality occurs. This state will preserve a split between the acceptance and the nonrecognition of the finality of death. The irreconcilability of these positions threatens the cohesiveness of the psychic organism and disables the ego's integrative function in all aspects of life.

We have arrived at a fitting moment to relate a pertinent piece of psychoanalytic history. Freud's (1905) "Fragment of an Analysis of a

Case of Hysteria'' is a time-honored specimen of oedipal pathology in a late-adolescent girl by the name of Dora. The very diagnosis of hysteria epitomizes a sexual conflict characteristic of this neurotic illness. The patient's symptoms—in this case conversion symptoms—reflect the pathological elaborations of an unresolved virulent Oedipus complex at adolescence. The case history portrays in greatest clarity how the affective and sexual conflicts of Dora's love for her father became fatefully interwoven with the life of a married couple, Mr. K and Mrs. K, who were friends of her family. Dora's father had started an affair with Mrs. K, whose husband, Mr. K, was enamored of Dora, then an adolescent girl of sixteen. At eighteen Dora started treatment with Freud. How ingeniously Freud pieced together the details of fact and fantasy, conscious and unconscious, in the course of the treatment is too well known to require any comment here.

When Dora suddenly disrupted the analysis after three months' duration, Freud searched for the emotional currents that had caused this impetuous action. What further puzzled Freud was the unsatisfactory relief from symptoms, despite the clarifications and interpretations he had offered the patient and which, undoubtedly, were correct. What was amiss in the work that left it incomplete on two accounts? As to the disruption, Freud concluded that "I did not succeed in mastering the transference in good time" (p. 118). Dora—a hysteric of eighteen—might well have responded to the objective detailed discussions of sexual matters of the greatest delicacy as she had done once before to the seductive intimacy of Mr. K, from whom she fled in panic and vengefulness.

Be this as it may, it is quite another aspect of the case history I want to bring to your attention. This aspect concerns the preoedipal fixation on the dyadic relationship which, on the oedipal level, lead to the revival and the subsequent repression of the negative oedipal tie. A fixation on this preoedipal attachment, when resuscitated at adolescence, is frequently silenced—in life as well as in treatment—by the diversionary display of heterosexual wishes, actions, conflicts, and agitations. I have alluded to both these issues in my antecedent discussion (1) of the normative homosexual conflict in relation to adolescent sexual identity formation, and (2) of a specific adolescent reaction which I have termed the oedipal defense. By quoting from the Dora case I wish to demonstrate the fact that Freud was fully aware of both these issues, but kept them confined in his commentary on the case. He never alluded to them in treatment, but pursued with single-minded pertinacity the positive oedipal theme, namely, the acting out of Dora's wish for and rejection of Mr. K's attempted seduction (p. 25). In fact, the case has been—and still is—read without attributing to preoedipal issues the general developmental validity which they deserve in adolescent pathology.

While working on the Dora paper, Freud wrote to Fliess (Freud 1954, letter 141, p. 326) that in the case at hand "the chief issue in the conflicting mental processes is the opposition between an inclination towards men and towards women" in an adolescent girl. When Dora declared (Freud 1905), after her conflict was thoroughly analyzed, that she "can't forgive him [father] for it [affair with Mrs. K]" (p. 54) and added "I can think of nothing else" (p. 54), Freud concluded that "this excessively intense train of thought must owe its reinforcement to the unconscious" (p. 54). This comment he clarified by saying: "For behind Dora's supervalent train of thought which was concerned with her father's relations with Frau K there lay concealed a feeling of jealousy which had that lady as its *object* [*sic*]—a feeling, that is, which could only be based upon an affection on Dora's part for one of her own sex" (p. 60). Freud concluded that the girl was jealous of her father and not of his mistress; in other words, she wished to be the object of the woman's love.

Freud views this attachment in the context of adolescent boys and girls who show "clear signs, even in normal cases, of the existence of an affection for people of their own sex" (p. 60). Once more, in the postscript, Freud returns to this crucial and central complex in Dora's pathology; here we read: "I failed to discover in time and to inform the patient that her homosexual (gynaecophilic) love for Frau K was the strongest unconscious current in her mental life" (p. 120). With these thoughts in mind, the two dreams, especially the second (pp. 94–111), in which the Sistine Madonna figures prominently as an association (p. 96), might be understood differently in terms of that "strongest unconscious current in her mental life."

The two women Dora had loved finally betrayed her. The girl discovered that "she was being admired and fondly treated by her governess not for her own sake but for her father's" (p. 61). As a repetition of this, Frau K, with whom "the scarcely grown girl had lived for years on a feeling of the closest intimacy . . . had not loved her for her own sake but on account of her father" (pp. 61–62).

Dora's thwarted love for both women became forcefully removed from her conscious affective life, while the heterosexual drive was histrionically pushed into the forefront of her mind. Freud refers to this as "noisy demonstrations to show that she grudged her [Mrs. K] the possession of her father; and in this way she concealed from herself the contrary fact, which was that she grudged her father Frau K's love" (p. 63). With scientific objectivity Freud states that he will not "go any further in to this important subject . . . because Dora's analysis came to an end before it could throw any light on this side of her mental life" (p. 60).

In a final opinion of this case, which for a long time has typified the psychopathology of repressed heterosexual libido, Freud stated that the mortification in the betrayal of the two women whose maternal love Dora craved "touched her, perhaps, more nearly and had a greater pathogenic effect than the other case, which she tried to use as a screen for it—the fact that she had been sacrificed by her father" (p. 62). These realizations came too late or were postponed too long to have benefited the patient.

I must confess that I myself did not read the Dora paper in the present light until I had become aware through my own clinical work of those concepts which I have presented earlier in this paper. Even though Freud has stated in the Dora case such contingent observations and conclusions which I endeavored to highlight, these were never systematically incorporated in the classical psychoanalytic theory of adolescence. While I present my own conceptualizations about adolescent development in this chapter, I also want to show that some of them were contained *in nuce* in the Dora paper. To do homage to Freud's genius, I have presented a neglected aspect of the Dora case, hoping to stimulate its rereading with an altered and broadened focus of attention.

The revisitation of the Dora case lends itself to the introduction of a topic which I have explored for many years. I refer to my efforts to trace the divergent developmental lines in male and female adolescence, sorting out, as it were, their inherent similarities and intrinsic differences. I shall not dwell on the male and female oedipal constellation because it is a topic so well known and so firmly established that it needs no comment here. However, some words about the preoedipal period of both sexes are in order, because the reverberations of these early object relations determine to such a large extent the adolescent-specific relations to male and female, to people generally, to the world at large, and to abstract thought and to the self.

From therapeutic work with adolescent girls and young women we know of the powerful regressive pull to the preoedipal mother, leading to symptom formation and acting out. Overeating and nibbling are common enough habits. When the girl goes through the preadolescent phase we recognize in her object relations the regressively revived imagoes of the good and the bad mother. The reflections of this phase appear in merger fantasies and violent distancing behavior. Their enmeshment with oedipal issues is always part of the clinical picture. However, the infantile tie to the mother remains for the girl a lasting source of ambivalence and ambiguity because it contains by its very nature homosexual components; these are bound to be reinforced by puberty. We always discover in the heterosexual behavior of the adolescent girl—especially the young adolescent girl—a twofold aim: one leads to the gratification of infantile tactile-contact hunger, while the other seeks to strengthen the girl's still infirm sexual identity. Both these aims are entangled in the young adolescent girl's—initially defensive—attachment to the opposite sex. Her advance to adult genitality occurs only gradually and often remains incomplete without, however, necessarily endangering the healthy personality integration of the woman.

The future capacity and pleasure in mothering is, to a large extent, facilitated by the mature female's unconflicted and open access to the integrated good-bad mother imagoes. Adolescent emotional development determines the outcome toward this end in a decisive way. In my opinion, there is no treatment of the adolescent girl in which the features of the regressive pull and the ambivalence struggle with the early mother are not issues of central importance. We can always detect in the woman the remnants of that primordial love in her relations to members of her own sex. The fact that the girl, but not the boy, has in later life to change the gender of the first love and hate object, the mother, renders the psychological development of the girl more complex than that of the boy.

In contrast, the boy's infantile tie to the early mother remains sexually polarized throughout the phase of adolescent regression and, consequently, is a source of conflict essentially different from that of the adolescent girl. The girl tends to extricate herself from the regressive pull toward merger by a forward rush into the oedipal stage. The small boy, on the other hand, normally goes through a stage when the fear of the archaic castrating mother—the original caretaker and organizer of all infantile body functions—forms the nucleus of the male's apprehensiveness vis-à-vis the woman. This is most convincingly demonstrated during male preadolescence, when we observe this apprehensiveness in either the avoidance of the opposite sex and hostility toward women in general or in the sexual bravado of juvenile machismo. These conflicts of early childhood and adolescence, universal as they are, never cease to affect the relations between the sexes throughout life. As an aside, I call your attention to the statistically well-known facts about adolescent incest. Besides oedipal components, incest for the adolescent girl is a defense against maternal merger, while incest for the adolescent boy represents merger and ego dissolution within the undifferentiated stage, namely psychosis. Here lies the reason for the fact that incest of the adolescent girl is a more frequent occurrence than incest of the adolescent boy. For the girl incest is not necessarily linked to personality disintegration, while incest of the adolescent boy remains a most rare occurrence and the boy proves invariably to be psychotic.

The preoedipal element in the Dora case, which I lifted from the larger context of Freud's reconstructions, has by now gathered enough clinical evidence to be looked at in the light of a typical adolescent regressive paradigm. We must attribute, therefore, a normative character to the reworking at adolescence of both preoedipal and oedipal stages of development. With the growing recognition that analytic work encompasses legitimately preverbal mental content, the intrinsic role of preoedipality in adolescent therapy or in the normative adolescent process has to be reconsidered as well. This is to say that in every oedipal pathology we will discover precursors from the preoedipal stage of development; these have to be identified and dealt with in therapy. This work is usually done in conjunction with oedipal issues and ego problems because they have all become enmeshed with each other in a comprehensive pathological formation by the time adolescence is reached. If we take for granted that preoedipal regression is normative for adolescence, this fact presents a particular problem for the clinician who treats adolescents.

Preoedipal fixations have become identified with borderline conditions, a diagnostic category of established validity. However, in the assessment of adolescent preoedipal regression, it seems to me, an essential differentiation must be established. Within the framework of adolescent regression we might recognize a belated developmental forward thrust toward the triadic or oedipal level, or, in contrast, regression might reveal a retrograde pathogenic pull to the dyadic stage of early infancy. The testing ground for these relativities which are of such critical consequence for the outcome of the adolescent process, and for adolescent therapy generally, lies in the realm of the transference. Speaking broadly, the dependent preoedipal needfulness of some adolescents can be of such elemental nature that only a limited developmental progression can be attained in treatment, and that mainly through identification. Such a benign alteration of an archaic introject is no minor achievement. In contrast, the adolescent who has become able, through trust and insight, to tolerate in the therapeutic situation the frustrations and thwarted expectations, with all their attendant affects of aggression and guilt, tells us by this very fact that he has reached the level of oedipal conflict. The differentiation between developmental arrest and developmental conflict is only too often not as clearly distinguishable at first sight during assessment and initial therapy as we wish it were. This ambiguity defines an area into which adolescent research might profitably move.

Earlier in this presentation I developed a clinical rationale for stating that the Oedipus complex, in its positive aspect, undergoes a resolution, normal or abnormal, before the latency period can set in, but that the negative Oedipus complex reaches a conflictual crisis and undergoes a resolution, normal or abnormal, not until adolescence. This is to say that we might speak of a two-timed or biphasic oedipal resolution, one in early childhood and one at adolescence. Of course, the influences of both on the ensuing nature of adult object relations are always interwoven and cannot be neatly isolated; the best one can do is to speak of preponderances, dominances, and idiosyncratic urgencies in relation to the respective residues from preoedipal and oedipal resolutions. Since the normality of adult object relations hinges fatefully on these resolutions and, since such basic elements of the personality as, for example, the adult sense of self, sexual identity, and the adult ego ideal are determined by the totality—that is, positive *and* negative oedipal resolutions—this issue deserves our most thoughtful attention.

The proposition that the totality of the oedipal crisis has not passed until the adolescent process is completed leads to the conclusion that the termination of childhood coincides with the closure of adolescence. It is not just a matter of speech to declare adolescence to be the terminal stage of childhood, after which the stage of adulthood asserts itself. Let me pursue just one line of reasoning that rests on the above proposition and has a bearing on our clinical work.

If—as we have postulated—the resolution of the Oedipus complex in its totality is biphasic, then we must conclude that the infantile neurosis represents a psychic formation which obviously excludes the adolescent-specific oedipal conflict with the parent of the same sex and its resolution as well. These considerations lead me to conclude that the "definitive neurosis"—using Freud's words—is a psychic formation that can only reach its final and lasting structure during the terminal stage of childhood, namely, during the consolidation stage of late adolescence. At this stage, then, the adult neurosis, the definitive neurosis, consolidates as an integral aspect of psychic structuralization which heralds the closure of adolescence.

These theoretical conclusions were derived from clinical observation in cases of late adolescents whose symptoms were due to internalized conflicts, therefore constituting, by definition, a neurosis. What I observed in the analysis of these older adolescents were stubborn resistances which failed to yield to any kind of intervention until they vanished without any cause for which I could claim credit. After having observed this problem for some time, I came to the conclusion that the patient's apparent disinterest in or retreat from the therapeutic engagement revealed a particular kind of psychodynamic which diverges from the standard definition of resistance. If this kind of psychological distancing or uncommunicative self-absorption is treated as a resistance, the effect is nil. In other words, if repeated interpretations, referring to so-called inner dangers of which the transference reaction is one, remain ineffectual, we might well look for other determinants. The distraction, so it seemed to me, was attributable to internal organizing processes structuring or consolidating the definitive neurosis. At such times it appears unavoidable that patient and therapist are at cross-purposes. The patient is engaged in the structuralization of his neurotic complexes, while the therapist is eager to cure the disturbance which brought the patient to his office. Paradoxically, analytic cure can be accomplished best with neurotic formations whose incubation time inhibits the therapist from keeping up his work. Resorting to resistance interpretations is a common attempt to overcome such stalemated situations. Of course, dynamic or genuine resistances never fail to appear alongside those I have set apart as typical of the consolidation period of late adolescence. I am far from suggesting that these developmental occurrences speak for a counterindication of analysis because, regardless of the silent work of neurosogenesis at late adolescence, therapy proceeds, working its way from the surface to the depth as usual. What I introduce here is a modification in the understanding of the resistance dynamics in the analytic treatment of the late adolescent.

Conclusions

The therapeutic issues outlined are typical for adolescence; they are quite familiar to us from child therapy. Due to the adolescent's physical status, desires, ambitions, and social roles we tend to align the adolescent, especially the older adolescent, with the adult and see him as an adult manqué. I can report from decades of supervision that the therapist who is at home in the treatment of children usually orients himself with greater ease in the world of the adolescent than the therapist whose therapeutic work has been preponderantly with adults.

One further thought, implicit in the foregoing developmental considerations, should be made explicit at this point. Speaking of the consolidation stage of late adolescence, it should be understood that at this stage psychic structures acquire a high degree of irreversibility. They lose, so to say, that unique fluidity or elasticity of childhood which facilitates, as late as adolescence, adaptive corrections of the past. The structural stabilization at the closure of adolescence is epitomized by the finality of character formation. This acquisition of the late adolescent personality marks the passing of childhood or, in common parlance, of adolescence. I assume, therefore, on the basis of all that was said, that adolescence cannot remain an open-ended developmental stage. Adolescent closure follows the epigenetic law of development; like all other stages of childhood, adolescence also loses its developmental momentum, regardless of whether the tasks or challenges of this period have been fulfilled. Adolescent closure occurs at a biologically and culturally determined time, be this in a normal or abnormal manner. It seems to belong to the laws of development that fixation points at any stage are carried forward into the next developmental stage, thus keeping alive an ongoing effort of the ego at the harmonization of sensitivities, vulnerabilities, and idealizations that make up the essence of each individual self. In this sense we can say, quoting Wordsworth, "The child is father of the man."

REFERENCES

Freud, S. 1905. Fragment of an analysis of a case of hysteria. *Standard Edition* 7:15–122. London: Hogarth, 1953.

Freud, S. 1914. On narcissism: an introduction. *Standard Edition* 14:73–102. London: Hogarth, 1957.

Freud, S. 1954. *The Origins of Psychoanalysis: Letters to Wilhelm Fliess, Drafts and Notes: 1887–1902.* New York: Basic.

Mahler, M. S.; Pine, F.; and Bergman, A. 1975. *The Psychological Birth of the Human Infant.* New York: Basic.

2   ISLAND IN THE RIVER: THE ANOREXIC ADOLESCENT IN TREATMENT

HILDE BRUCH

Anorexia nervosa is an extremely complex illness, much more than merely dieting out of hand. Its true beginning is a child's passive participation in life, absorbing from the world without actively integrating anything. The relationship to the parents appears superficially to be congenial; actually it is too close, without necessary separation, individuation, and differentiation. This harmony is achieved through excessive conformity on the part of the child.

When, with adolescence, positive self-assertion becomes unavoidable, when an attitude of fitting-in is no longer appropriate, the severe deficiencies in the core personality become apparent. These youngsters fail to take the step toward more independent cognitive operations and continue to look at the world with the preoperational, concrete views of early childhood. They interpret the cultural demand for slenderness and dieting in concrete terms, expecting that it would earn them the respect and admiration they have yearned for all their lives. The weight loss accomplishes much. The parents are drawn back into being protective, not demanding, toward the child. The tragedy is that the very attention they demand reinforces old abnormal patterns, making development of true independence impossible.

The longer the illness lasts, the more isolated the victims become, the greater the danger of their becoming completely self-absorbed, overpowered by bizarre and abnormal ruminations. The state of star-

William A. Schonfeld Distinguished Service Award address presented at the 1978 annual meeting of the American Society for Adolescent Psychiatry, Atlanta, May 6, 1978.
© 1979 by The University of Chicago. 0-226-24052-5/79/1979-0002$01.30

vation itself creates psychological problems that are biologically, not psychodynamically, determined, and a certain nutritional restitution is necessary before meaningful psychotherapeutic involvement is possible. For effective treatment, changes and corrections must be accomplished in several areas: the abnormal nutrition must be improved; the stagnating patterns of family interaction must be clarified and unlocked; most of all, psychotherapeutic help is needed to correct the underlying erroneous assumptions that are the precondition for this self-deceptive pseudosolution.

Anorexia nervosa has the reputation of offering unusually difficult treatment problems. On principle, these patients resist treatment; they feel that in their extreme thinness they have found the perfect solution, that it makes them feel better. They do not complain about their condition—on the contrary, they glory in it. They are reluctant to let go of the security of their cadaverous existence.

The therapeutic task is to help an anorexic patient in her search for autonomy and self-directed identity by evoking awareness of impulses, feelings, and needs that originate within her. Therapeutic focus must be on her failure in self-expression, on her defective tools and concepts for organizing and expressing needs, and on her bewilderment in dealing with others. An anorexic's life is based on certain faulty assumptions that need to be exposed and corrected. Deep down every anorexic is convinced that, basically, body and soul, she is inadequate, low, mediocre, inferior, and despised by others. All her efforts are directed toward hiding the fatal flaw of her fundamental inadequacy. She is convinced that the people around her—her family, friends, and the world at large—look at her with disapproving eyes, ready to pounce and to criticize her. The image of human behavior and interaction that an anorexic constructs in her smooth functioning home is one of surprising cynicism and pessimism.

Therapy aims at liberating patients from the distorting influences of their early experiences and from the errors of their convictions so that they can discover that they have substance and worth and do not need the strained and stressful superstructure of artificial perfection. This is a difficult task, since the false reality with which they have lived represents their only way of having experiences. Patients will cling to their distorted concepts and will let go of them only slowly and reluctantly. I shall attempt here to illustrate some of these problems through description of one treatment session. The title of this chapter reflects the image used by the patient to describe her anorexic way of life.

Case History

Annette, now twenty-four years old, has been anorexic for nearly nine years. She has been in treatment for a little over two years (approximately 220 therapeutic sessions). She was a late-born, youngest child in a large family, nearly seven years younger than the next older sister who plays an important role in the discussion. She is five feet, six inches tall, and her highest weight had been 106 pounds at age fifteen. From then on there was a gradual but persistent weight loss with cessation of menses. She weighed approximately ninety pounds on graduation from high school, and was down to the low seventies when graduating from college. At the time she was seen in consultation, her weight was seventy-two pounds with visible edema; it dropped to sixty-nine pounds when her protein intake was increased. She was hospitalized twice to improve her nutrition. After discharge she would lose again, but during the last year her weight has gradually risen to about 105 pounds. She has maintained this weight now for several months but has been unable to reach a normal weight, although she says that she is tired of looking like a child and would like to weigh more. As far as I know she is a true abstainer, without vomiting, binge eating, or use of laxatives or diuretics. Though from a wealthy background, she has always been exceedingly frugal, buys only inexpensive food, without any indulgences or even variation, dresses very simply, uses no cosmetics, and keeps her house during the winter months at sixty-one degrees "to save energy." She has kept a responsible job as a research assistant and takes part in several group activities.

When first seen in therapy, she was exceedingly rigid and reserved, giving the impression of a walking marble statue who would answer questions politely and appropriately but with a minimum of spontaneity. With improved nutrition she relaxed somewhat, but each time her weight dropped below ninety pounds, she became rigid and uncommunicative. She has been very slow to open up, and several topics had been discussed over and over again. One was a part of the family saga: that when quite young she sweetly and patiently waited to be picked up after a nap, never calling that she was awake. To Annette a question such as "Why didn't you shout that you were through napping?" was like being incited to riot. It was inconceivable to her that any child would do something so daring.

Her submissive attitude was also expressed in an often repeated statement: "I know that I can't help feeling anger, but I can keep from showing it." This restraint applied to all expressions of feelings and emotions—most of which she was not even aware of. She also did not believe that other people ever showed their true feelings. Her childhood had been a constant state of worry about what her parents really felt behind what she considered only their facade of friendly and devoted encouragement.

On the other hand, she was unstinting and unrestrained in describing her own shortcomings, her mediocre inefficiency, and she would frequently speak of herself as "the scum of the earth," not even worthy to give herself proper care. Like other anorexics, she was exceedingly dependent on the opinion of others and was deeply convinced that the people around her were forever condemning her. She felt as though she had grown up in a puritanical village where everybody was just waiting to tear each other down for any violation of rules. Conformity and living by the rules had been the maxims of her life.

A particular difficulty in treatment was that any acknowledgment of something positive in herself was immediately condemned as being boastful, as revealing her as "full of herself," which then became further reason for self-condemnation. Nevertheless there was gradual progress, and only rarely did she speak in belittling terms about herself. She could even accept that eventually she might be able to lead a self-respecting, meaningful life. One day when she was rather depressed she confessed that she still had a feeling that there was something "embarrassing and black" about her, something I labeled in my mind as needing elaboration when she was in a more positive state of mind.

In the session preceding the one to be reported, she had talked about an unusually enjoyable weekend where she had felt in good rapport with other people. I felt this was a good time to examine the "black" inside feelings with the implication of unacceptable impulses which she had probably not even dared to admit to herself. Even this pleasant rapport had ended up with her comparing herself, unfavorably, to Josie, her next older sister, in whose presence she had always felt uncomfortable and continued to even now as an adult. I explained to her, using Sullivan's concept of malevolent transformation, that after having been hurt repeatedly, children tended to approach new situations with a certain expectation of rebuff. What seemed to be going on in her relationship with Josie was that whenever she had any dealings with her sister she expected to get hurt, that she had to constrain the hostile feelings this aroused in her, and that this might be the basis for the dark feelings she had about herself. Instead of defending her sister as she had done in the past, since Josie had never done anything wrong to her and it was unjust to blame herself, Annette went along with the inquiry and this time enlarged on several points; how angry, hurt, and vindictive she had felt. I intended to continue the theme. In the past she had repeatedly disclaimed such revelations, but not this time; she opened the next session with this same theme.

Recorded Session

When she entered the office, Annette looked more animated than usual and began immediately: "It's amazing. What you said yesterday about my not really knowing Josie, always approaching her expecting to be hurt, has made me now very curious. It is almost as if I want to go and meet her, you know, like a new person—who are you?" This "it's amazing" reflects a real loosening up, a greater spontaneity than usual. It is my custom to acknowledge any signs of change and I commented on the way she expressed herself as something new. The important point was that she now could conceive of herself as relating differently to her sister, like a grown-up person, no longer the hurt and frightened child who kept her vindictiveness a secret.

Annette continued, "Well, it's almost like meeting a stranger. I mean the way I feel. As if I had been told about this person, and now I am curious to meet her and see what she is like in the flesh rather than what somebody else has told me." I remined her that the "somebody who told her" was her own disturbed and distorted memory. To this she agreed: "I guess I am saying I want to meet her as a stranger because in the past I was dealing with a person I was looking for."

I referred back to the previous discussion when she had spoken of "the shameful black" in herself, which we had related to unacceptable hostile feelings. "The way you responded tells us that it makes sense to you, that you had been approaching Josie in expectation of defending yourself against her, but also that you had to control your own angry impulses so that you would not hurt her." Annette elaborated on how she had always related to this sister in terms of superiority and inferiority, that she had always compared herself to Josie and always came out second best. "I mean, really I was looking for things where I could make myself feel rotten because of how good she was. In a way I was always doing the reverse of getting even; I was making it worse for myself.''

With such an intelligent, educated patient I use at times theoretical concepts by way of explanation. I do this for a variety of reasons. There is the practical one of having a short-term expression for certain complex situations. More important is conveying to a patient that, however distressed she might feel about her reactions and confusion, this is not completely out of the ordinary, but that psychiatrists at least have a word for it. The intent is to make her experiences less unheard of, neither wicked and inhuman nor unique or absolutely superior. I explained to her at this point the meaning of the *double bind*, how children may find themselves confronted by insoluble dilemmas. Whatever they do, there is danger of getting hurt. If they let it be known how upset and hurt they feel, they might be faced with the greater danger of losing the love of the people on whom they are most dependent. "Yesterday you said not once but twice that one cannot squash a sister, indicating a double bind dilemma. When you experienced her rejection you must have felt extremely angry at her; but you lived also with the rule that one must love a sister. Therefore you were unable to protest or make your own demands."

The way she continued showed that this explanation was meaningful to her: "At the same time I was working so hard to get any approval from her, anything she could give me." Then she mentioned the "dress incident," referring to a discussion quite some time back during which I had asked something like "but why didn't you get even with her and cut up her best dress?" She had answered spontaneously, "She would have hated me even more." Avoiding her sister's hatred had been a dominant theme in her life. She elaborated, "I never wanted to give her real cause that she might call me the bratty little sister, or that I would be an obnoxious kid to whom she can say 'go away, I don't want you around.' I mean I never wanted knowingly to put myself in this position even though I often felt like it." In response, I elaborated on the many double bind dilemmas she must have encountered and added: "Probably the most important question is whether you can recognize how much real cause you had for anger, rage, and vindictiveness and how you then accounted for your having such bad feelings against yourself. Or do you have any other ideas or explanations about what you called 'the shameful black' in you?"

She was not ready to pursue my idea but continued with her own train of thought, something quite unusual for this overproper and conforming girl. ''Well, I did but that's changing the subject. I want to answer the question that you put up first. I almost don't know what to think about my own perceptions of Josie, knowing now that they were so incorrect. I mean I almost don't feel the need for having to blame her for being a mean sister; I don't even know if she was a mean sister.'' I tried to make a comment about the differences between events that take place and the way an individual experiences them, but again she went on with her own reexamination. ''Now, today—it may change tomorrow—I sort of have the feeling—well, I don't really care what she was and what I felt. That's what I call settling myself in regard to the members of my family. I have done it with the others, in particular with father and the older ones. When I say 'I want to meet her as a stranger' I feel I want her to know I'm new too. If she doesn't like me, well that's too bad, that's not my problem anymore. It's her problem. If she doesn't like me, well, tough beans—I don't have to worry about her problems, I have enough to worry about myself.''

Since I felt it was important to learn how it affected her self-concept, I went back to my earlier question: ''Does it help you to handle your self-punishing attitude better? Are you kinder to yourself if it makes sense that you have these angry feelings and that they are justified?'' This time she agreed, ''Yes, because I no longer have to feel guilty about having felt guilty. Because I no longer have to feel that I have to worry about her. My worry about her was all this putting me down, wanting to get even. I meant she is no longer representing something that everytime I look at and think about means I feel very antagonistic; the antagonism has gone out of it.'' I confirmed this by adding, ''And it was the antagonism which you felt you had to hide. Can you imagine now how it will be if Josie and you meet as new people?'' She responded by elaborating how she had become more at ease with the rest of her family. ''I feel almost the same now with Josie, as if I hadn't known her before. She is related by blood, but I had been basing my whole knowing about her on just a tiny fraction of what she is.''

I continued my theme about whether she could see the difference in her self-concept. ''In a way you have looked at Josie through distorting, black, ugly-making glasses but you looked at yourself with the same ugly-making glasses.'' She eagerly said, ''I looked at her like that because I felt I was wrong, that there was something the matter with me, and that made me feel so angry toward her.'' This I confirmed:

"As if your feelings toward her were proof of your own wrongness," and she elaborated, "I mean a civilized human being who has basically been brought up to be a nice person, how can she really express her feelings?" A few sessions earlier she had described how she had always felt that every friendliness that was shown to her by anyone in the family had been really a fraud, that Josie was the only one who expressed how negatively they really felt. "It's almost as if this whole weight has been taken away from me. It was what I was doing to myself in relation to thinking about her. It is no longer of importance because she is not in charge of my life, and I don't have to judge myself thinking she is judging my life, which is all very complicated. And until now whatever was going on and when I would think of anything I had done I would say automatically, 'it's not so great. Look at what she can do.' It was often like that—as long as I don't think about her I feel fine about myself, but as soon as I refer to her then I cut myself down. Because in comparison I could always make Josie look better." I confirmed what she had said: "If that is really so, that this is how you feel now, then we can say that we made a great step forward yesterday. You recognized how such a misdirection of one's view of somebody else comes about." This she further confirmed:

And you look at the other person only to find her always in a hurtful context. I mean I really couldn't see Josie, I mean emotionally—intellectually I can say this and that about her—but I didn't ever feel very much warmth toward her because all I saw were my own clouded glasses. I see now the whole thing is so childish, the way I have carried anything I may have experienced through all this time. Maybe when I was little and didn't think about what I was seeing. When you are two and in a crib you aren't consciously saying "what is she doing, what am I thinking about her and all that." But I carried on through life and made it the only thing I ever saw. Up until yesterday, at three o'clock it changed. It's incredible, it's just wild. The most liberating thing I can see and say is "I don't care about her; I don't care about what she thinks, or I don't care what I think she thinks." What had been ruining me was my not being able to step out of my age level, ten, twelve, fourteen, sixteen, up until now—carrying all that stuff around with me, all the way back and not permitting anything else to be different.

During this whole discussion Annette had been unusually lively and self-assertive. She had used the word "liberating," and she acted much freer. Proof of this is the fact that she opened up a new theme, eager and willing to enlarge on something she had mentioned before but only in an offhand way: "I don't know if you remember what I said a few weeks ago. I was talking about how I felt about the rest of the world, as if I were on an island." Now she went into details: "Josie was standing on the bridge and would not permit me to get off my island. It's all the same thing—she was the one I saw standing on the bridge. I always had the feeling, 'it was her or me.' If I wanted to get over I'd have to chuck her over the bridge and she would drown. And for her to be acceptable to the rest of the world, she had to make sure that I stayed on the island."

I made a comment that one could understand why she had hesitated to talk about such vindictive images, adding "no child is born to be a murderer or to hurt her sister." She confirms, "I know—that's why I was so reluctant to approach her or to talk about her. The only way I could save myself was to get rid of her." I related the guilty concept of her inner blackness to this attitude. Now that her secret feelings were in the open one might expect that she would look at herself and the world differently. I asked: "Isn't it a better world?" to which she eagerly replied: "Gosh, yes." She added that it had always been a problem. "No matter how much antagonism I felt, I could not commit sistercide or whatever it is." I helped her with the word, and we made it "sororicide," an expression of the intensity of her hostile feelings, which she had kept rigidly controlled.

She opened up another theme: "The other thing I wanted to say about the word 'black' and the associations I have to it was the feeling of being different, of knowing the attitude of myself toward myself. The worst is that I really feel I am not myself and this is really sick, this is not being myself, my body or person, not really a human being. And that, that is what is really weird." This was the first time that she talked in such terms about herself. I asked: "So you too have suffered from such feelings? I know it is weird; I have heard from so many others about this fear of not being really human." Annette admitted: "And this was the hardest to come out. It is sort of an opener that if you don't see yourself or your body as everybody else considers themselves to be, then you are not really human." I explained that in my contact with other patients, fat people on rigid diets and other anorexics, I had learned about the fear of being at the edge of being human. Though many anorexics suffer from it when their weight is very low, they don't seem to be quite aware of it at that time. Annette stated: "Well, I have become much more aware of it now that I have this consistent desire to be a person. I almost feel that the way I was with the skinniness, with the whole attitude of not wanting to be a woman or an adult or to have a full figure and all the rest, was related to the body and my perception of it."

I inquired directly how she had seen herself when she was at her lowest weight (a question that had been frequently asked), and she reacted with her old evasiveness. "I didn't really look at myself very much—I didn't have a long mirror so I didn't have an image. And I think it was pretty much not wanting to see what I looked like." I wondered how this avoidance of looking at herself was related to this fear of nonhumanness. In the old literature, in the very first description, 300 years ago, the anorexic was called "a skeleton only clad with skin." Then I referred to a recent article in *The New Yorker* (Lang 1977) called "A Backward Look," which dealt with the way German people remembered the Hitler time. Most denied having known anything about concentration camps except one man who, when still a high school student, had been assigned to guard duty. He reported, "There suddenly came a number of skeletons—hundreds of them, unburied skeletons—shrouded in striped uniforms, carrying shovels and they were running." The image of the running cadavers had appeared later in many of his nightmares. He did not speak of them as thin people, only in dehumanized terms, as if the way they looked was a caricature of the human shape. Annette listened intensely and added: "And it's not only a caricature. It is worse. It's the desire to be so thin. I mean there is the desire not to be like ordinary people, not to look like the rest of the world."

When asked about the island image she explained: "Looking at myself on the island, I am still a skinny nonperson; in a way, it doesn't matter if I am isolated and different. I mean in that image it is all right that Josie is on the bridge because she is more in touch with humanity than I am. As long as I remain so far away from being an acceptable or an accepting compatriot with people in the world, I might as well stay on the island." I took up this theme: "So you did experience your skinniness as a great alienation, that of being different?" Her answer was: "Well, I do now." I explained to her that many other anorexics speak about it only after they are nearly well, though they had felt dehumanized, not part of the human race while skinny.

I continued: "You reacted as if Josie didn't let you off the island, that she had condemned you to your isolation and didn't offer you a place in the world." Annette enlarged on this point: "But it was also that I didn't deserve to approach her for a place because I had made myself into this phantom on the island. There is no point in blaming her because society dictates that unless I can be civilized there is no reason to try and get in. And I have made myself into this uncivilized being, if not a cannibal on the island at least something so out of touch and out of tune with the rest of the world that I need to be kept isolated on an island." This led to the question of out of what inner necessity her development had led to this extreme isolation. She explained, "I think, going back to what I see as the blackest of the black, it is my own self-possessed desire not to be a person. I mean there's that, it is acknowledging that anorexia doesn't just happen, it is my own attitude that very strongly said, 'I still don't want to be normal.' I mean that is the ultimate in guilt, it really is the active volition."

I reminded her that she has often complained that even if she were of normal weight her figure wouldn't be perfect. She explained: "And I see my body as distorted—really distorted. All right, one day I will weigh 120 pounds, but I am still perfectly flat on top. That's a real freak for the circus." I explained again that it is a child's exaggeration that rates any variation as being put apart, and that these same distortions had made her think of herself as unworthy. She still clung to the basic anorexic attitude with the self-depreciating conviction that whatever she was and did was not good enough. She agreed that now that she no longer blames her sister for being on the bridge, it is the question of whether she herself is socialized, civilized, or human enough to walk over the bridge. "Now I see it very clearly, as me standing on the island looking at the bridge, and it is no longer the question of anything else or anybody else or any other circumstances. It is me, and the bridge is there and what do I do?" I summarized the session by reminding her that life would be easier when she stopped thinking of herself in this complete isolation. I referred to *I Never Promised You a Rose Garden* (the film of which was being shown at that time) and that it would be hard to say what expressed more inner disturbance, creating a different world of fantasy or her having created a different body. There can be no promise of a garden of roses, but I can state definitely that it will be easier and more rewarding to live in the real world than staying on the skeleton island.

Discussion

A session like this is a far cry from the tedious rigidity that characterized the early part of therapy. Though anorexics deny that they are sick and in need of treatment, most go along after a treatment program has been outlined. As a matter of fact, one of the difficulties in therapy is the anorexics' tendency to be overconforming. They might agree with everything that is being said, elaborate on it, even to the point of fabricating material to please the therapist, while at the same time cherishing the secret knowledge that things as they are being discussed are not so. The pseudo-agreeing is often a way of avoiding the real issues. The basic attitude is one of deep mistrust, and this is expressed in their rarely if ever volunteering anything. A true therapeutic alliance, with agreed on treatment goals, develops only slowly. In this session Annette elaborated on her feelings and observations, and she corrected me when I too one-sidedly focused on her negative self-concept. Her opening up of new themes—one described as "this was the hardest to come out"—reflects reliable trust in the therapeutic relationship. Like other anorexics she had asked repeatedly how much longer treatment would last, feeling that nothing new was being discussed. A remnant of this old mistrust was her evasiveness when directly questioned how she had seen herself during the starvation period. What she then brought up on her own was much more meaningful.

Such changes in attitude occur over and over in therapy. Without this, there would be no progress. Usually such changes occur in small steps, often so inconspicuous that they are not always recognized. What happened during this session was a large and quite dramatic step forward. During and following the preceding session she had not only accepted but truly integrated what had been suggested, that her belittling and self-accusing attitude might be related to unacknowledged and unexpressed hostile feelings. Having considered this possibility during the session, she had a flash of insight afterward, with sudden recognition that she had been mistaken in the way she had looked at her sister. During the reported session, this issue and its many implications were further explored. Annette acknowledged a feeling of liberation for giving up the erroneous childhood conviction, feeling free now to meet her sister as a new person, whereby she too would be a new person, truly an equal.

With this new sense of liberation she was ready to discuss and explore her concept of her position in life. She saw herself isolated on an island, excluded from joining the mainstream of life, and the power excluding her was a sister whom she had always felt was intimidating and forbidding. After the error of this conviction had been clarified, she proceeded to look at her own role in this isolation, that she had withdrawn as if she were a nonperson, on her own volition. This change from seeing herself as a passive victim to acknowledging herself as an active participant in the whole development, in particular the development of the anorexia illness, is an important turning point in treatment. At the onset, the anorexia syndrome is presented as something that has just happened; that a sinister fate befalls the patient and the family. For a true resolution of the underlying problems, the patient needs to become aware of her own role in the development of the illness. The pursuit of excessive thinness needs to be recognized in its various aspects. During the early part of the illness it represents an effort to feel better through a special accomplishment that supposedly compensates for her depression and low self-esteem. Yet it leads to greater isolation and further falling behind in maturation and individuation. Working toward alternative solutions becomes possible only after their active participation has been recognized.

However, coming to a new understanding is not enough. For effective changes in actual living, each point needs to be clarified in its many ramifications. About six months have passed since this session, and it is of interest to consider what has happened since. The change in Annette's relationship to her sister has persisted, and she has stopped continuously devaluating herself in comparison to Josie. There is also a decided change in her excessive preoccupation with what she calls "her image in the eyes of others." The recognition that she could have been so wrong in relation to one person made it possible to look at other relationships in a new way. This working through involves reexamination of many different experiences and relationships.

In the beginning of treatment she spoke in glowing and admiring terms about the superior features of her family. It was exceedingly difficult for her to acknowledge that there had been experiences within her home that had interfered with her developing a positive self-concept, a sense of her personal worth and value, but had left her with a profound basic mistrust about the people around her, and even more about her own worthwhileness. She is still struggling with the conviction that it is not the child's fault to have arrived "as an afterthought" (to use her expression) and therefore always in danger of being made to feel like an unwanted nuisance who was in the way. She is decidedly more convinced of her right to live her own life and to acknowledge her own feelings and desires, though she still is skeptical of whether she will ever be able to trust her own genuineness.

During the reported session she was evasive when asked direct questions but then spoke spontaneously about her anorexic self-image. Being isolated on an island expresses the central theme of her whole illness; she was unable to cross to the mainland. Though self-created, the extreme thinness makes her feel unhuman, both in her basic make-up and also in her actions. During the following weeks the theme of the island came up repeatedly, and she related her sense of isolation and unconnectedness to experiences in real life. One day, after some unpleasantness at work, she expressed her extreme isolation as feeling like the Lady in the Harbor (the Statue of Liberty), cold like the statue, untouched and untouchable, on a little island in the gray ocean, with no relationship to anybody or anything. She also expressed open regret about the many wasted years in which she had kept away from human contact.

In this context she began to speak of her excessive thinness as something truly undesirable. About a week after the reported session, she had a dream in which she saw herself as the skeleton-thin anorexic she had been, what she had always said that she had not really seen. This time she felt real horror looking at this creature, an inability to believe that she could ever have been like that. For the first time she spoke about the utter despair of this time in her life, the terror of being caught in a trap of her own making. This is an important criterion of progress in treatment. I feel no anorexic is safe from relapse until she has looked at her illness with real emotion, with fear and horror of all the pain and hunger she has suffered, and for having reduced her body to that of an unhuman creature.

No single insight or understanding removes the symptoms and problems. Each new formulation is a step forward, an opening for a new evaluation of the underlying factors. Gradually it becomes apparent how the body and its functioning had been misinterpreted with childish anxiety and how its maturing with the new sexual demands had been experienced as dangerous and unacceptable, and thus had led to a withdrawal from life. It is the therapist's task to be guide and mentor during this self-exploration, assisting not only in defining past errors but also in uncovering positive steps toward an active participation in life.

REFERENCE

Lang, D. 1977. A backward look. *New Yorker* (October 3), pp. 55–56.

3 ADOLESCENTS, BELIEVING AND BELONGING

SAUL V. LEVINE

This chapter presents a simple thesis, one that is not entirely novel but which has only recently begun to be substantiated empirically and through research. It has implications for understanding adolescent behavior in general—especially so for the youngster who is alienated and, in particular, for therapeutic or rehabilitative efforts with the antisocial adolescent, for whom all corrective attempts have failed miserably.

The thesis is that adolescents have two basic psychosocial needs which, when fulfilled, enable them to cope better with those critical years and thereafter. These are, simply put, (1) *a belief system*, something intense to believe in, and (2) *a sense of belonging*, of community.

We adopt Rokeach's (1969) view that a belief system represents an all-embracing set of attitudes, values, and beliefs which essentially define an individual's perception of and relationship with his or her external world. Social bonding has been shown by anthropologists, ethologists, and psychiatrists to be as inherent a need of individuals as more biological drive reduction. Yet, in contemporary society these two phenomena have been at least as decimated as any other. The litany of detrimental effects that rapid change has wrought on the Western world has been well documented (Slater 1970; Toffler 1971) and need not be repeated here. Suffice to say that Leighton's components of psychosocial disintegration are in evidence (Leighton 1973). Families who maintain a strong belief system and traditional family structure seem best able to shield their youth from alienation, anomie, and destructive antisocial behavior, including drug use (Blum 1970;

© 1979 by The University of Chicago. 0-226-24052-5/79/1979-0022$01.16

41

Keniston 1965). Yet both elements seem to be waning in contemporary society: the family is no longer sacrosanct, and common belief systems are less in evidence than ever before (Braungart 1976).

Consequently, we find that there are literally thousands of adolescents and youths across North America who have for a variety of reasons become immersed in social systems different from, or in conflict with, traditional family structure or dominant social values. These living arrangements may be on a voluntary basis (religious ashrams, communes, therapeutic communities, drughouses, drop-in or runaway centers—crash pads, political groups, free clinics, alternative schools, etc), or they may have been imposed upon the young people (group homes, halfway houses, training schools, hospitals, therapeutic or corrective work farms, detention centers, pioneer programs, etc.), or a combination of the two may pertain. The particular adolescents in the latter group may have been in conflict with the law, societal values, or labeled as disturbed by professionals or lay individuals. Even in the voluntary group, however, the members were at some level in overt conflict with mainstream middle-class social values and life-styles. Whatever the basis for their departure or extrusion from the family, these young people felt outside the system and saw themselves, and were seen by others, as not belonging. They fit Seaman's (1959) definition of alienation: feelings of normlessness, powerlessness, isolation, self-estrangement, and meaninglessness. In Frank's (1973) terms, because of their obvious demoralization many of the readers of this chapter would conclude that these young people were prime candiates for various types of psychotherapy.

In a series of studies on contemporary youth that I have been involved with over the past few years—on urban communes (Levine, Carr, and Horenblas 1973), fringe religious movements (Levine and Salter 1976), and the drug scene (Levine, Lloyd, and Longdon 1972), and in work with normal adolescents, adolescents in therapeutic communities, group homes (corrective and therapeutic), and in psychotherapy, it has become abundantly clear that the proposition postulated earlier is not only valid but bears a lot more scrutiny than our field has been devoting to it. I will go so far as to say that the extent to which an external belief system and a sense of belonging to a participating community exist in any social system will by and large determine the success or failure of the program, the future direction of the young person, and even acceptance by the dominant society. This conceptual framework is not in contradistinction to the developmental issues of this age group as elucidated by Erikson (1968), Kohlberg (1970), Piaget (1967), and others—rather, this is a somewhat more psychosocial approach than the primary intrapsychic orientation of these theoreticians.

Normal Adolescent Needs

We have learned much about the mythology of contemporary youth (Levine 1975). Rather than paragons of virtue or purveyors of iniquity, they are much more like their parents than we have acknowledged (or liked to believe), even in terms of values, attitudes, and aspirations (Mead 1970; Offer 1969). Furthermore, those values they espouse which are engendered by their peer group turn out to be more superficial and transient than those fostered by their parents, another surprise to many of us (Conger 1977; Douvan and Adelson 1977). Adolescents are (and always have been) phenomenally susceptible to ideologies, belief systems, and mass movements (Braungart 1976; Toch 1965; Adelson 1976). We are not here talking necessarily about disturbed adolescents. Numerous studies have shown that while most adolescents seem to be resilient, adaptive, and enthusiastic about life, many others harbor feelings of alienation and demoralization (Masterson 1967; Pasamanick 1959) to varying extents and are especially vulnerable or receptive to easy answers. Adelson (1976) has shown us that we must make a clear distinction between younger and older adolescents; that the former are much more concrete, rigid, absolutist, inflexible, and intolerant than the latter. Both groups are vulnerable to "cults of unreason" (Evans 1973), but for different reasons. In the younger group, belief systems and action-oriented movements serve to accommodate the disillusionment with parents, confusion, and antisocial impulses. In older adolescents, feelings and experiences of alienation and demoralization are much more common. Identity-related issues are clearly manifested in both (Erikson 1968).

We have found in our studies, and others in theirs, that voluntary membership in socially dissonant cults or group belief systems and subsequent behavior patterns are most often a result of these latter feelings (Levine and Salter 1976). Loneliness, or rather aloneness, we have also seen to be a prerequisite. Rosenberg (1976) has shown that susceptibility to beliefs and indoctrination is increased in adolescents with low self-esteem. Conversely, self-esteem rises in those who believe in their cause and feel as an integral part of a group. The young adolescents are strikingly authoritarian, but as opposed to Adorno, Fendel-Brunswick, and Levinson's (1950) relating this characteristic to particular types of families or personalities, the authoritarianism here is seen almost as a developmental stage that they must pass through.

Adolescents as Believers, and True Believers

It has always been relatively easy to indoctrinate the young (Toch 1965). Throughout childhood they have been dependent, presented with a narrow perception of the world; have idealized their parents; have been inexperienced, naive, and relatively ignorant. Adolescence suddenly appears. The body changes, autonomy looms, impulses bedevil, choices must be made. In this zeitgeist—this era of unpredictability, frenetic change, rapid technological advances, changing values, and multiple options—any group, individual, or philosophy which can provide stability, immediate answers, and like-minded peers is inherently attractive.

The answers may be simplistic, devoid of logic, or destructive, but, given the prerequisites (e.g., alienation and loneliness) in the proper predisposing context, they will be adopted as dogma and then proseletyzed as gospel. We have seen this occur especially in the various fringe religions we studied (Levine and Salter 1976), but the same phenomenon has been reported in other situations like political movements, psychotherapeutic fads, chemical cults (Greeley 1974; Group for the Advancement of Psychiatry 1976), etc. What often goes along with the consonant context for this phenomenon are paradoxical issues such as a rigid superstructure, a clear hierarchy, puritanical morality, and mysterious ritual; paradoxical because in this supposedly permissive era, these constricting elements are said by many to be pariah to adolescents. On the other hand, the major recent trends of communalism and anti-intellectualism that Yankelovich (1974) has cited have been substantiated in those true-believing young people we have looked at. There is no doubt that many of our youth, especially those lacking in inner resources, are searching for a belief system which will enable them to cope with perceived or real external stresses (Coelho, Hamburg, and Adams 1974).

These adolescents have a great need for absolutes, to counter ambiguity, fluidity, and the indeterminable. The playwright Pirandello (1922) captures this need beautifully in the following passage: "Don't you see what they are after? they all want the truth—a truth that is: Something specific, something concrete. They don't care what it is. All they want is something categorical, something that speaks plainly! Then they'll quiet down."

The "conversion" experience is as close to "ah hah!" as one ever gets—it is accompanied by a sense of relief, a clarity, even at times an altered state of consciousness (Greeley 1964; Group for the Advancement of Psychiatry 1976). It is also a closed system, blinding to other sources of information and contradicting ideas. It encourages ethnocentrism and intolerance of others, especially of competing movements (Rokeach 1960). The centrality of the belief, the all-embracing nature of the "Answer" and not the specific content of the belief, determines the perception of the believer's reality (Hoffer 1951; Koestler 1952). Their sense of being alone is alleviated by group membership, a warm feeling of communality with shared goals and values (Levine et al. 1973; Levine et al. 1972; Levine and Salter 1976). There is also a phenomenal centripetal group pressure which enhances the unity of perceptions, attitudes, and behavior.

While we might disagree somewhat about what constitutes mental health, there is little doubt that most criteria would be met, at least for a time, in any of the voluntary social systems cited above. That is, many adolescents who were just not succeeding in traditional society, given the correct environment (for them) sprang to life in a relatively short time (Levine and Salter 1976). Aside from alienation, demoralization, and loneliness, some adolescents prior to joining social movements were in poor physical health, anxious, sleepless, abusing drugs, confused, or antisocial. Quite a few had been seen by a variety of mental health professionals to no avail. Their conversion was followed by vastly improved physical and emotional health. Even if we invoke cognitive dissonance to explain their uniformly positive reports (Festinger 1957), they looked and felt better, and on any self- or other reporting scales, most were doing very well indeed. Our dismay about the source of their improvement should not lead us to dismiss it as an invalid psychotherapeutic effect. The same criticism has been leveled at our results. And we should be wary of falling into the trap of automatically inferring exploitation on the basis of indirect evidence (Toch 1965).

Clinical Implications

Assuming that the proposed premise is correct, that believing and belonging form the potential basis of indoctrination and winning over of alienated youth, then we wonder whether that same basis could not be utilized in rehabilitative, correctional, and therapeutic work with many uncontrollable adolescents. We must face the possibility that concentration wholly on psychodynamics in therapeutic work with these youngsters is possibly doomed to failure, except perhaps as an academic exercise. For example, antisocial adolescents may have reached their behavioral pattern through a variety of derivations, but the end result is always a conflict with, and a threat to, society. The motivation for engaging in these acts and the performance of them often develop their own functional autonomy (Allport 1950), irrespective of the psychodynamic basis. And without utilizing belief and belonging in a rehabilitative milieu (be it via corrections or mental health professionals), we and other helping professions have failed miserably (Jesness 1971–72; O'Neal and Robins 1968; Palmer 1971). Follow-up studies show few if any benefits derived from traditional approaches— recidivism rates remain high (Dixon and Wright 1975; Elinson 1972). As a matter of fact, there are those who feel that nonintervention is superior to any kind of therapeutic endeavor (Schur 1973). This is not a diatribe against traditional psychotherapy. That it has limited usefulness in the area we are discussing is no longer even debatable. But even in psychotherapy the elements of belief and belonging may play a larger role than we have been prepared to recognize. There are some who feel that the spiritual aspects of psychotherapy (belief, susceptibility, answers, etc.) are fundamental to its success (Frank 1973; Kiev 1964; Prince 1968; Torrey 1972).

The question is whether we can put these powerful tools to work for us—to reach young people and get them to adopt socially consonant values and behaviors. As it is at present, when the voids of belief and belonging are spontaneously filled in alienated youth their needs and society's are often mutually contradictory. We are not saying that there is a single approach to all young people who are either in conflict with the law or who are disturbed—far from it. A variety of intentional social systems tailored to meet diverse individual needs must be set up (Daniels and Kuldau 1967), with built-in, prospective, controlled evaluation. But without a central focus on the belief system and the sense of participatory community, our feeling is that the social systems cannot succeed. Conversely, with these concerns as central foci and intrinsic parts of the program, their chances for success may be greatly enhanced.

There are ongoing attempts to make use of both the susceptibility of young people and the strengths inherent in belief systems and belonging in therapeutic, correctional, rehabilitative, or alternative living programs (Doherty 1974). These young people may be particularly vulnerable because of their experience with failure, their sense of futility and low self-esteem (Levine and Salter 1976). The initial results are tentatively encouraging and are certainly as impressive—or considerably more so—than what traditional psychiatric theory and practice have been able to accomplish. Synanon, for example, in its pioneering work with drug addicts, has now developed into a large, intentional social system with the two suggested basic ingredients included (Rothchild and Wolf 1976). Others (Langrod 1972; Robbins 1964) have recommended the use of belief systems in rehabilitative work with drug users. In their work with disturbed and antisocial adolescents, the Achievement Houses (Phillips, Phillips, and Fixsen 1973) and Vision Quest (Petroni and Gurgevich 1977) utilize the milieu, peer pressure, and responsibility to the group and sense of community, all of which are subsumed under the term "belonging." In our opinion, however, they do not go far enough in inculcating something to believe in, a cause, if you will, which may be vital (except inadvertently, perhaps, with charismatic leaders).

And with young adolescents in particular, based in part on Adelson's work, we would have no qualms about incorporating in a treatment or corrective program a highly structured milieu, with firm rules, consequences (positive and negative), high expectations, and demands. This must be accomplished in a humane, warm context—the two approaches are not mutually exclusive. In fact, either alone is insufficient. Human dignity, respect, emotional nurturance, and support are prerequisites in any program (Phillips et al. 1973), both from a civil and a therapeutic point of view. Coupled with education, vocational training, psychotherapy, relationships, and other approaches, we would have a much better chance of succeeding in both the short and the long run. At the least, this hypothesis should be put to the empirical test. We await the findings of one such ongoing, controlled, prospective study.[1]

In these corrective instances we have been discussing alienated adolescents who have started on the path of society's losers and have been labeled by professionals as sick or bad. If left to their own devices, this group will either end up as rejects, institutionalized, or with significant emotional problems (O'Neal and Robins 1968). The unemployment, school dropout, crime, and welfare statistics are largely dominated by youth (Moynihan 1973) who are out of the mainstream of society. What of these alienated adolescents who manage to escape the labeling process? They may well join their own "cults of unreason" in their pursuit of the millennium (Cohn 1957). Their older, educated, and relatively affluent collegiate brethren might find and join activist movements (Smith, Haan, and Black 1970) like the antiwar movement of the late sixties. But we have a mandate in society to provide alternatives for those increasing numbers of young people who are floundering and who cannot achieve belief and belonging by themselves; or for those who might find their salvation, their meaning in life, their relationships, from groups which might have less than salutory effects on the young people or society.

This latter possibility poses a danger that the movements the young choose might be exploitative (some fringe religions—Lefkowitz 1971; Levine and Salter 1976), or even destructive (Bugliosi 1974). Adolescents have achieved belief and belonging in large social movements which can be seen to be bad (or good) depending on what side of any fence you happen to be on (e.g., Red Guard, Hitler's Yugent, Mussolini's Brown Shirts, or the U.S. antiwar movement, the civil rights movement).

Conclusions

Another danger exists in this entire thesis. If we learn how to maximize or exploit belief and belonging in youth, are we not also controlling and programming youth? And who is to say that our choices of values and behavior are superior? Are we to encourage communality, noncompetitiveness, and anti-intellectualism, or espouse individuality, acquisitiveness, and competition?

Belief and belonging are not novel issues—references to the concepts in these or other works are legion throughout literature. It has been most apparent to us in looking at youngsters in grossly diverse circumstances, in all our studies or in therapeutic environments, that these two recurrent themes, or voids, were ubiquitous. When these were filled by socially consonant or dissonant beliefs and groups, as long as the adolescent perceived them as beneficial dramatic improvement ensued. Surely we must at least be aware of the potential force inherent in this process.

This is submitted as a provocative presentation in the hope that it stimulates discussion, even criticism or disagreement. But more importantly, we are interested in heuristic effects. We now have the tools to put the concepts of belief and belonging to the test in treatment facilities and other intentional social systems. Group-living atmospheres and belief systems are now amenable to measurement, documentation, and evaluation (Bucholz 1976; Moos 1974). These issues are becoming increasingly vital in a society where many normal adolescents are significantly alienated and vulnerable.

NOTE

1. R. Jones, personal communication.

REFERENCES

Adelson, J. 1976. The development of ideology in adolescents. In S. Dragastin and G. Elder, eds. *Adolescence in the Life Cycle.* New York: Wiley.

Adorno, T. W.; Fendel-Brunswick, E.; and Levinson, D. J. 1950. *The Authoritarian Personality.* New York: Harper.

Allport, G. W. 1950. *The Individual and His Religion.* New York: Macmillan.

Blum, R., and Associates. 1970. *Society and Drugs.* San Francisco: Jossey-Bass.

49

Braungart, R. 1976. Youth and social movements. In S. Dragastin and J. Elder, eds. *Adolescence in the Life Cycle*. New York: Wiley.

Bucholz, R. A. 1976. Measurement of beliefs. *Human Relations* 29(12): 1177–1187.

Bugliosi, V. 1974. *Helter-Skelter*. New York: Norton.

Coelho, G.; Hamburg, D.; and Adams, J. 1974. *Coping and Adaption*. New York: Basic.

Cohn, N. 1957. *The Pursuit of the Millennium*. New York: Essential Books.

Conger, J. J. 1977. *Adolescence and Youth, Psychosocial Development in a Changing World*. New York: Harper & Row.

Daniels, G., and Kuldau, J. 1967. Marginal man, the tether of tradition and intentional social system therapy. *Community Mental Health Journal* 3(1): 13–30.

Dixon, M. C., and Wright, W. E. 1975. Juvenile delinquency prevention program: an evaluation of policy related research on the effectiveness of prevention programs. Nashville, Tenn.: Office of Educational Services, Peabody College for Teachers.

Doherty, G. 1974. Teaching acting out youth acceptable ways of exerting control over their environment. *Canada's Mental Health* 22(June): 9–10.

Douvan, E., and Adelson, J. 1977. Adolescent friendships. In J. J. Conger, ed. *Contemporary Issues in Adolescent Development*. New York: Harper & Row.

Elinson, J. 1972. Effectiveness of social action programs in health and welfare. In C. Weiss, ed. *Evaluating Action Programs*. Boston: Allyn & Bacon.

Erikson, E. 1968. *Identity: Youth and Crisis*. New York: Norton.

Evans, C. 1973. *Cults of Unreason*. London: Harrop.

Festinger, L. 1957. *A Theory of Cognitive Dissonance*. Evanston, Ill.: Row, Peterson.

Frank, J. 1973. The demoralized mind. *Psychology Today* 6(11): 22–28.

Greeley, A. 1964. *Ecstasy, a Way of Knowing*. Englewood Cliffs, N.J.: Prentice-Hall.

Group for the Advancement of Psychiatry (Committee on Psychiatry and Religion). 1976. *Mysticism: Spiritual Quest or Psychic Disorder?* New York: Group for the Advancement of Psychiatry.

Hoffer, E. 1951. *The True Believer*. New York: Harper & Row.

Jesness, C. F. 1971–72. Comparative effectiveness of two institutional treatment programs for delinquents. *Child Care Quarterly* 1:119–130.

Keniston, K. 1965. *The Uncommitted: Alienated Youth in America.* New York: Dell.

Kiev, A. 1964. *Magic, Faith and Healing: Studies in Primitive Psychology.* New York: Free Press.

Koestler, A. 1952. *The God That Failed.* New York: Bantam.

Kohlberg, L. 1970. Moral development and the education of adolescents. In E. Evans, ed. *Adolescent Reading in Behavior Development.* Hinsdale, Ill.: Dryden.

Langrod, J. 1972. The role of religion in the treatment of addiction. In L. Brill and L. Leibman, eds. *The Treatment of Drug Abuse.* New York: Behavioral.

Lefkowitz, L. 1971. *Attorney-General's Report on the Children of God.* Albany: State of New York.

Leighton, D. 1973. The empirical status of the integration-disintegration hypothesis. In B. Kaplan, ed. *Psychiatric Disorder and the Urban Environment.* New York: Behavioral.

Levine, S. 1975. The mythology of contemporary youth. *Canadian Medical Association Journal* 113:501–504.

Levine, S.; Carr, R.; and Horenblas, W. 1973. The urban commune: fact or fancy, promise or pipe dream. *American Journal of Orthopsychiatry* 43(1): 149–163.

Levine, S.; Lloyd, D.; and Longdon, W. 1972. The speed user: social and psychological factors in amphetamine abuse. *Canadian Psychiatric Association Journal* 17:3:229–241.

Levine, S., and Salter, N. 1976. Youth and contemporary religious movements: psychosocial findings. *Canadian Psychiatric Association Journal* 21:411–420.

Masterson, J. F. 1967. *The Psychiatric Dilemma of Adolescence.* Boston: Little, Brown.

Mead, M. 1970. *Culture and Commitment: A Study of the Generation Gap.* Garden City, N.Y.: Doubleday.

Moos, R. H. 1974. *Evaluating Treatment Environments: A Social-Ecological Approach.* New York: Wiley.

Moynihan, D. 1973. Peace—some thoughts on the late 1960's and 1970's. *Public Interest* 32:3–12.

Offer, D. 1969. *The Psychological World of the Teenager.* New York: Basic.

O'Neal, P., and Robins, L. N. 1968. The relation of childhood behaviour problems to adult psychiatric states: a 30-year follow-up study of 150 subjects. In H. C. Quay, ed. *Children's Behaviour Disorders: Selected Readings.* Toronto: Van Nostrand.

Palmer, T. B. 1971. California's community treatment programme for delinquent adolescents. *Journal of Research and Crime and Delinquency* 8:74–92.

Pasamanick, B. 1959. A survey of mental disease in an urban population. In *Epidemiology of Mental Disorder.* New York: American Association for Advancement of Science.

Petroni, F., and Gurgevich, S. T. 1977. Vision Quest: the kid nobody wants: an innovative treatment program for youthful offenders. Paper presented at American Orthopsychiatry Association 54th Annual Meeting, March 1977, New York.

Phillips, E. L.; Phillips, E. A.; and Fixsen, D. L. 1973. Achievement place: behavior-shaping works for delinquents. *Psychology Today* 7:75–79.

Piaget, J. 1967. *Six Psychological Studies.* New York: Random House.

Pirandello, L. 1922. "It is so! (if you think so)." In *Three Plays.* New York: Dutton.

Prince, R. 1968. Religious experience, youth and social change. *Montreal Review* 3:1–3.

Robbins, T. 1964. Eastern mysticisms and the resocialization of drug users. *Journal for Scientific Study of Religion* 8(2): 308–317.

Rokeach, M. 1960. *The Open and Closed Mind.* New York: Basic.

Rokeach, M. 1969. *Beliefs, Attitudes and Values.* San Francisco: Jossey-Bass.

Rosenberg, M. 1976. The dissonant context and the adolescent self-concept. In S. Dragastin, and G. Elder, eds. *Adolescence in the Life Cycle.* New York: Wiley.

Rothchild, J., and Wolf, S. 1976. *The Children of the Counterculture.* New York: Doubleday.

Rutter, M.; Graham, P.; and Chadwick, O. In press. Adolescent turmoil—fact or fiction? *Journal of Child Psychology and Psychiatry and Related Disciplines.*

Schur, E. M. 1973. *Radical Non-Intervention: Rethinking the Delinquency Problem.* Englewood Cliffs, N.J.: Prentice-Hall.

Seaman, M. 1959. On the meaning of alienation. *American Sociological Revue* 24(6): 783–791.

Slater, P. 1970. *The Pursuit of Loneliness: American Culture at the Breaking Point.* Boston: Beacon.

Smith, M. B.; Haan, N.; and Black, J. 1970. Social-psychological aspects of student activism. *Youth and Society* 1(3): 261–288.

Toch, H. 1965. *The Social Psychology of Social Movements.* New York: Bobbs-Merrill.

Toffler, A. 1971. *Future Shock.* New York: Basic.

Torrey, E. F. 1972. *The Mind Game: Psychiatry and Witchcraft.* New York: Emerson Hall.

Yankelovich, D. 1974. *The New Morality: A Profile of American Youth in the 1970's.* New York: McGraw-Hill.

4 RUNNING AWAY: REACTION OR REVOLUTION

JAMES S. GORDON

The Reaction

Young people who left their homes during the colonial era were regarded as a loss to the family's economy as well as defectors from its morality. Like single older people, orphans, and bastards, these runaways were quickly placed in family settings. The justification was biblical, "God settleth the solitary in families" (Ps. 68:6), but the arrangement also had its political and economic advantages: the community was spared the danger of a potentially seditious force and the labor of these young people became available to the families which took them in (Bremner et al. 1970).

This view of the young person as a potential economic asset and of running away as a social and economic disruption as well as an offense against God continued through the seventeenth and much of the eighteenth centuries. In the late eighteenth and early nineteenth centuries an accelerated rate of immigration, the importation of large numbers of young servants, and the nation's gradual secularization, industrialization, and urbanization combined to decrease the economic utility of American children and to increase the numbers of those who did not live with their parents. Large numbers of young people ran from rural areas, where they had been supplanted as laborers by immigrants who were stronger and no more expensive, and flocked to the cities. Some found work in newly opened factories. Others, along with the children of impoverished Irish and German immigrants, wandered the streets.

By the beginning of the nineteenth century these homeless young people had come to be regarded as a special and serious problem, "The class," according to Brace (1880), "of a large city most dangerous to its property, its morals and its political life" (p. 11). Some were confined in almshouses with the poor, the mad, and the chronically ill; others were transported by Brace and his fellow reformers to serve as laborers in "the best of all asylums, the farms of western settlers." By the middle of the century deviance had become delinquency; informal arrangements for the care of runaways had been supplanted by prison-like institutions, "schools of reform," and "houses of refuge."

The increasingly rapid decline of the social and economic role of young people in the late nineteenth century paved the way for a new conceptualization of and a new name for their stage of life. The belief that particular young people, among them the runaways and the homeless, needed to be reformed began to yield to the view that this stage of life, now called "adolescence," was itself a particularly treacherous one. Laws prohibiting child labor, enforcing compulsory education, and creating a separate juvenile-justice system provided a structure which protected the vulnerable young from some adult exploitation while it restrained them from replacing their elders in the job market. At the same time the developing fields of psychiatry, psychology, and psychoanalysis offered tools for understanding and treating the more recalcitrant members of this group.

The chief ideologue in this creation of adolescence was G. Stanley Hall (1904). Though many of his theoretical contributions have since been repudiated, and though anthropological data such as those gathered by Mead (1928, 1930) contradicts it, Hall's view of adolescence as a stage of development characterized by continuous crisis has persisted. For the last seventy-five years many of those who have written about or been responsible for the treatment of adolescents have continued to make the effect (the difficulty of being a young person in twentieth-century America) into the cause (adolescence is a time of great stress).

At its best this psychological perspective has been useful in palliating the isolation and objectification of the young; in helping their parents and those charged with their care to understand the subjective experience, motives, feelings, and conflicts of adolescents as well as their behaviors. Over the last fifty years it has enabled researchers like Armstrong (1932), Gordon (1975a, 1975b, 1978b), Minehan (1934), Outland (1934), Shellow, Schamp, Liebow, and Unger (1967) to understand running away as a response to familial, social, and economic situations which young people can neither understand nor change. It has also encouraged therapists, caseworkers, and probation officers who work with individual runaways to see the commonalities among those who stay at home and those who leave and to subordinate the strong arm of discipline to an inquiring mind and a compassionate heart.

Sometimes, however, the burgeoning influence of a pathologically oriented medical perspective distorted the clinical view of runaways and obscured the larger social, economic, and familial factors which shaped the lives and behavior of adolescents and pushed them from their homes. Riemer (1940), for example, noted the "extremely negative character of young runaways" and went on to describe them as antagonistic, surly, defiant, somewhat assaultive, destructive young people who are at times oversubmissive and docile. Later psychiatric studies have generally been less vituperative, but they too have been narrowed by a perspective dominated by notions of psychopathology and delinquency that seemed sometimes to fuse. Foster (1962), Jenkins (1969, 1971), and Jenkins and Boyer (1968) emphasized behavioral factors common to runaways and "other delinquents," while other investigators, including Leventhal (1963, 1964), focused on the individual psychopathology which running away was presumed to reflect. In their thirty-year follow-up study of child guidance clinic patients these latter authors suggested that running away was indeed a "predictor" of both delinquency and psychopathology; they noted among other findings that runaways had "an adult incarceration rate that was four-fold that of other patients" and that they were one of the groups "most likely to show psychotic signs as adults."

In 1968 running away was a "status offense" in more than half our States (Beaser 1975); it was a behavior like truancy or an attribute like incorrigibility which was a punishable crime for people under eighteen but not for adults. In that same year running away also became an official category—the "Runaway Reaction of Adolescence," in the *Diagnostic and Statistical Manual* of the American Psychiatric Association (1968). The vocabulary had become scientific rather than religious, moral, and economic, but the stigmatization of earlier descriptions and the forced incarceration of earlier treatment remained.

Teenagers on their own continued to be summarily returned to their families. Poor young people who persisted in running were generally sent by judges to detention centers and reform schools while their middle-class sisters and brothers were diagnosed and committed by psychiatrists to indefinite stays in mental hospitals. The treatment both groups received was in many ways similar; in penal and mental institutions attempts were made to reform their behavior, to improve their character and attitudes, and to shape their future—at times with drugs and/or behavior modification. No longer a slipped gear in the economic machinery, a public shame, or a nuisance, runaways were now a species of involuntary patient requiring diagnosis, treatment, and cure.

The Revolution

In the 1960s their shared isolation from the concerns and lives of adults and the tendency of adults to label and stigmatize their particular stage of development had helped to make the young skeptical of the dominant values of American society. The civil rights movement inspired some of them to see their own powerlessness as a mirror of black people's, to begin to think about youth rights as well as civil rights.

Soon the contradictions between the American ideals of truthfulness, peace, democracy, and self-determination and the American actions in Indochina began to alienate large numbers of young people who had been only marginally touched by the civil rights struggles. Revolted by the televised slaughter of the Vietnamese and terrified by the hypocrisy of its justification, many of them came to fear that the powerful weapons of the American military establishment might some day be turned on them (Gordon 1972).

In this climate disputes about politics, sex, drugs, and grooming tended to escalate to bitter and implacable confrontations. In their wake large numbers of young people left—or were told to leave—their homes.

Young people had always hoped to find a better, or at least a less dismal and confining, life on their own. In the city or on the road they looked for comrades to keep them company, to strengthen them in their quest. Only in the 1960s, however, did large numbers of young people begin consciously to regard running away as a political protest and their fellowship as the basis of a culture and a movement. While psychiatrists were discovering a new behavior disorder and debating their long-term prognosis, young runaways and their advocates publicly declared that their departure—voluntary or forced—was a legitimate rebellion against a restrictive family and a dangerously oppressive society.

By the mid 1960s a small number of runaways had begun to gather with the beatniks and their hippie descendents, and antiwar and civil rights activists in the centers of what soon came to be called the counterculture. In the Haight-Ashbury district of San Francisco, in Manhattan's East Village, Washington, D.C.'s Dupont Circle, and in college communities like Ann Arbor, Madison, and Cambridge they created new styles of dress and music, politics and art, interpersonal relations and intoxication—amalgams of past and present, technological innovation, economic necessity, and imaginative fantasy. The relaxed and sensual way in which they lived together, their opposition to materialism, competitiveness, hypocrisy, and war, and, not least, the intensity of media attention, soon drew tens of thousands of other young people after them.

Local groups formed to respond to the immediate needs of the thousands of homeless and penniless young people who flocked to their communities. Building on the interests and talents of natural helpers, drawing on the skills and energy of the young people who came for help, they swiftly constructed a network of human services. In San Francisco the Diggers, borrowing their name from sixteenth-century English egalitarians, improvised daily bread and soup kitchens for thousands of Haight-Ashbury residents. Switchboard operators directed telephone callers to crash pads, free clothes, and legal services. The Haight-Ashbury Free Clinic, staffed by street people and local physicians, dealt with the ailments of a young and transient population that was experimenting with its limits of physical and mental endurance.

Once the excitement of living on the street wore off, many young people found themselves desperately looking for a place to live, sympathetic attention, and a caring community. Few turned to mental health professionals for help. Most mental health professionals seemed hopelessly incapable of sympathizing with or even understanding the rebellious young. Even those who were genuinely sympathetic were still unable to offer the concrete help—the food, housing, and supportive community setting—that the young needed.

Runaway houses were swiftly created to fill the gap left by traditional mental health and social service facilities. In these settings runaways found not only a refuge but also a redefinition of their situation. Older people who wore the same kinds of clothes and listened to the same kind of music helped them to see running away not as an illness or a criminal act but as part of a process of personal growth and social struggle. They helped young runaways to understand that they had the right to—and inevitably did—make the decisions that would shape their lives and their futures. Living and working together in a runaway house, runaways and their counselors forged a cross-generational alliance of older and younger brothers and sisters.

Running Away: A New Synthesis

By the early 1970s the Vietnam War and the movement which grew to oppose it, the huge urban counterculture, and the economic boom which sustained it all began to dissipate. The numbers of runaways did not, as many expected, decline. Each year approximately 750,000 young people continued to run from their homes.

In earlier eras runaways tended to come from families or sectors of society made perilously vulnerable by poverty, death, or the cultural, social, and economic dislocation attendant on immigration, rapid industrialization, and economic catastrophe. Urban poverty, cultural anomie, and broken homes have continued to be significant causes of running away. According to the *National Statistical Survey on Runaway Youth* (Youth Development Bureau, DHEW 1976) children who run are more likely to come from one-parent families and young people who live in rural areas leave their homes half as often as their urban or suburban peers. On the other hand, broken families, poverty, cultural dislocation, and their sequelae have become pervasive facts of life for all Americans. Kenniston and the Carnegie Council on Children (1977) note that almost 17 percent of all our children live below the official poverty line and as many more are in fact poor, while Bronfenbrenner (1976) adds that 40 percent of all marriages end in divorce, that parents are spending less and less time with their children, that all adults and their children move from city to city and house to house at an ever-accelerating rate, and that child abuse and running away are endemic among the rich as well as the poor.

Few of the young people who now leave their homes are consciously trying to find a movement or a counterculture to shape their disillusionment to social change or communal satisfaction. Many of them—30 percent among the predominantly black youth who now run to the Washington, D.C., Runaway House and fully half of the teenagers who come to the Youth Service Bureau in white, middle-class Huntington, Long Island—report that they are leaving because they have been physically abused by their parents or guardians. Others simply feel angry, depressed, and isolated at home. They speak freely of their boredom and unhappiness at school, or being bewildered and dismayed by their inability to find a job or a place in the world, of their anger at being labeled as the family problem. Though these young people are called runaways and have indeed left their homes, the majority of them feel as though they have been "pushed out" or "thrown away" by their parents and society.

By the early 1970s it had become clear that many of these young people were staying in or near their own communities and that they had the same kinds of needs as those who left for the big cities. Concerned citizens in middle-class suburbs, urban ghettos, and rural areas were soon meeting to plan their own runaway programs. These new runaway houses drew their inspiration from programs in Haight-Ashbury and on the Lower East Side but their particular style and substance from life in the community. Some were started by young college graduates who hoped to bring the spirit of the antiwar and civil rights movement to their own communities, to bring the politics of human liberation down to a personal scale. Increasingly, however, these projects were sponsored by establishment organizations, sanctioned by municipal governments, and staffed, at least in part, by workers with advanced degrees and expertise in counseling, social work, and psychology.

In 1972, thirty houses struggled on seed grants, borrowed money, and benefit suppers to provide short-term lodging, food, and supportive counseling to runaways. By 1978 there were some 200 runaway houses, 150 of which are funded through an $11 million program of HEW's Youth Development Bureau (Youth Development Bureau, DHEW 1977). Last year these homes provided food, housing, and comprehensive crisis-oriented, individual, group, and family counseling to 50,000 runaways, and nonresidential services to approximately 250,000 young people and their families.

As these programs have grown in numbers and matured, they have tried to combine the responsiveness and flexibility of the first runaway houses with the close critical attention to the details of individual and family situations which characterize the work of mental health professionals and the wider social and political activism of community organizers. In the context of the programs that have emerged from this synthesis, young people and their counselors have the opportunity to redefine the meaning of running away; to transform a stigmatized act into a catalyst for individual, familial, and community change.

THE CONTEXT OF RUNNING AWAY

The physical existence of runaway houses provides a necessary context for redefining running away. Earlier, runaways who came to the attention of authorities were summarily confined as deviants, criminals, or mental patients. In contrast, young people who come to runaway houses are welcomed as guests in a household. They come on their own and are free to leave when they wish. The rules of these households are not created to reform them or to modify their behavior but rather to ensure the house's survival and the comfort of all those who live and work there. The counselors in the houses are older friends and advisers, not warders and judges. The young person is ultimately responsible for whether or not he will return home, work, go to school, or continue running.

In this context young people who have been running for weeks or months are able to relax and consider their situation. Knowing they are not confined, they stay. Feeling they are trusted and respected, they begin to trust and respect. Some young people continue to disobey the rules that have been established to insure the house's survival, but many of those who were said to be hopelessly impulsive find it easy enough to live within limits that seem neither capricious nor arbitrary.

THE MEANING OF RUNNING AWAY

Historically, running away has been seen by adults in power as a defection from the family and the social order, a crime against the community, and a sign of mental illness. The perspective of the young people who run has been ignored and their right to define their situation denied. Law-enforcement and mental health agencies have tended to perpetuate, not remedy, this process of isolation and labeling. If a psychologist or probation officer declares a child to be sick, delinquent, or in need of supervision, and insists on testing or confining him, these actions and attributions outweigh any references to family problems or social and environmental influences.

In the context of a situation where they feel comfortable, in the company of people who are willing to credit their perspective, young people can begin to disentangle themselves from others' definitions of them and explore the reasons why they really did leave home. For some it is simply a matter of escaping from unbearable, humiliating, physical punishment or sexual abuse. For many more, running away feels like a desperate assertion of selfhood. Many young people no longer can be or wish to be the good child their parents seem to insist on. Others are furious that their attempts at independence seem always to be defined as a species of behavior or thought disorder. In running away, these young people are escaping as much from familial definitions as they are from physical control. It is these definitions that they describe and experience as murderous or prison-like.

From their first hours in a runaway house young people are encouraged to see that running away is neither pathological nor heroic but a temporarily necessary and positive act. Counselors encourage runaways to look carefully at the situations from which they have come and the way they have behaved; to reverse in the very process of recollection, analysis, and narrative the passivity to which their role and status as adolescents constantly urges them. In daily groups with other runaways, these young people find that even their most unhappy experiences and desperate insights may be of use to others who are having similar problems as well as to themselves.

Howell, Emmons, and Frank's study (1973) of young people in one program suggests that in the context of a runaway house this process of redefinition is successful. Though they had experienced "major difficulties during their run," 66 percent of the young people who stayed at Project Place in Boston "believed in retrospect that running away has been a positive growing experience for them." My own work at the Washington, D.C., Runaway House and elsewhere (Gordon 1975a, 1975b, 1978a, 1978b; Gordon and Houghton 1977) confirms Howell's statistics. Their time spent at the runaway house is the first opportunity that many young people have to think and act for themselves. Some of them who had come to believe they were hopelessly stupid, inadequate, or impulsive have patiently worked out solutions to complicated personal and family problems. Others, habitual runaways and diagnosed schizophrenics, have discovered that in the context of a respectful setting they can behave sanely and responsibly.

RUNNING AWAY AND THE FAMILY

Running away is a communication to the rest of the family as well as an act of self-assertion. It is impossible for parents—even if they deny the importance and meaning of the behavior—not to know that their child is missing. Whether they accuse the young person of betrayal, belabor themselves with guilt, or are secretly pleased, they feel a loss and an uncertainty. In the struggle the balance between parent and child has shifted. If they wish to continue their contact with their children, the parents must pay attention to their children's point of view and their wishes.

Ten years ago runaway-house counselors saw the family from which young people fled as oppressive and unworkable. Many thought of themselves solely as youth advocates and restricted their contact with parents to the negotiation of family truces. By the early 1970s counselors had realized the necessity of working intensively with families which the young could neither leave, nor change, nor adapt to. They turned for assistance to family systems therapy and to mental health professionals who were accustomed to working with families. This therapeutic perspective avoided the deprecation and scapegoating which seemed inevitably to befall runaways who were involved in individual psychotherapy and emphasized mutual relatedness and collective responsibility for family difficulties. The work of Haley and Hoffman (1968), Laing and Esterson (1971), Minuchin (1974), and Satir (1964) helped runaway-house counselors to understand the forces which propelled young people from their homes and encouraged them to work therapeutically to try to reverse destructive family patterns.

Instead of treating the departure of the young as a rebellion or a disaster, runaway-house counselors began to use it as a lever to urge families toward confrontation and change. While parents were wondering why their children had left, counselors were helping runaways to look critically at their situation and to explore their options for the future. In the course of this process many young people quickly saw the need for meeting with their families. They realized they could not return home if things were unchanged; nor, given their legal status and earning capacity as minors, could they survive on their own without the support of parental resources or at least the protection of parental permission. Even foster placement was dependent on their parents' signatures. After a few days or a week in a runaway house young people who had always hated and feared counseling were urging their parents to come to family therapy in order to communicate better and attempt to work things out.

Sometimes even in the first session with a family runaway-house counselors are able to help the young person articulate the content of the protest that has been expressed in running away, to help the parents and other siblings hear its meaning. Sometimes the family arrives at a mutual understanding which facilitates practical compromise and a swift return home. More often the counselors must begin by simply trying to create a safe place for the family to be together in all its mystified contrariness. Slowly they try to help family members to find the common language of understanding in which habitual, often incoherent, quarrels become mutually intelligible; they hope to show them concretely how each of them affects the other and how all are enmeshed in repetitive and counterproductive behavior.

Sometimes runaway-house counselors are able to help a family to resolve the immediate crisis and then work to reach a new, more mutually satisfying equilibrium (Gordon 1975a). Sometimes formal counseling lasts for only one session; understanding for just a moment. Over the years those of us who work with the families of runaways have learned to value that moment as an example of the possibility of communication and closeness, one that may later be referred to and enlarged upon. Sometimes there is only a sharpening of conflict. Here the session provides a safe place for disagreements and the opportunity to clarify them. The family discovers that impasses may be broken, that choices are possible, and that differences do not necessarily spell disaster.

After several sessions, many runaways begin to gain a perspective on family conflict which helps them to grow free of it. They realize that the pressures which have been brought to bear on them are not unlike those their parents feel. They are able to see that their families either are or feel socially marginal and that their parents lack both intimate friends and close ties to an extended family. In time it becomes clear to many of the young people that their parents' angry and confused imprecations are reflections of their own bewilderment and betrayal, that their own flight from home and the struggles which led up to it are far less catastrophic and far more remediable than their parents' alienation.

Long-Term Needs and Long-Range Perspectives

Instead of trying to make young people fit into programs that were once successful, runaway houses have tried to change their programs to meet the expressed and changing needs of the young people who use them. Early in their evolution, for example, a number of programs realized that even after a two-week cooling-off period, even after intensive individual and family counseling, some runaways would neither be able to return home nor live on their own. Skeptical of the need for hospitalization and dissatisfied with foster homes which refused to take or deal successfully with acting-out, borderline, or psychotic young people, runaway houses began to create their own long-term alternatives to institutions (Gordon 1976, 1978b). At present more than forty such programs—evenly divided between group homes and individualized foster placement services—are operating.

The very existence of such facilities simplifies the work of the runaway houses which sponsor them and forestalls the disastrous alternatives which hover over many initial family sessions. Since an appropriate long-term alternative is available, neither runaways nor their parents need feel compelled to make decisions immediately. For the small group of young people who eventually do need to live in them, these group and individual foster homes offer the same kind of respectful and responsive living situations that they have grown to appreciate at the runaway house.

At the same time that they have improved their ability to deal with troubled young people and their families, runaway programs have also recognized the need to try to remedy some of the conditions which have helped produce these troubled young people: an adversarial position vis-à-vis the larger society has been tempered to an advocacy within it. Ten years ago runaway house workers tended to condemn the nuclear families from which the young fled. Today—through outreach to intact families, lectures to churches and adult education programs, and efforts to organize civic improvement associations, day-care centers, block parties, etc.—runaway houses are helping to augment and strengthen community supports for families they perceive as vulnerable and isolated. Counselors who once helped runaways escape from social workers and police are now helping social workers and police to understand and work with young people and to direct them to runaway houses.

As they have become sensitive to other needs, runaway houses have been quick to improvise other services. The particular problems of female runaways—41 percent of all those who leave home but 60 percent of those who seek shelter and counseling at runaway houses—have prompted a number of runaway houses to offer special programs for young women. In girls' groups they have the opportunity to explore the conflict between the pride and the hope that the women's movement has helped them to feel and the pressures toward conformity and passivity which continue to pervade our society; to discuss their feelings about their sexuality and its implications for their relationships with parents, boyfriends, and girl friends. More recently, runaway houses have created specialized counseling programs and residences for rape victims—as many as two-thirds of the young women at some urban houses—for young prostitutes of both sexes, and for young people who feel or fear they might be gay.

Similarly, runaway centers in large cities have become acutely aware of the needs of the minority-group young people who live around them. With the abolition of many programs, the deepening of the recession, and the decline in employment and increasing fragmentation of families, more and more young people have had to come out of the ghettos to seek help elsewhere. Urban runaway programs which once housed no more than 10–15 percent minority-group youth are now working with a population that is overwhelmingly black or Hispanic, with a group of young people whose handicaps—material, educational, and vocational—are enormous. These houses have hired a proportion of minority-group counselors to match the numbers of young people and have made efforts to address their specific cultural identities and economic needs.

In the last several years a number of runaway houses have tried to institutionalize their responsiveness to young people's needs and to allow themselves to evolve into ongoing living and working communities to which the young can continue to belong long after they have ceased to be formal clients. This informal aftercare permits young people who have returned home to continue to draw strength from the house. Some come back for formal counseling sessions, others just to visit. Virtually all of these programs also give young people the opportunity to participate actively in the house's work as members of boards of directors, participants in peer counseling programs, and counselors in training.

In recent years this concern for reversing the social and economic passivity of young people has also prompted runaway houses to create programs designed to help young people to prepare themselves for useful work. At a time when as many as 60–80 percent of the young people in some inner-city communities can find no work at all, when many teenagers are bewildered and uncertain about their future, runaway houses have begun to try to provide a bridge to an adult livelihood for their young clients. Some train young people to work as counselors, maintenance people, administrators, office help, etc., in their own and similar programs. Others have tried to extend the feeling of community and the intimate personal learning that pervades their own project to shopkeepers, crafts people, and local community businesses in which they place young people as apprentices.

Conclusions

For three centuries in America running away was regarded as a sign of deviance, a symptom of delinquency, and a reaction against unquestioned and largely unexamined social norms. Young people who could were to be swiftly reintegrated into their families and their society. Those who could not were to be isolated from the larger society and reformed through institutionalization.

In the 1960s young people and their allies in and out of the mental health professions began to reverse this process of labeling and coercion. In the context of a supportive counterculture, in the shelter of runaway houses created to meet their needs, young people began to take their marginal status as a badge of revolutionary honor, to see their extrusion as a critique of their families and their society.

In the 1970s running away is neither heroic nor deviant. The experience of the 1960s and the continued high incidence of running away has helped runaway-house workers to see the voluntary or forced separation of the young from their families as a reflection of widespread social disorganization and familial fragmentation, as a potential catalyst for family change and an opportunity to reverse the passivity and victimization to which our society urges the young.

Runaway houses cannot, of course, reverse the economic and social conditions which profoundly affect families and propel young people from their homes or singlehandedly alter the contemporary treatment of adolescents. They can, however, continue to offer the 750,000 young people who each year leave their homes a time and a place for themselves, a chance to take a critical and often compassionate look at the families with which they have been hopelessly struggling, and an opportunity to make the difficult transition to adulthood in the company of older people who care. Their stubborn insistence on supporting the independence and strength of young people whom others would stigmatize and institutionalize, their ability to adapt mental health skills to their programs, their willingness to change to meet the changing needs of their clients, and their insistence on creating a community capable of dealing with the larger social and economic conditions which affect those who come to them for help, combine to offer us, as mental health professionals, a new and vigorous model for working with the young.

REFERENCES

Armstrong, C. 1932. *660 Runaway Boys*. Boston: Badger.

Beaser, H. 1975. *The Legal Status of Runaway Children*. Final report for a study conducted for the Office of Youth Development, DHEW, by Educational Systems Corporation. Washington, D.C.: Government Printing Office.

Brace, C. L. 1880. *The Dangerous Classes of New York*. New York: Wynkoop & Hallenbeck.

Bremner, R. H., et al., eds. 1970. *Children and Youth in America: A Documentary History*. Vol. 1. *1600–1865*. Cambridge, Mass.: Harvard University Press.

Bronfenbrenner, U. 1976. The disturbing changes in the American family. *Search* 4:4–10.

Diagnostic and Statistical Manual of Mental Disorders. 1968. 2d ed. Washington, D.C.: American Psychiatric Association.

Foster, R. M. 1962. Interpsychic and environmental factors in running away from home. *American Journal of Orthopsychiatry* 32:486–491.

Gordon, J. S. 1972. The Vietnamization of our children. *Washingtonian* 8(2):78–81.

Gordon, J. S. 1975a. The Washington, D.C., runaway house. *Journal of Community Psychology* 14(2): 68–80.

Gordon, J. S. 1975b. Working with runaways and their families: how the SAJA community does it. *Family Process* 3(1): 235–262.

Gordon, J. S. 1976. Alternative group foster homes: a new place for young people to live. *Psychiatry* 39(4): 339–354.

Gordon, J. S. 1978a. Group homes: alternative to institutions. *Social Work* 23:300–305.

Gordon, J. S. 1978b. The runaway center as community mental health center. *American Journal of Psychiatry* 135(8): 932–935.

Gordon, J. S., and Houghton, J. 1977. *Final Report of the National Institute of Mental Health Runaway Youth Program.* Washington, D.C.: National Institute of Mental Health.

Haley, J., and Hoffman, L. 1968. *Techniques of Family Therapy.* New York: Basic.

Hall, G. S. 1904. *Adolescence: Its Psychology and Its Relation to Physiology, Anthropology, Sociology, Sex, Crime, Religion, and Education.* Vols. 1 and 2. New York: Appleton.

Howell, M. C.: Emmons, E. B.: and Frank, D. A. 1973. Reminiscences of runaway adolescents. *American Journal of Orthopsychiatry* 43(5): 840–853.

Jenkins, R. L. 1969. Classification of behavior problems of children. *American Journal of Psychiatry* 125(8): 1032–1039.

Jenkins, R. L. 1971. The runaway reaction. *American Journal of Psychiatry* 128(2): 168–173.

Jenkins, R. L., and Boyer, A. 1968. Types of delinquent behavior and background factors. *International Journal of Social Psychiatry* 14:65–76.

Kenniston, K., and the Carnegie Council on Children. 1977. *All Our Children: The American Family under Pressure.* New York: Harcourt Brace.

Laing, R. D., and Esterson, A. 1971. *Sanity, Madness and the Family.* New York: Basic.

Leventhal, T. 1963. Control problems in runaway children. *Archives of General Psychiatry* 9:122–126.

Leventhal, T. 1964. Inner control deficiencies in runaway children. *Archives of General Psychiatry* 11:170–176.

Mead, M. 1928. *Coming of Age in Samoa.* New York: Morrow.

Mead, M. 1930. *Growing Up in New Guinea.* New York: Morrow.

Minehan, T. 1934. *Boy and Girl Tramps of America.* New York: Grossett & Dunlop.

Minuchin, S. 1974. *Families and Family Therapy.* Cambridge, Mass.: Harvard University Press.

Outland, G. E. 1938. The home situation as a direct cause of boy transiency. *Journal of Juvenile Research* 22:3343.

Riemer, M. 1940. Runaway children. *American Journal of Orthopsychiatry* 522–528.

Satir, V. M. 1964. *Conjoint Family Therapy.* Palo Alto, Calif.: Science & Behavior.

Shellow, R.; Schamp, J. R.; Liebow, E.; and Unger, E. 1967. *Suburban Runaways of the 1960's.* Monographs of the Society for Research in Child Development, vol. 32, no. 3. Chicago: University of Chicago Press.

Youth Development Bureau, DHEW, 1976. *National Statistical Survey on Runaway Youth.* Washington, D.C.: Government Printing Office.

Youth Development Bureau, DHEW, 1977. *Annual Report on Activities Conducted to Implement the Runaway Youth Act.* Washington, D.C.: Government Printing Office.

5   THE ADOLESCENT IDENTITY CRISIS REVISITED

ROBERT L. ARNSTEIN

Adolescent identity crisis is a clinical and developmental concept that has been much discussed and written about in the last twenty-five years. As more thought is given to stages in adult development, it is clear that it both forms a backdrop for future mid-life crises and actively influences the dynamic family interactions that occur between adolescent children and their mid-life parents. Furthermore, it involves the process of moving from adolescence to adulthood. F. Gottlieb (personal communication, 1977) points out that there are actually several adolescent identity crises: pubertal, mid-adolescent, and late adolescent. However, it is only the late adolescent period that will be addressed here.

Although more than one college student has arrived at our service, obviously upset, and announced, "I'm having an identity crisis," I realized when I thought carefully about the subject that I never really had resolved to my own satisfaction four troubling questions: (1) What was really meant by an identity crisis? (2) Was an identity crisis, however defined, a necessary part of maturing? (3) If so, how could one describe it in psychological terms to account for not only those individuals who have overt and relatively visible crises, but also those who matured or developed without any major apparent crisis? (4) If such a crisis was a necessary aspect of maturing, what caused a crisis to occur in one individual's development and not in another's, and were there likely to be specific later consequences in either case?

It is not uncommon to see students at college who are quite uncertain about their life and career direction. Talking with such individuals, one has the distinct feeling that they are in an unsettled state and not really in a position to make decisions that will be lasting and lead to a more definitive identity. Many young people recognize this problem and take some action that postpones such decisions. During the days of the draft the postponement was often involuntary, whereas now it is more likely to be a stint in the Peace Corps or a job that is clearly temporary. If one talks with these same individuals two to three years later, one often has an entirely different feeling about their emotional state; all sorts of issues in addition to career choice seem to be resolved.

This led me to consider the problem in terms of definitions and the historical development of the concept. A review of the literature made it apparent that there exists a confusing and overlapping mass of related terms—such as identification, maturing, autonomy, emancipation from the family, bisexual resolution, epigenesis, self, character, normality, self-cognizance, social role, commitment, and ego ideal—culled from references to anthropology, sociology, philosophy, religion, natural sciences, poetry, psychology, and psychoanalytic theory (Erikson 1945, 1946, 1950, 1953, 1956, 1968; Lichtenstein 1977). The very broad range of the elements that have been related to identity makes it difficult to discuss the adolescent identity crisis in any orderly fashion because it has many different meanings depending upon who is using the phrase and from what reference point.

Adolescence is a period of life that has long been written about both in personal terms and in fiction (Kiell 1964). It has been recognized as an important period in an individual's development, but in early psychoanalytic writing its importance was clearly subordinated to the period of childhood because of Freud's discovery of infantile sexuality and the consequent emphasis on early psychosexual development. The publication of Anna Freud's (1936) *The Ego and the Mechanisms of Defense* and the subsequent development of ego psychology served to focus new light on the adolescent period. There then followed a series of studies by Blos (1962), Spiegel (1958), and, again, Anna Freud (1958) which discussed the changes that occurred in the psychic equilibrium as a result of the drive intensification associated with puberty.

Concurrently, other clinicians less concerned with psychoanalytic theory observed the changes that occurred during adolescence, and those mental health workers associated with colleges focused on the events of late adolescence. Fry and Rostow (1942) wrote about this period: "detachment from the family is a necessary step toward the emotional maturity of an individual; it is a prerequisite to the smooth development of other growth processes," and "as the individual gets older he must seek to establish some measure of independence in his system of living; the achievement of detachment from the family becomes a necessary step in conforming to the mores of society and in helping to insure the emotional balance and well-being of his own personality."

Lidz (1968) said: "The major tasks of late adolescence concern the achievement of an ego identity and capacities for intimacy. When the young person has liberated himself from his family sufficiently and gained enough latitude and security to permit sexual expression he pauses before undertaking definitive commitments. The expansiveness of mid-adolescence gives way to the need to consolidate and to try out imaginatively and realistically various ways of life . . . ." and "The transition from adolescent to adult behavior involves becoming a person in one's own right, not simply someone's son or daughter, and one who is recognized by the community in such terms. . . . It is concerned not simply with inner organization but also with how that organization permits the individual to move properly into the social roles permitted an adult and expected of him in a given society and its subsystems."

In a psychoanalytic panel (Buxbaum 1958) on the psychology of adolescence, there was general agreement that adolescence can be separated into three phases, during which the individual is expected to reach genital primacy and to make a nonincestuous object choice. Early adolescence and mid adolescence seemed to be fairly well-defined periods, but late adolescence could not be defined so easily. It was felt that "when an adolescent is considered an adult depends to a large degeree upon the society in which he lives . . . society imposes on him the length and duration of adolescence."

The term "identity" in the special sense that it is usually used today in mental health circles seems to have been introduced by Erikson (1945), and he, of course, is largely responsible for its subsequent elaboration. The concept was initially developed as a result of his observations of two Indian tribes, and in his earliest articles he seems more concerned with social identity, how the Indian child learns the appropriate identity that he or she is expected to have as an adult member of the culture. But from the beginning he recognized the dual nature of the identity concept, which has both an internal and an external component. Thus, one of his early definitions (Erikson 1946) is as follows: "The conscious feeling of having a personal identity is based on two simultaneous observations: the perception of one's self-sameness and continuity in time; and the simultaneous perception of the fact that others recognize one's sameness and continuity.'' This concept appears as ''Identity vs. Identity Diffusion,'' the fifth stage of Erikson's (1950) eight stages of the life cycle.

The concept of identity was broadened by several psychoanalytic theorists, notably Mahler, Greenacre, and Eissler, who attempted to trace its origins back to the earliest mother-child relationship and to relate it to body image, individuation-separation, and development of object relations (Rubenfine 1958). This is a much more fundamental vision of the identity problem having to do with what makes an individual conscious of himself or herself as a unique being and able to say ''I am I.''

Eissler (1958) talks about the ''prestages'' of identity formation that occur prior to puberty, which do not include the full sense of identity but are related to ''the ego's capacity to experience itself as a continuum.'' Greenacre (1958) conceptualizes ''the sense of own identity as coming into some kind of preliminary working form in the phallic-oedipal period,'' but it ''is subject to various changes and modal points of development, roughly following stages of body and maturational achievement with their accompanying emotional problems. Consequently, no sense of adult functional identity can be completed until after adolescence is well past and assimilated.''

Mahler (Rubenfine 1958) differentiates two important periods relating to integration of feelings of identity. The first is the period of separation-individuation, from one to three years of age, and the second is the period from three to latency, which she relates to the phase of resolution of bisexual identification. Although obviously not unrelated to Erikson's identity concept, which also had roots in infancy, these ideas differ rather markedly from his definition (Erikson 1956) of ''a configuration gradually integrating constitutional givens, idiosyncratic libidinal needs, favored capacities, significant identifications, effective defenses, successful sublimations, and consistent roles.'' This clearly tries to define adult identity in all its constituent parts, and is certainly all-inclusive—so all-inclusive, in fact, that it is difficult to know how it can be used—but it does make clear that he feels identity is a conglomerate with both unconscious and conscious elements and with interactions, both internal and external, between these elements. The individual may feel a coherence and consistency, but the fact that there are many elements included in the totality suggests to me that aspects of identity may change over time without necessarily disrupting the internal sense of consistency and continuity.

A brief digression is in order to consider the epigenetic principle on which Erikson's (1968) life-cycle concept is based. He states, "Whenever we try to understand growth, it is well to remember the epigenetic principle which is derived from the growth of organisms in utero." He postulates a ground plan and says, "Personality, therefore, can be said to develop according to steps predetermined in the human organism's readiness to be driven toward, to be aware of, and to interact with a widening radius of significant individuals and institutions."

The concept of epigenesis becomes significant when one considers the term "crisis." As far as I can determine, Erikson (1951) first used this concept when he stated, "As a therapeutic method psychoanalysis is occupied with disturbances in mental development. As a method of research it has made possible the delineation and the study of certain crises in the development of total personality," and "Each crisis in our growth and development brings with it new drives and new anxieties, new possibilities for development, and new limitations, new achievements, and new frustrations." In his paper (Erikson 1956) it is somewhat unclear whether he means crisis in the literal sense of the word, but he later states, "Crisis is used here in a developmental sense to connote not a threat of a catastrophe, but a turning point, a crucial period of increased vulnerability and heightened potential, and, therefore, the ontogenetic source of generational strength and maladjustment."

In her consideration of adolescence, Anna Freud (1958) asks, "Is the adolescent upset inevitable?" She answers affirmatively, stating that the equilibrium between the id and ego forces achieved at the end of latency is disrupted by the pubertal increase in drive activity, and, "consequently, it has to be abandoned to allow adult sexuality to be integrated into the individual's personality." If, however, one reads her paper carefully, one finds that she seems to be talking about earlier crises because she comments that some adolescents reach fourteen, fifteen, or sixteen years without having shown any overt signs; thus, the crisis she refers to directly seems more akin to Gottlieb's pubertal or mid-adolescent crises and not the Erikson identity crisis, which seems clearly to occur in late adolescence and to relate to the transition from adolescence to adulthood. On the other hand, this is less clear when later in her paper she describes details of "normal" adolescence in words that could well apply to the late adolescent period:

I take it that it is normal for an adolescent to behave for a considerable length of time in an inconsistent and unpredictable manner; to fight his impulses and to accept them; to ward them off successfully and to be overrun by them; to love his parents and to hate them; to revolt against them and to be dependent on them; to be deeply ashamed to acknowledge his mother before others and, unexpectedly, to desire heart-to-heart talks with her; to thrive on imitation of and identification with others while searching increasingly for his own identity; to be more idealistic, artistic, generous, and unselfish than he will ever be again, but also the opposite: self-centered, egotistical, calculating.

Thus, I think it is correct to say that Anna Freud seems to believe that some kind of crisis and resolution is necessary for healthy psychological development, while Erikson leaves it rather open. Certainly, in general parlance, I think, the term "identity crisis" is used to suggest a period of turmoil and uncertainty rather than an orderly process of decision making.

With the publication of the *Problems of Ego Identity*, Erikson (1956) developed and elaborated many of his earlier concepts, including identity formation, identity crisis, and psychosocial moratorium. He refers to different connotations of identity: "At one time, then, it will appear to refer to a conscious sense of individual identity; at another to an unconscious striving for a continuity of personal character; at a third, as a criterion for the silent doings of ego synthesis; and, finally, as a maintenance of an inner solidarity with a group's ideals and identity."

In summary, Erikson (1968) states:

Young people must become whole people in their own right, and this during a developmental stage characterized by a diversity of changes in physical growth, genital maturation, and social awareness. The wholeness to be achieved at this stage I have called a sense of inner identity. The young person, in order to experience wholeness, must feel a progressive continuity between that which he has come to be during the long years of childhood and that which he promises to become in the anticipated future; between that which he conceives himself to be and that which he perceives others to see in him and to expect of him.

Two other approaches to the problem need to be discussed. Offer and Offer (1976) reported a ten-year research project on a group of "normal adolescent males," studies by various interview, rating scale, and projective test techniques. The results delineated three major types of growth patterns, which they described as "continuous growth," "surgent growth," and "tumultuous growth." The continuous-growth group had a smooth transition through adolescence, an intact family that fostered independence, no serious clash of value systems, good interpersonal relationships including appropriate progress toward heterosexual intimacy, and a general sense of contentment. The surgent-growth group functioned equally adaptively but experienced more emotional conflict and a pattern of progression and regression with more conflict over values, concern about control of sexual impulses, and more difficulty in maintaining peer relationships. The tumultuous-growth group showed marked inner turmoil and some overt behavioral problems. For this group, adolescence was experienced as a discordant period with family conflict and some overt clinical problems, and although "less happy with themselves, [they were] just as successful academically or vocationally." Offer concludes that "there is more than one normal developmental process from childhood to adulthood." Discussion of his work by a psychoanalytic group raised questions about his criteria for "normality," however, leading to questioning of his conclusions (Sachs 1977).

A further and more complex phenomenon is the interaction between individual development and the particular culture in which a given individual is growing up. As already noted, Erikson's (1945, 1946) earliest comments on identity were related primarily to the specific culture of the individual and dealt with the issue of transition to adult status within that society. This brings to mind historical and anthropological observations on rites which mark this transition in formal and ritual ways. It is my impression that these rites usually occur at an earlier age, before full physical growth and development have occurred. One wonders, however, whether, at the time that the rite originated in a given society, emotional and psychological development were in consonance with the relevant cultural definition of adulthood.

77

In contemporary Western society, such rites have largely disappeared or are clearly unrelated to adulthood, and we tend to mark the end of adolescence at a later age. This raises the question whether psychological development has been actually retarded by the complexity of our culture or whether it has been arbitrarily delayed by the increased length of education, which, of course, is not unrelated to the complexity of the culture. In this connection, Prelinger (1974) feels strongly that adolescence is a culturally created stage of life.

If one believes, then, that society has an impact on psychological development, one must ask whether U.S. or Western European cultural values have had a fundamental influence on the psychological qualities that we feel are a necessary part of maturing. I have cited references that list independence from the family and formation of a separate identity as necessary tasks (Fry and Rostow 1942; Lidz 1968). Prelinger (1974) suggests that this description of maturity is the result of a society which stresses individualism and in which social and geographical mobility and freedom of choice as to career and marital partner are highly valued privileges. If one lives in a socially stratified society with little geographical or social mobility, arranged marriage, and a tradition of family-determined occupation, adulthood might not require the same qualities. In such a society the dependent individual might achieve a more successful adaptation, and one might talk about maturing and identity formation very differently.

With this as background, what can be said about a current view of late adolescence? I am convinced that, at least, in our contemporary society the transition to adulthood requires some degree of emancipation from the family; the establishment of a satisfactory sexual identity; the choice of a career, occupation, or work role; and the consolidation of a personal identity which includes all of the foregoing plus aspects that may be related to intellectual, social, interpersonal, religious, and moral functioning. Furthermore, the formation of identity incorporates both conscious and unconscious elements. The latter relate back to childhood and may define and limit the eventual shape that the adult identity of the individual takes. But as I have already indicated, I believe that a definition of identity such as Erikson's admits of partial identities, many of which have a component of conscious choice. To me, late adolescence is distinguished by the degree of conscious experimentation possible with a series of such partial identities, and by the opportunity to choose deliberately, at least within limits, the mix that will comprise the adult identity.

In this chapter I would like essentially to ignore the unconscious elements and discuss the simpler conscious elements considered by the late adolescent. These are not actually so simple because, as has been stated, even the conscious elements must be viewed from two points of references: the internal and external representations. The internal reference point describes how the individual sees himself, and the external describes how others see him. The internal representation of identity, then, consists of the sum of the roles that the individual sees himself as fulfilling plus the personality traits or qualities that he feels he possesses. The external representation consists of those roles and traits that others perceive him as fulfilling and possessing. Obviously, internal and external identity representations may sometimes be congruent or may be quite divergent. If one accepts the notion that identity consists of an amalgam of partial identities, which are capable of change, then it follows that the partial identities are not necessarily static but are in a kind of dynamic balance within the individual. They are constantly interacting, and there may also be interaction between internal and external so that the individual's sense of his own identity may be affected by others' perception of, and reaction to, him.

I have already mentioned the issue of choice. The opportunity for choice has been a goal of our society and, at least for those adolescents who are able to go to college, there is a bewildering array of choices all or any of which may have an impact on the kind of person he or she is going to become. Although I rather doubt that any individual consciously sets out to find "An Identity," most, I think, have some sense of the potential for new and broadening experience, and some quite deliberately experiment with all kinds of experience in the pursuit of personal development. One student expressed this feeling by saying that she heard a great deal about identity in high school, but she never understood what was meant. After a time at college, however, she recognized that it meant the opening of new possibilities to which different parts of her responded.

But the opportunity for choice which is so sought after and eulogized as a by-product of a free and mobile society has a negative side. During late adolescence, almost simultaneously with the opening of possibilities, the considerable pressure to choose has the effect of closing off some options. The most obvious choice of the period concerns occupation or career, but to choose one career inevitably means giving up many others. This narrowing of possibilities frequently has symbolic as well as practical meaning to the individual. For the first time he is forced to recognize that anything may be possible, but not everything. S. Sarason (personal communication, 1974) has suggested that the choice of major for some college students creates great psychic difficulty because the individual unconsciously associates this closing off with the final closing off of death, and consequently, the individual for the first time is brought face to face with his own mortality. Erikson (1968) has alluded to both the necessity for choice and the difficulty of making it as follows: "The sense of identity then, becomes more necessary (and more problematical), wherever a wide range of possible identities is envisaged." Conversely, the existence of very few choices may eliminate the dilemma of choosing, but simultaneously it may impose on the individual one or more partial identities which may make for considerable unhappiness. This paradox probably is most evident in areas having to do with career. If one graduates from college and is faced with getting a job—any job—an identity may be forced on one, and one isn't necessarily pleased with the result. The student who finds herself selling sandwiches door-to-door may have an identity as a peddler, but it is not satisfactory as a partial identity of a permanent nature, and she will in all probability give it up. Or, if one chooses to be a historian and no positions for teaching history exist, it may be difficult to maintain the identity.

I would like to discuss briefly three subareas of identity: educational, interpersonal, and ethical. In the educational sphere I include vocational choice, which in our society perhaps has an inordinate bearing on identity. What one does is a common question, and consequently, what one decides to do becomes an important part of a final identity. For many, the choice may be a relatively clear one even though the source of the decision is unclear. It may represent a field in which based on preliminary experience one feels one can excel, it may bear the clear-cut impress of family preference and/or pressure, or sometimes it is initially no more than a vague interest in a field which is generally acceptable, for example, business or teaching. For some, the decision is not so clear, and several shifts may occur before a final choice is made. Others may have no direction whatever during late adolescence, and the decision is postponed until the individual has had a variety of life experiences or until an outside fate intervenes.

The second area includes interpersonal, social, and sexual experience. As one reaches late adolescence, one has opportunities to broaden one's social contacts through attendance at college, job contacts, or travel. The experience of meeting new people may well open to the individual new vistas or possibilities through the interests of friends and through love relationships. In addition, sexual experience contributes to the establishment of a sexual identity which, obviously, is an important component of identity.

The third area, which I have called ethical, includes religious and moral considerations. Religion, defined most broadly, includes some inner conviction about the purpose of life. For many individuals this may not be a conscious concern, but for someone who is trying to make important decisions that will affect his or her future, it often is. In addition, an important partial identity that is derived from one's family experience often involves one's feeling about organized religion, and this feeling frequently is reassessed during this period. Within the moral sphere I refer to the overall goal of achieving some sense of inner acceptability of oneself as a person, operating in a social context, and including the development of a personally viable code of behavior. One has to live with oneself and one's identity for the rest of one's life, and the ultimate test of identity formation is the ability to do so relatively comfortably and within the confines of behavior tolerated by the social group in which one lives.

Although I have so far addressed the topic in very general terms, there are three current factors that I feel are influential, because I do believe that societal influence can be important in defining identity issues for any given generation.

The women's movement of the last twenty years is a good example of how an external force can affect an individual's feelings of identity. One can argue that such a movement would not have taken hold had there not been many individuals in whom it touched a responsive chord. Once in existence, however, I think it has a profound effect on many individuals who would not necessarily have developed their identity in a particular way in its absence. Some of the current mid-life concerns of women, I believe, are the result of the fact that the women's movement did not exist when they were adolescents. Presumably, they would have continued with their previous identity, perhaps unhappy and dissatisfied without quite knowing why, but not viewing the problem as a dilemma of identity and attempting a resolution.

Second, I have noted (Arnstein 1977) the impact of new attitudes toward relationships and sexuality that have influenced identity concepts. These include the expansion of friendship patterns to include cross-sex, nonerotized relationships; the greater acceptance of living-together relationships, which unquestionably bears on issues of commitment and career choice; a greater openness about homosexual orientation, which faces individuals more directly with the possibility of accepting an overt identity as homosexually oriented; and the possibility of a bisexual orientation, which introduces a new dimension to the traditional view of sexual identity. All four attitudinal shifts affect identity formation, I believe, by increasing the options available in relationships, and to a certain extent one's identity is defined by one's relationships.

Third, there currently is an interesting and paradoxical trend related to sexual development. As educational programs have increased in length and have postponed the age of adulthood, defined as assuming the full adult social role, there has been a tendency for genital sexual activity to start at earlier ages so that the establishment of sexual identity as evidenced by genital experience and adult sexual behavior is occurring for many closer to puberty when the capacity develops biologically. Although this may always have been the case for certain social groups, it is becoming more evident in just those groups for whom other aspects of adolescence are being prolonged by education and training. I have no clear idea what the psychological consequences are or will be, but I think they warrant consideration. One possible consequence could be that with greater opportunity for sexual release outside of marriage, the sexual drive to settle the partial identity of commitment to a particular marital partner is less intense, and that aspect of identity may remain open longer.

Finally, to return to my four questions: Although there is considerable difference of opinion, I feel that the term "identity crisis" is often used in misleading fashion. I do believe that late adolescence is a critical period in which important decisions, primarily conscious, will be made by every individual in the process of forming a more or less adult identity. This identity is still subject to later change, but usually postadolescent changes are of less significant magnitude. I do not feel able to say much about the psychological nature of the process except to say that some self-awareness may help in the conscious process of choosing. During the period there is often considerable turmoil, both internal and overt, but I have very little understanding of why individuals vary so much in the extent of such turmoil, and I can only cite Offer's work (Offer and Offer 1976) as a possible explanation. I think, however, this is still a relatively open question and deserves further study. The turmoil often involves stormy relations with parents and is followed by a changed relationship within the family. I further believe that the turmoil can reach pathological extremes and be expressed as an emancipation disorder of adolescence or an identity disorder.

Conclusions

Still unanswered are many other questions and many facets of the four questions I initially posed. For example, is there a normative adolescent psychological development? Is the critical period for identity formation in late adolescence age specific? If so, is this determined biologically or socioculturally? And what are the implications for an individual if it comes earlier or later than is usual for a given society? Some of these questions bear not only upon the adolescent's transition to adulthood but also on the potential impact of the late adolescent on his or her parents. If crisis and resolution are necessary parts of achieving maturity, parents who have somehow reached mid life without experiencing such a crisis may be more susceptible to identification with, or more upset by, an adolescent child grappling with this problem. Similarly, if one accepts the idea that critical periods of identity concern are affected by specific ideas or beliefs predominant during a particular era in society, parents and adolescent children may be vulnerable to, and affected simultaneously by, the same contemporary cultural climate or events. In summary, one can conceptualize three periods of identity formation: the child establishes that "I am I"; the adolescent asks "Who am I?"; and the adult is the "who" the late adolescent has consciously chosen to be within the limits unconsciously set up in childhood.

REFERENCES

Arnstein, R. 1977. Friends, lovers, and other more complicated relationships. *Journal of the American College Health Association* 25:232–236.

Blos, P. 1962. *On Adolescence: A Psychoanalytic Interpretation*. New York: Free Press.

Buxbaum, E. 1958. The psychology of adolescence. Panel Report. *Journal of the American Psychoanalytic Association* 6:111–121.

Eissler, K. 1958. Notes on problems of technique in the psychoanalytic treatment of adolescents. *Psychoanalytic Study of the Child* 13:223–254.

Erikson, E. 1945. Childhood and tradition in two American Indian tribes. *Psychoanalytic Study of the Child* 1:319–351.

Erikson, E. 1946. Ego development and historical change. *Psychoanalytic Study of the Child* 2:359–397.

Erikson, E. 1950. *Childhood and Society*. New York: Norton.

Erikson, E. 1953. On the sense of inner identity. In R. Knight and C. Friedman, eds. *Psychoanalytic Psychiatry and Psychology*. New York: International Universities Press, 1954.

Erikson, E. 1956. The problem of ego identity. *Journal of the American Psychoanalytic Association* 4:56–122.

Erikson, E. 1968. *Identity: Youth and Crisis*. New York: Norton.

Freud, A. 1936. *The Ego and the Mechanisms of Defense*. New York: International Universities Press, 1946.

Freud, A. 1958. Adolescence. *Psychoanalytic Study of the Child* 13:255–279.

Fry, C. C., and Rostow, E. G. 1942. *Mental Health in College*. New York: Commonwealth Fund.

Greenacre, P. 1958. Early physical determinants in the development of the sense of identity. *Journal of the American Psychoanalytic Association* 6:612–628.

Kiell, N. 1964. *The Universal Experience of Adolescence*. New York: International Universities Press.

Lichtenstein, H. 1977. *The Dilemma of Human Identity*. New York: Aronson.

Lidz, T. 1968. *The Person*. New York: Basic.

Offer, D., and Offer, J. B. 1976. Three developmental routes through normal male adolescence. *Adolescent Psychiatry* 4:121–141.

Prelinger, E. 1974. Crises of identity. In M. D. Keys, ed. *The Identity Crisis*. New York: National Project Center for Film and the Humanities.

Rubinfine, D. 1958. Problems of identity. Panel Report. *Journal of the American Psychoanalytic Association* 6:131–143.

Sachs, D. 1977. Current concepts of normality. Panel Report. *Journal of the American Psychoanalytic Association* 25:679–693.

Spiegel, L. A. 1958. Comments on psychoanalytic psychology of adolescence. *Psychoanalytic Study of the Child* 13:296–309.

6 COMPREHENSIVE MENTAL HEALTH CONSULTATION IN HIGH SCHOOLS

HENRY O. KANDLER

Nearly all children go to school. For children between the ages of five and eighteen, school provides the most influential experiences in their lives, next to their homes. Their successes, problems, and conflicts occur in school, and they spend more time doing school work than any other activity. Children complain about having to go to school, but the school community is a major organizing institution and usually the source of their social lives. By learning about other children and their families they obtain information which enables them to deal better with their own lives.

It is striking that many youngsters in a big city high school who are marked absent are, in fact, around the school—playing cards in the study hall, meeting friends in the lunchroom, hanging around the school steps when the weather is nice or in the luncheonette across the street when it is raining. At times such an "absent" youngster will attend the class of a favorite teacher, keep an appointment with the guidance counselor, or work on the yearbook. For these teenagers, and there are many of them, something is awry. And there are many more, sitting in their classrooms, daydreaming, unable to learn, anxious or bored.

Too often in the history of education, children with real social, psychological, or psychiatric problems are labeled as "badly be-haved." When this occurs, the parents may be called to school, subtly or directly blamed for their child's deviant behavior, and told to correct the situation. They fear that their child might be suspended and the world will assume that they are failures as parents. At times the child is taken to the family doctor for a physical checkup which is only useful when a contributing medical illness is found. Rarely is professional psychiatric or psychological help sought or obtained.

Today, more than ever, it is important that the various disciplines encompassing mental health—especially psychiatry, psychology, and social work—provide their knowledge to education. This chapter will explore various aspects of providing comprehensive mental health consultations to schools.

History and Current Practices

In the 1920s and 1930s, Anna Freud was a pioneer in discussing the relationship between psychoanalytic psychology and education. This was a natural evolution of psychoanalysis's concern with the development and upbringing of children. Freud described how aggressive and sexual drives and the development of the ego and superego affect a child's behavior in the classroom and his or her ability to learn (Freud 1930). In other papers (Freud 1949, 1952) she clarified how the role of the teacher must change from nursery school to grade school and beyond. She advocated that teachers teach different grades in order to develop perspectives on normal growth and to learn how to respond differentially, depending on a child's emotional and cognitive development.

Klein (1949) reviewed the psychoanalytic papers dealing with school-related problems and discussed clinical examples from his own practice. He stated:

School experiences are the first important experiences outside the family circle that involve systematic separation from the home and where the child is confronted with the need to adjust to strange children and adults, and at the same time to perform tasks from which escape is difficult. The attitudes of the teacher, the classmates, and the schoolwork are an important bridge between early attitudes to the parents, siblings and the self, and their later expression in adult life. The component instinctual drives, sado-masochistic trends, scoptophilic and exhibitionistic impulses, oral and anal strivings, and narcissistic attitudes play basic roles in the learning process and its impairment.

It was not until after the Second World War that psychological causes for poor school work became widely accepted. Guidance counselors, social workers, and psychologists began to be hired by school districts. Outside consultants, ranging from educational specialists to psychiatrists, were engaged. It was recognized that some children have emotional problems which prevent learning (Pearson 1952, 1954). Teachers became concerned with mental health (Smith 1956; Spache 1955). They were taught about early recognition of psychological problems, and the classroom was seen as a place for the prevention of future emotional difficulties. Techniques were developed for evaluating and helping children with reading and writing problems (Winkler, Tiegland, Munger, and Kranzler 1965). Teachers started to look at themselves and how they functioned as adult models and classroom leaders.

In the late 1950s and 1960s concepts derived from the theories of the psychology of groups, systems analysis, and community psychiatry began to be applied in some schools. Professionals concerned with education began to appreciate that there could be something wrong with the school itself, viewed as a dynamic system, which could prevent children from learning. It became apparent that teachers, administrators, and even the community in which the school was located could be major contributing factors to educational failures.

Newman (1967) described a philosophy of consultation based on the psychology of the interaction between two people, somewhat like the traditional supervision used in programs teaching psychotherapy. Newman defined the method of school consultation she and her staff developed as "based on certain principles of a psychodynamic approach to learning. It is centered on the relationships of consultant to staff members, and of staff members to the children they serve." The consultants are available "for continuous and regular consultation," not just for crises. Further, she stated "that continuing relationships and familiarity form the basis for trust, and that only with such trust, skillfully worked with, can one open new pathways of behavior and the new understandings that make possible desired changes of a lasting nature." She also felt that "there should be more emphasis on working with groups—applying knowledge of group behavior—in consultation with school staffs."

Caplan (1970) defined mental health consultation as a "process of interaction between two professional persons—the consultant, who is a specialist, and the consultee, who invokes the consultant's help in regard to a current work problem." In this type of consultation the consultant accepts no direct responsibility for implementing remedial action; rather, responsibility "remains with the consultee just as much as it did before he asked the consultant for help." Furthermore, Caplan described an educative function, "to add to the consultee's knowledge and to lessen areas of misunderstanding, so that he may be able in the future to deal more effectively on his own with this category of problem." He emphasized that consultation is not psychotherapy and that the personal problems of the consultee are never dealt with directly.

These models—individual evaluation and treatment of students, psychoanalytically oriented supervision of school staff, and consultation based on expert knowledge and education—are not mutually exclusive. All three approaches can be used by a team of mental health consultants in a school setting.

Description of School Mental Health Services

Schools are the natural meeting places for children, parents, educators, and mental health professionals. While the main purpose of school is to educate children, children, teachers, and schools often have problems which interfere with this process. Although schools should not be psychiatric clinics, they are the best environment for the early recognition of developmental, social, and psychological problems and an excellent setting for the rapid provision of help. Children and parents who would never go to a clinic or social agency will see the mental health professional at their school. Many children with less severe but, nevertheless, disabling problems can be helped directly, while others, who need more extensive help, can be referred to an appropriate agency or specialist.

A school consultation service established as an extension of our clinic has for over ten years provided teams which go into schools as a more effective and efficient way to deal with requests for help.[1] During a typical week at one of the high schools, the following services were provided: psychiatric and psychological evaluations, brief psychotherapy sessions, consultations with school staff, a seminar for guidance personnel, classroom discussion with students, and group therapy.

Requests for help usually start as a referral of a specific child. This may then lead to requests for help ranging from weekly conferences with a guidance counselor and discussions of staff problems with a principal to monthly seminars with a group of teachers interested in learning more about their interactions with their pupils. The adolescent students are another group often seeking consultation. They not only want help in coping with personal problems, but they also want to find better ways of dealing with other students, teachers, and the school system. Our school consultation service developed from these requests and from the schools' needs for psychological knowledge in dealing with students' and staff problems, and for training of students and professionals in school consultation techniques.

Any successful program of mental health in a school depends on the persons assigned to deal with those students referred by teachers and advisors. Usually these are guidance counselors, sometimes an assistant principal, and in more affluent school districts a social worker or psychologist. They should begin with a brief evaluation of the problem in order to decide what could be done. They might recommend brief counseling, a discussion with the teacher, or a conference with the parents. A more serious problem may require a fuller evaluation, perhaps with psychological tests and certain physical examinations. If a youngster is retarded, mentally ill, or physically handicapped, the law requires that he receive help to enable him to be educated to the full extent of his abilities. Nearly all school districts have special classes for the emotionally disturbed, retarded, and physically handicapped. If the school districts cannot provide these services themselves, they are required to place such students in private schools and pay for them. Some school districts have combined to provide specialized classes in regional centralized facilities. The degree of social and psychological services available to these youngsters varies considerably. For the most part they are inadequate. Virtually all of these children and their parents need psychological counseling and advice in dealing with many social and economic problems.

However, these youngsters with a specific, diagnosed condition represent only a part of the overall problem. Most children who have difficulties in school do not require special classes but need treatment and support so that they can learn to cope better with the everyday occurrences of school life. They need services in the school itself or in their community.

These services can be broken down into six broad, often overlapping areas: (1) evaluation of, referral of, and psychological support for those students who need special programs or classes; (2) counseling and brief therapy with students in regular school; (3) consultation with teachers, guidance counselors, and administrators; (4) training of staff; (5) teaching students about mental health issues; and (6) working with parents.

In the first area are services to children with obvious mental or physical disabilities. These are usually recognized when a child first enters school or often before. These children require careful diagnosis followed by a thorough educational evaluation. If such a child needs to be in a special class, there is usually some certification procedure and, more recently, a hearing and appeal procedure available to parents if they disagree. More typically, however, parents find themselves in the position of requesting special services which are not readily available.

Mental health specialists should provide counseling and, when needed, specific psychological treatment to students in special classes. They should be able to work with teachers, especially to translate for them a child's particular needs. These specialists should also work with parents to help them understand their child's strengths and disabilities and the parents' reaction to them. Further, they should promote optimal cooperation between parents, teacher, and child. It may be essential to help families of handicapped children with specific social problems such as housing, transportation, and finances. Psychological support and advice must also be available to those teachers within a regular school who do remedial work with such specific problems as learning disabilities, dyslexia, and speech problems.

The second area involves the major day-to-day contact between the mental health professionals and the rest of the school community. Students are usually referred by the guidance personnel or an educational administrator. In some schools teachers can refer students directly, students can make appointments for themselves without being referred, and parents may request that their child receive help.

After a preliminary evaluation the mental health consultant may do one of several things: (1) give advice to the person making the referral on how to help the student (if the student is self-referred, the consultant will advise the student on how to proceed in finding help for the problem presented); (2) confer with the student's family to clarify the issues further; (3) counsel or give brief psychotherapy; and (4) refer for further evaluation or therapy, within the school if available, to a social agency, clinic, or private practitioner in the community.

Because of the nature of consultative relationships, an evaluation or therapy can only be successful if it is based on the kind of candid information that is only obtainable in a relationship based on confidentiality and mutual trust. If the promised or implied confidentiality is ever betrayed, the consultant will no longer be trusted by the students, and he will no longer be effective. Therefore, any of the treatment-plan choices must be made with the student, and only with his permission may any of the evaluation's content be shared.

Often a three-way conference including the referral source, the student, and the consultant is the best way to give some information to a teacher or guidance counselor. If a family conference is indicated, the student and consultant should first decide what is to be told to the parents. At times feeling that he has the consultant in his corner, a student will be surprisingly open with his parents, telling them things he had hidden from them previously. If the problem the student presents is of a personal nature, the consultant may just say to the referring guidance counselor, "I saw John today. He is concerned about a personal matter which we will try to work out and I will see him once a week for a while." When a referral is necessary this often requires the joint efforts of the consultant, the school staff, and the parents. It can usually be done on the basis of the presenting symptoms or behavior without revealing any confidential material from the evaluation except, of course, to the professional to whom the referral is made.

Such referrals can be for special psychological evaluations, for longer-term psychotherapy, for medical and neurological examinations and treatment, for vision and hearing tests, and to social agencies and public assistance programs.

Therapy conducted in the school itself is usually brief in nature. It includes counseling of up to four sessions, brief psychotherapy (perhaps once a week from six to ten sessions), supportive therapy once every two weeks for twenty minutes, or group therapy—the latter being particularly well suited to a school setting.

The third area covers those instances when a consultation by the mental health specialist does not involve students directly. For example, a principal, dean, department head, or director of guidance may wish to discuss some general issues such as alcohol use by students or staff, relations with parents and the community, or intrastaff conflicts or administrative problems. The consultant may also be called upon to give advice to members of the faculty for their own personal problems or to arrange referrals for them.

The fourth area for the mental health consultant is that of the teaching and supervision of school staff, primarily to help them improve their skills in the area of human relations. This can include seminars for teachers, perhaps with credit through an in-service training program, and conferences with guidance personnel oriented around the discussion of particular students. This area includes consultations with teachers about teaching and interpersonal relationships in the classroom. Videotapes of actual classroom sessions have been very successful when discussed in small groups. Discussion following the viewing of these videotapes helps to make teachers more aware of mental health principles as they apply to the group interactions within the class. Berlin (1962, p. 671) stated:

> The Mental Health Consultant in a school system often has a unique opportunity to communicate and sometimes to demonstrate mental health principles to teachers.
>
> Perhaps the most important principle he can communicate to school people is the fact that all human feelings can be talked about without shame, blame or passing judgment on the teacher as a "bad" person. . . . He demonstrates in many ways that his job as an expert in interpersonal relations is to help the teacher understand himself in terms of the job he is doing, and, in particular, to help him be consciously aware of his feelings about the particular child who is a problem for him. The purpose is always to enable the teacher to do his work more effectively.

The fifth area is that in which the consultant teaches classes of students mental health topics such as sex education, psychology, and certain social issues.

A sixth area for the mental health consultant is working directly with parents. This may include talks to PTA organizations, training of school volunteers, and seminars and discussion groups about child and adolescent development and parenting issues.

Parents in culturally and economically deprived inner city areas are faced with special problems. Many have had bad experiences in school when they were children. As adults they are often afraid of any institution which represents authority, and they have never learned to understand the complexities of the school system. The mental health consultant can be most helpful to these parents by working with them to be able to deal with school authorities so that their children can take better advantage of what education has to offer.

Types of Consultations

The difficulties which usually bring a child to the attention of the guidance counselor and the mental health team are deviant behavior, disturbing behavior in the classroom, antisocial behavior in the schoolyard, failing grades, cutting classes, and absences. From the student's point of view the reasons are somewhat different. In the lower grades the child often presents well-defined problems: learning difficulties, physical disabilities, and mental illnesses ranging from the neurotic to the psychotic. In children who are in junior or senior high schools, by far the most frequent presenting complaint is related to the child's family, especially family conflicts and broken homes. Other complaints include failing marks due to lack of motivation and various other difficulties in school work; complaints about the school, teachers, and classes; peer problems; difficulties in making friends; fears and questions relating to sexual, aggressive, and dependent feelings; questions about cutting classes, drug use, violence, and run-ins with the law; and, finally, anxiety over plans for the future, phobic reactions, and various physical complaints.

Obviously these are only symptoms, usually representing some intrapsychic or developmental problem, although we also see the effects of tragic social problems ranging from inadequate housing and lack of money and jobs to such personal misfortunes as illness and death. If there are such psychological, personal, or social problems, coupled with a lack of communication at home, youngsters may turn to the guidance counselor at school.

The following are some examples of the types of problems dealt with by a team of school mental health consultants.

CASE EXAMPLE 1

Julie, a fifteen-year-old sophomore in high school, asked to see the psychiatrist as suggested by her health education teacher because she wanted some information for a paper she was writing. When they met, she explained that she was writing a paper about psychiatric hospitalization and asked the psychiatrist if he could recommend some articles. He said he would look some up and get the references to her but asked her how she had decided to write about this topic. Julie explained that her cousin had been hospitalized recently because of certain religious ideas. She asked the psychiatrist the difference between a belief and a delusion, and they discussed this for a while. She seemed quite anxious. The psychiatrist asked her if she ever worried about anything. Hesitantly, she told him that she was afraid of heights, water, and especially bugs. The previous summer she had been on a vacation in the country and had felt quite disabled. He explained the differences between phobias and delusions, and she seemed relieved. He suggested that they meet again the following week so that he could give her the references she had requested.

The following week, after discussing the articles, Julie told him that she had felt better after talking to him about her phobias. She had been worried that she might have a breakdown like her cousin. They discussed what kind of therapy might help with phobias. She pointed out that her fear of bugs was only a problem in the country. She said that she was not interested in treatment at the moment but would keep in touch with him.

CASE EXAMPLE 2

Bob, a fourteen-year-old tenth grader, was referred by his guidance counselor because he had been absent for many days with asthma. He told the consultant that he had had asthma since he was five. His parents divorced when he was four years old and he had not seen his father in two years. He had a sister, age twelve, and a brother seventeen who had been getting into trouble with the police. Bob tried to help his mother, who was on welfare and often ill. He complained that his mother did not understand him, his asthma, or his need to have some time for himself. It was suggested that a meeting with him and his mother might be helpful. He readily agreed.

The mother was a pleasant woman but without many resources and quite helpless as a parent. There was much more conflict at home than

Bob had indicated. Mother was seductive with Bob and fought with the older brother. Bob tried to protect her and was very competitive with his brother. The mother complained that Bob would not do his homework and she felt resentful when he wanted to go out and play with his friends. In addition, Bob was not getting any medical care for his asthma.

He was referred to the pulmonary clinic of a teaching hospital in his neighborhood, where psychiatric services were also available. In the meantime, Bob agreed to make an appointment with his guidance counselor to work out how he could catch up with the work he missed during his absences.

CASE EXAMPLE 3

Betty was a fourteen-year-old freshman in high school. The principal asked that someone on the consulting team see Betty because she had failed three out of five subjects in the first marking period of the year. Her teachers described Betty as defiant, unable to concentrate, self-destructive in her relationships with her classmates, and uncoordinated. Although she did well in mathematics, she could not spell.

At the meeting, to which she came reluctantly, she said she had no problems and refused to give the consultant a sample of her writing. She said she did not want help and would not make another appointment. The consultant, a psychologist, discussed the situation with the principal and guidance counselor. It was agreed that the consultant and guidance counselor should meet with the parents.

The parents were very concerned about Betty. She had always had trouble with reading and spelling. As long as they could remember, Betty had been uncoordinated. They felt guilty and wondered how they were responsible for Betty's difficulties. Recently she had been in much conflict with them, getting into violent arguments about smoking, staying out late at night, and failing to do her homework.

The psychologist suggested to the parents that Betty might have a learning disability and should have a neurological and psychological evaluation. The parents readily agreed. The consultant insisted on another meeting with Betty, during which she told her what had been discussed with her parents. Betty seemed somewhat less antagonistic and agreed to go for the evaluations. The consultant helped with the referrals to the specialists and arranged to discuss the results with the guidance counselor after the evaluations were completed.

CASE EXAMPLE 4

Joe, a senior in high school, was referred by his guidance counselor for cutting classes. He was bright, had always done well in school, and had won a scholarship to college, but now he was in danger of not graduating. Joe said he had "this problem" which caused him to miss classes, and he was too embarrassed to return.

Joe told the consultant that he was born in Europe and had come to this country when he was ten years old. He said that he had a very good family but they were formal and old fashioned. "They have different values," he said, "they don't understand me or my interests." He wanted to be a writer; he loved poetry. He read a lot and had just finished reading all the novels of Dickens. Joe said he had many friends but did not date. He denied that he had any problems with his family. He said that he would try to return to his classes and agreed to see the consultant again. As he was leaving, he turned and said, "By the way, I need to have a lot of work done on my teeth. It's just for cosmetic reasons. I can't make up my mind—I guess I'll have it done, I know then I'll be able to go back to my classes." The consultant had not noticed Joe's teeth up to that point, but with a closer look saw that they were moderately prominent.

They met again the following week. Joe reported that he was back in most of his classes. He said that he had made arrangements to have the dental surgery over the Christmas vacation and added that he was afraid girls would not look at him unless he had the dental work done.

The consultant saw Joe five times over the remainder of the school year. The dental work was almost completed. Joe began to express some criticism of his father; he described him as too rigid and felt that his father was not really interested in him. He talked about his apprehension at leaving home and going away to college. Joe finished the year with good grades and by the last session was looking forward to attending college in the fall.

CASE EXAMPLE 5

Alfred was referred by his guidance counselor as a very bright student who was flunking French. The father, who had been in touch with the counselor, thought that this might be related to the recent death of Alfred's mother. Alfred had always had problems adjusting socially and in the past had been briefly in psychotherapy.

The consultant described him as a "gnome-like, hypomanic, over-intellectualized genius" who had no idea why his counselor had suggested the consultation. Alfred explained everything in terms of physics and mathematics. He stated that he had no patience with people, that emotions were useless, and that "society must find a way to get rid of feelings so that the world can be run by computers." He was sure he could pull up his French grade to an A. He said that he spent most of his time when not at school reading in his room or working on his collections of stamps, postcards, and maps. He said that he did not want to see the consultant again and did not believe in psychiatry, but he agreed to have the consultant talk to his father on the telephone.

The father was quite concerned about Alfred. The mother had died of cancer two years previously. Alfred refused to talk about his mother's death. The father described the boy as being lonely and without friends. "At times he gets into a panic at home. Then he can't do his work, especially his French."

Alfred was discussed at the weekly guidance staff meeting. It was decided that his guidance counselor, a woman who spoke fluent French, would arrange to see him twenty minutes a week, ostensibly to discuss his French. His English teacher, who attended the conference, agreed to spend some additional time with Alfred and would try to get him interested in joining the Debating Club, for which he was the advisor. The consultant met regularly with the guidance counselor to discuss Alfred. Alfred never missed an appointment with her. After two months, they began to discuss some of his difficulties. He accepted a referral to a nearby psychiatric clinic, where at the suggestion of the consultant, he was assigned to a woman therapist. Alfred continued to meet weekly with his guidance counselor for the rest of the school year.

CASE EXAMPLE 6

In a minischool for drug abuse-prone youngsters, the director of the consultation service led a monthly meeting of his staff and the teachers, principal, and psychologist of the school. The teachers began this meeting by requesting that Natalie be discussed. Although she was bright and at times did superior schoolwork, she was often angry, volatile, foul mouthed, suspicious, and provocative, causing disturbances which made learning impossible for the other children. In a general discussion about her, it turned out that the teachers knew a great deal about her life and family. Natalie had always had trouble in school. She never knew her father; her mother worked and was often ill. Natalie and her mother could not stand each other, and Natalie often stayed with an aunt or neighbor. She felt rejected and abandoned, and it was clear that her mother would rather live without her. Her story and that of her siblings, half and stepsisters and brothers, was a long saga of abuse and neglect. One teacher mentioned that Natalie had told her she would soon be transferred to another school. "She's paranoid, she's always saying something like that." However, the principal apologetically acknowledged that he had been making plans to request the mother to come to a meeting at the district office, the purpose of which was to transfer Natalie. He had not discussed this with the rest of the staff. The teachers were upset. One said he had felt guilty when he got angry at Natalie and because he thought that they had not tried hard enough to help her. In the discussion which followed, two points of view developed. The view of the principal was that she was disrupting the education of the other children in her class and not learning anything herself, while she deprived another youngster of a spot in this special program. The teachers, on the other hand, liked her and wanted more time to figure out how to help Natalie. A compromise was reached which included the following: The teachers involved with Natalie would draw up a new, individualized program for her; the social worker from the consultation team would evaluate Natalie's family and living arrangements and, if possible, begin working with the mother; the psychiatrist on the team would investigate treatment possibilities for Natalie; the principal would agree to postpone any plans for transferring her, but a specific date was set for reevaluating her progress; and the head teacher of the minischool would discuss these plans with Natalie and, while making it clear that her behavior had been unacceptable, would express the staff's interest and concern about her.

CASE EXAMPLE 7

At times a school as a complex community is in crisis. For example, recently the director of Pupil Personnel Services of a nearby school district called the psychiatric clinic for an evaluation of an intermediate school student who lived in the area. She described him as making overt sexual advances, and she thought he was having a "sexual identity problem." She explained that the teachers liked him and wanted to work toward keeping him in the school but wanted to know "if this is an extreme form of normal adolescence."

On examination he was found to be acutely psychotic, grossly confused about his sexual identity, and delusional, and he had to be hospitalized. The psychiatrist of the school consultation service, whom the director of Pupil Personnel Services had called, became intrigued with the diagnosis the director had given him. In a further telephone discussion she said there were lots of problems in this new school, and she invited him to visit there with her. The following week the consultant met at the school with her, the principal, the guidance counselor, and the boy's teacher. It became clear that the staff at the school had denied the obvious seriousness of this student's illness. They blamed his upset and the many other problems at the school on the general "bad" behavior of the student body. This was a brand new intermediate school in a run-down ghetto area. Two-thirds of the teachers had previously taught at elementary schools in much better middle-class neighborhoods. They had had no experience teaching adolescents. They had not wanted to be transferred to this new school and they were upset about teaching in this run-down area where many of the families spoke only Spanish. Obviously this was an institutional identity problem of the school itself.

Therefore it was planned that groups of ten teachers meet for six consecutive weeks for a series of lunchtime seminars. The group, led by the psychiatrist, began by considering several case presentations of classroom problems. They discussed how to get the administration to respond more quickly when a teacher asked for help with a student who was having difficulties or disturbing the class. They then talked about normal adolescence and how the teachers felt about having to deal with youngsters who were more aggressive, challenging, and sexually provocative. The consultant presented some examples of variants of normal adolescent behavior based on different ethnic and socioeconomic backgrounds. They began to confide their personal misgivings about the move to this new school and community, especially their fears of violence. And finally they talked openly about their own reactions to these older youngsters when they were a disturbance in their classroom. They concluded that "if we got rid of the ten biggest troublemakers in the school, they'd only be replaced by ten more. We'll just have to work together and figure out how we can handle things better."

Social Structure and Administrative Power

In the past decade there has been a growing literature documenting that many public schools are "oppressive and joyless" (Silberman 1970), while advantages and disadvantages of "permissiveness" have been debated. Other authors have written that our schools tend to suppress initiative, imagination, and curiosity, and foster mediocrity, conformity, and rote thinking. Of more particular interest to mental health professionals, it is suggested that the schools tend to bring out latent pathology in children and generally retard even normal children's maturation, hindering children from understanding and solving the most ordinary and common psychological problems by themselves. Even in the best of schools youngsters learn the lessons of caste, class, and power.

To maximize what a consultant can do in a school setting, he has to understand the social structure, methods of administration, and personalities of the staff, especially of those in positions of power. The consultant must also know something about the parents and the community in which the school is situated and must be aware of the different criteria in various schools for determining what is a problem for referral to the guidance counselor or mental health professional and what requires disciplinary action. He must know how the power is distributed, who dispenses help, and who gets credit for it.

For example, in a series of meetings with a district administrator, a mental health team was trying to work out an agreement about how it might help a particular program of special education classes. It soon became apparent that the administrator wanted to use the team as a "present" to various other schools in order to make up for recent budget cuts, unrelated to what the team wanted to do, what it could do, or how it could contribute its expertise most effectively.

Consultants must be aware of issues of job security and who feels threatened by an outside expert. And finally, mental health professionals must know what the parents and community will allow, what they think of psychiatry, what they think of psychological testing, and what they think of social workers.

It is most important that there be a clear understanding between the consultant and the school concerning the responsibilities of each profession. This must include such issues as the amount of time the consultant will be available each week, what kind of office space the school will provide, and the length of the agreement (usually the school year). At times a written agreement, which may include the PTA and the superintendent of the school district as cosigners, has been helpful in defining the responsibilities of the parties involved.

It is obvious today that schools beset by lack of funds, overcrowding, crime, and open conflict often do not allow for maximal learning. It is also well documented that children coming from deprived environments begin school with a tremendous handicap few overcome. There are, however, less visible factors which determine how a school functions. For example, when a principal is hired, experience and training are carefully scrutinized, but psychological makeup may be neglected. Yet the personality of the principal influences how teachers and students relate to each other and often determines what is considered a mental health problem and who is to receive help. The following are three brief vignettes to illustrate how various high school principals function.

CASE EXAMPLE 8

In the first school, the guidance counselor had to request permission from the principal before referring a student to the consulting team. In effect the principal alone decided the criteria for a psychiatric consultation. He reviewed all such requests from teachers to the guidance counselors. Students and teachers had no direct access to the psychiatric consultant.

CASE EXAMPLE 9

A consultant began working in the second school one May; he did not meet the principal until January of the following year, and then only at his request. This principal delegated authority to the point of withdrawing from the everyday affairs of the school. She only intervened when there were crises which came to her attention. Referrals to the consultant were therefore made directly by teachers and counselors alike. Students were also free to make appointments directly. No records were kept of these referrals and no questions were asked.

CASE EXAMPLE 10

In a third school few students were referred. One morning a social worker on the consulting team was sitting with the assistant principal, a well-meaning, anxious, rather ineffective man who was complaining about the lack of discipline at the school. Just then a youngster about sixteen years of age passed by the glass-windowed door and waved cheerily. The assistant principal said to the social worker, "Now there's an example," and motioned to the boy to enter his office, which he did, saying with a smile, "How are you, Mr. F?" The assistant principal answered, "You know you're not allowed to wear your coat in school, why are you breaking the rules? If the principal catches you, you'll be in trouble. He doesn't even want you to wear those hats." The student just smiled, said, "O.K." and went on his way, still wearing his coat and hat. The social worker asked the assistant principal why there was this rule, and he explained that it was to prevent students from leaving school in the middle of the day. He added that the principal was very strict about this and was upset that the parents association had recently insisted that students be allowed to wear hats in school, a symbol of status among the local youth groups and gangs.

These three styles of leadership helped to shape a different emotional climate in each of the three schools. In the first school, the principal and guidance counselor felt competitive with and threatened by the consultant. As a result, the teachers felt restrained from making their own judgments about students' needs and therefore refrained from becoming involved with the problems of their students. In the second school, the principal's attitude was seen as encouragement and approval of the way things were going in the school. In the third school the students had the feeling that the staff was an enemy against whom they had to be constantly on guard, while the teachers blamed the considerable difficulties in this school on the principal and the other administrators.

The presence of a consultant in a special education program, in the mind of some, validates the view that these children are "crazy." Similarly, when children are referred to the consultant it often reinforces their feelings that they are different. It is always the first task of the consultant to get himself accepted by both teachers and children. When that has taken place, the consultant is usually welcome in any class and can see any child any time. In such a milieu, the consultant can quickly be helpful when a crisis occurs. As a recent example, in a minischool where we had a consultant, a teenager died when he fell off the back of a bus where he was hitching a ride. The consultant was immediately able to meet with each class and its teacher to talk about the tragedy and to discuss the feelings it aroused. In addition, several children met with him privately the same day.

Besides using knowledge to provide consultation, education, and service to a school, the mental health professional can help improve a school by looking at the school from a systems point of view. From this vantage point he can try to influence the persons with power to make constructive changes by advising the principal or other staff members who have administrative power. The consultant can give advice on solving faculty problems and changing administrative structure or procedures, and he can recommend changes in staff or staff function. Sometimes changes in the physical environment within a school can also help to improve the learning environment.

Staff Of the School Mental Health Team

When reference was made to the specialists providing mental health services in schools, a general descriptive title was used, such as "mental health professional" or "consultant." Most important are the personalities of consultants. They must be sensitive to both the ethos of the school as a whole and to the needs of the individuals who function within it. Teachers must be able to trust the consultants' expertise and at the same time accept them as equals so that they can be a part of the daily informal conversations which take place in the staff lounge, corridors, and lunchroom. Consultants must also respect the knowledge and experience of the school staff. Often one of the most important functions of a consultant is to help teachers have confidence in their own observations and judgments about children.

The training of these specialists usually includes one of the following: education, guidance, counseling, social work, psychology, or psychiatry. However, as the report of the Joint Commission on Mental Health of Children (1969) points out, "professionals frequently have too rigid a view of their own particular specialized roles and functions. A broader, more flexible way of working is preferred, one which is based on the concepts of child development approach." The report goes on to state:

> A mental health service related to the school needs to include people who are capable of bridging the gap between the community and the school, bringing together the child and the curriculum, consulting on the learning and behavior of children with other school personnel, communicating and translating mental health concepts to the teacher, working with the teacher so that he can function in his classroom more effectively, and working with parents on a variety of child-rearing problems. Knowledge of ways of performing these functions does not need to be the particular specialty of any one professional group. They can be performed or shared by all, depending on the person's individual skill, experience, and training.

Of course, there are particular skills which training in a special area provides: for the guidance counselor, an intimate knowledge of the school system and how it works; for a psychologist, psychological testing and evaluations of learning disabilities; for a psychiatrist, the relationship between physiological and neurological states and mental functioning; and for a social worker, a knowledge of the morass of social agencies and their interrelationships. Therefore, a mental health team composed of specialists with a variety of training and backgrounds serves a school best.

Similarly, there are different advantages and disadvantages when such a specialist is a regular member of the school staff and when he or she is an outside consultant. The insider has the advantage of being a part of the system, where his power, or lack of it, is well established. The insider is on an equal basis with the teachers, which also makes him susceptible to favoring a teacher's point of view and to protecting his own rights within the system. Outside specialists have the advantage that they can be more independent in their judgments and counsel. In times of dwindling budgets, they can bring the resources of an outside agency, clinic, or university to a school. The outsider is at a disadvantage in that he or she has no direct power within the system and must often spend much time promoting service planning. The outsider can more easily be eliminated, at times for being right and for shaking up the system.

Boards of education are mandated to provide special education and hence must do the evaluation and certification of students who may need it. They must also provide the psychological and social services needed by the children in these programs and their families as part of the educative process. This usually falls to full-time staff in these special settings.

Whatever the services are that are being provided, they must be located at the school. The best arrangement is one that uses both permanent staff of the school system and a team of outside consultants who work together.

Within the regular schools, the key member of the mental health team is the school guidance counselor. Besides doing evaluations, counseling, and referrals, the guidance counselor is in the best position, together with the teacher in the classroom, for the early recognition of psychological and social problems. The guidance counselor is also the person who can most easily bring together administrators, teachers, students, parents, and mental health professionals, either by a formal referral, conference, or casual conversation in the lunchroom.

Local clinics, social agencies, universities, medical schools, and private physicians, psychologists, and social workers provide a wealth of expertise to the school in addition to being the recipients of referrals. They can make invaluable contributions by staffing a multidisciplinary mental health team within a school. Many of the services outlined can be provided by outside consultants and the permanent staff hired by the school district. Each group can contribute what is best from its vantage point.

Problems in the Provision of Services

Providing psychological services in public schools—especially by a team of experts from local agencies, hospitals, and professional schools—brings with it certain problems. The most important issue is that of confidentiality. Without complete trust a youngster being seen in consultation may withhold information without which it would be difficult, if not impossible, to do a proper evaluation or therapy. Whatever the purpose of the consultation, the issue of confidentiality must be discussed from the start. The consultant and the student must clarify what information can be shared with a guidance counselor, teacher, or parents (if there is to be a meeting with them). If the matter under discussion is entirely personal the consultant must assure the student that it will not be revealed to anyone. Similarly, all consultations with school staff must also be strictly confidential.

It is good clinical practice to keep records of all contacts made by a mental health team. This is useful in many ways: it allows for review when an opinion is in doubt; it makes it possible to pass along clinical records when there are staff changes; and, with proper permission, it enables the giving of information to outside professionals, agencies, and clinics when a referral is made. These records must be kept confidential and apart from the regular school files, which are usually open to parents and to anyone in the school system. Even so, these arrangements are threatened today by new right-to-information laws and regulations. Records can be protected by considering them as clinic visits and can be kept in the clinic or agency files.

A concomitant issue is that of parental permission. Can a psychologist talk to a child with a possible learning disability without permission from a parent? Can he test a child? Can he do brief therapy or counseling without permission? And what about high school adolescents who seek help for themselves but will only do so if their parents are not informed? Hofmann and Pilpel (1973) state that:

Nowhere has there been more vigorous movement toward according minors adult rights than in the matter of medical care.
Within the past six years nearly every state has enacted legislation
enabling certain groups of minors to consent to some or all of their
own health care, and the trend to expand the scope of such
statutes seems to be accelerating. These laws have arisen in part
out of the recognition that many adolescents do have the capacity
to make a valid informed consent.

Regarding the medical and psychiatric needs of teenagers, it would be
preferable if teenagers confided in their parents, but, even in intact
families, normal adolescent development conflicts often make this
difficult. It is in just those families where parent-child communications
have broken down that the youth will be most apt to act out and will
often seek medical and psychiatric help only if they can secure it on
their own consent and can be assured of confidentiality (Hofmann and
Pilpel 1973). Despite this, clinic administrators, school district
superintendents, and professionals of all kinds are ambivalent about
treating adolescents without permission, even though Pilpel (1972)
found that as yet no instance has occurred in which a physician or
health facility has been held liable for failing to secure parental consent
for medical treatment of a minor.

In most school districts there is increased structuring in the schools
which interferes with the kind of informal discussion among teachers
and with consultants which allows for solving problems in the
classrooms. Lunchtime seminars may not be allowed under some
union contracts and there are rigid procedural rules for the handling of
disturbing youngsters. As teachers look for more security and better
working conditions, decisions have been taken out of the hands of
teachers, school boards, and parents. Cheng (1976) points out that
issues are now negotiated by labor relations specialists hired by school
administrators, on one side, and teacher unions, on the other. He
recommends strategies for teachers and community groups through
which they can take a more active and creative part in these proceedings.

The main purpose of a mental health consultation team in a school
setting is to help provide better education for the students. Too often
the consultants lose sight of this purpose and function like a clinic in

the school. This may help some of the children, but it negates the unique aspects of on-site consultation.

A concomitant problem is that, with decreasing funds leading to loss of guidance staff, often only the most seriously disturbed youngsters in a school are seen, and they take up all the available time of the consultants. Mumford, Balser, and Rucker (1970) studied psychiatric services in secondary schools provided to a sample of the most seriously disturbed students in these schools. The treated group actually did worse than the control group, with both having a very high dropout rate. Students with diagnosable psychiatric conditions are best referred for intensive and prolonged treatment to clinics and private therapists. Similarly, it is not appropriate for school-based services to prescribe and supervise medication. Children requiring medication should be followed by a clinic or a private physician. Consulting teams should spend more time doing preventive work in the schools and dealing with those problems caused by developmental interruptions.

Research

There has not been enough research directed to the question of what makes a good school. Coleman and others (1966) reported that family background was the only important factor in determining pupil achievement and that parameters that the educational system can control, such as teacher-pupil ratio, were barely significant. Fleischmann (1973) corroborated this finding. Jenks and Brown (1975), in a study involving ninety-eight high schools and 12,000 students and conducted for nine years, found that no characteristics of seventeen variables tested—such as class size, teacher education, and family background—had any consistent effect on test scores, educational attainment, or occupational status after graduation. They concluded that chance was the most important factor in determining a student's achievement and future income.

These findings are misleading. Schools and teachers may have a reputation for excellence or mediocrity, and often test scores support these views. What is needed are studies which analyze how schools differ dynamically and how the attitudes of teachers and students affect the learning process.

Another shortcoming of the studies cited above is that they assume that all children are alike. Obviously this is not so. Perhaps only six children in a class of twenty-five need a smaller class to be able to learn. To ignore such considerations distorts the implications of the findings of these studies.

Even less has been studied about the effects of mental health principles on education. In the study by Mumford, Balser, and Rucker (1970), in spite of the fact that no improvement was found, the school staff found the consultants helpful. More promising have been studies like that of Comer (1976) which focused on a particular aspect of education—the length of time a child spends with the same teacher.

Escalona (1967) called on specialists in mental health to do more research to improve the effectiveness of education. She pointed out that "the experience of learning, and the perception of the self as one who can learn, generates a sense of the self as an active being, and a sense of the self as the carrier of power and competence." She goes on to state that "children who have learned to learn stand a better chance of surviving even serious trauma than do those who never had a chance for mastery on an intellectual level."

Conclusions

A mental health team can consult and provide service in a variety of ways in a school. To do disparate tasks requires a continuous dialogue between the consultants and the school staff so that each has a clear understanding of the abilities and needs of the other.

Consultation teams can provide evaluation and limited individual and group treatment for students and their families within the school setting. Mental health professionals can consult with teachers, guidance counselors, and administrators about specific issues and provide education for both students and their parents. And finally, consultation teams located in the schools can help teachers more effectively recognize and deal with mental health issues in the classroom. These include the early recognition of social, psychological, and psychiatric problems and the utilization of knowledge about personality and awareness of group dynamics to making the classroom a better environment in which children can grow and learn.

1. School Consultation Service of the Child and Adolescent Psychiatric Clinic, Bronx Municipal Hospital Center and the Albert Einstein College of Medicine, New York.

REFERENCES

Berlin, I. N. 1962. Mental health consultation in schools as a means of communicating mental health principles. *Journal of the American Academy of Child Psychiatry* 1(4): 671–679.

Caplan, G. 1970. *The Theory and Practice of Mental Health Consultation*. New York: Basic.

Cheng, C. W. 1976. Community participation in teacher collective bargaining: problems and prospects. *Harvard Educational Review* 46 (2): 153–174.

Coleman, J. S.; Campbell, E.; Hobson, C.; McPartland, J.; Mood, A.; Weinfeld, F.; and York, R. 1966. *Equality of Educational Opportunity*. Washington, D.C.: Government Printing Office.

Comer, J. P. 1976. Improving the quality and continuity of relationships in two inner city schools. *Journal of the American Academy of Child Psychiatry* 15(3): 535–545.

Escalona, S. K. 1967. Mental health, the educational process and the schools. *American Journal of Orthopsychiatry* 37:1–4.

Fleischmann, M. 1973. *On the Quality, Cost and Financing of Elementary and Secondary Education in New York State*. New York: Viking.

Freud, A. 1930. The relation between psychoanalysis and education. *The Writings of Anna Freud* 1:121–133. New York: International Universities Press, 1974.

Freud, A. 1949. Nursery school education: its uses and dangers. *The Writings of Anna Freud* 4:545–559. New York: International Universities Press, 1968.

Freud, A. 1952. Answering teachers questions. *The Writings of Anna Freud* 4:560–568. New York: International Universities Press, 1968.

Hofmann, A. D., and Pilpel, H. F. 1973. The legal rights of minors. *Pediatric Clinics of North America* 20(4): 989–1004.

Jenks, C., and Brown, M. 1975. Effects of high schools on their students. *Harvard Educational Review* 45(3): 273–324.

Joint Commission on Mental Health of Children. 1969. *Crisis in Child Mental Health: Challenge for the 1970's*. New York: Harper & Row.

Klein, E. 1949. Psychoanalytic aspects of school problems. *Psychoanalytic Study of the Child* 3/4:369–390.

Mumford, E.; Balser, B.; and Rucker, M. 1970. Ambiguities in a secondary school mental health project. *American Journal of Psychiatry* 126(12): 1711–1717.

Newman, R. G. 1967. *Psychological Consultation in the Schools*. New York: Basic.

Pearson, G. H. 1952. A survey of learning difficulties in children. *Psychoanalytic Study of the Child* 7:322–386.

Pearson, G. H. 1954. *Psychoanalysis and the Education of the Child*. New York: Norton.

Pilpel, H. F. 1972. Minors rights to medical care. *Albany Law Review* 36(3): 462–487.

Silberman, C. E. 1970. *Crisis in the Classroom*. New York: Random House.

Smith, D. E. P. 1956. Reading improvement as a function of student personality and teaching method. *Journal of Educational Psychology* 47:47–59.

Spache, G. D. 1955. Appraising the personality of remedial pupils. *Education in a Free World*. Washington, D.C.: American Council on Education.

Winkler, R. C.; Tiegland, J. J.; Munger, P. F.; and Kranzler, G. D. 1965. The effects of selected counseling and remedial techniques on underachieving elementary school students. *Journal of Consulting Psychology* 12:384–387.

PART II

DEVELOPMENTAL ISSUES: ADOLESCENT PROCESS, SEXUALITY, AND CHANGE

EDITORS' INTRODUCTION

The essence of adolescence is that it is a phase of psychic growth. The developmental processes that are characteristic of the transition from puberty to early adulthood involve the development of sexuality and the acquisition of a sexual identity. In contrast to childhood where infantile sexuality is the product of psychic forces and represents attachments to parents based upon self-preservative and self-esteeming needs, the sexuality of the adolescent has also acquired a biological impetus due to the maturation of the genital apparatus.

Never is the interplay of sociocultural forces and biological maturation so emphasized as it is during puberty and postpuberty. Repressive attitudes about sex seem to have disappeared; at least, this seems to be the case. Parents who have been raised nonpermissively regarding sexual attitudes have become liberated. They accept their children living with their boyfriends or girl friends without the legal bond of marriage. How comfortable such parents are is an open question. In view of the sudden sweeping changes in sexual mores, it would be difficult to believe that they have basically revised their deep characterologically ingrained attitudes. Clinical studies have demonstrated that the family has raised children according to the mores the parents accepted and then, when the child reaches puberty, suddenly switches to contemporary standards. This, of course, has its effects on the adolescent's confusion and construction of a sexual identity.

Sexual theories and formulations, in the past, have usually referred to masculine development. Girls have been relatively neglected and pushed into the background. Here, two papers refer to factors that are specific to the achievement of femininity, and they are discussed in their own right rather than as vicissitudes of male sexuality.

Roger L. Shapiro finds that character pathology in the adolescent is related in specific ways to the characteristics of defenses, regression, and consequent distortions in the relationships between the parents and the developing child. Evidence has been found that these families have shared unconscious fantasies which militate against change of repetitive behaviors and interfere with development and individuation of the child. He writes that it is possible to characterize the level of family regression, to define with precision shared unconscious fantasies and assumptions, and to describe the characteristics of shared and complementary higher-level or lower-level defensive behaviors between and among family members.

Albert Bryt examines the developmental task of adolescence, the impact of social conditions on the eventual goal of personality integration, as well as the influence of youth on society. He questions the concept of normative adolescent rebelliousness and believes young people are critical of the preservation of a democratic society. Bryt sees the role of psychiatry as facilitating the achievement of adolescent developmental tasks and discusses dissent, experimental role playing, individual emancipation, rights of young people, adolescent sexuality, and group conformity. He concludes that youth are interested in the pursuit of higher goals and in the preservation of social institutions rather than their destruction.

Clarice J. Kestenbaum studies the effects of current sexual attitudes on midadolescent girls. Still in the process of development, the midadolescent is in a vulnerable position regarding her self-concept and role in society. Kestenbaum believes that young adolescents are thrust prematurely into structureless sexual situations because of a growing societal permissiveness. She presents clinical illustrations to describe the use of maladaptive defense maneuvers in an attempt to handle the resulting stress.

Lynn Whisnant, Elizabeth Brett, and Leonard Zegans explore menarche and menstruation as an indicator of developmental attitudes toward a girl's body-image formation. In their clinical research they conclude that the use by adolescent girls of a tampon rather than a sanitary napkin may serve an important role in female psychosexual development through coming to terms with the maturing body, loosening childhood ties to mother, developing a positive body image, and making a positive identification as a mature female beginning heterosexual experiences.

Special Editor Sidney Werkman introduces a special section on the Effects of Geographic Mobility on Adolescents. This section, based on a series of meetings held by the American Society for Adolescent Psychiatry, examines the developmental aspects of moving and radical geographic cultural change.

Sidney Werkman describes his experiences with adolescents who have lived overseas with their families and as students at overseas school programs and focuses on their styles of adaptation, character, and attitudes. Overseas adolescents were found to be searching and open, but less secure and with vulnerability for experiencing adjustment reactions. They are candidates to become restless, possibly rootless, with a constant need to be on the move. Interferences with stable development at critical periods is postulated as the fundamental cause resulting in affective, separation-individuation, and self-concept difficulties.

Jon A. Shaw studies the adolescent's self-perception and hypothesizes that frequent family moves interfere with the adolescent process, with its movement toward consolidations of an ego-identity and capacity for intimate relationships, and may leave the adolescent with a negative perception of himself.

John G. Looney reports about the responses of refugee adolescents brought to the United States. He was struck by the differences between Vietnamese and American adolescents. The Vietnamese teenagers were generally stable, cooperative, caring, and committed to their family. The factor most highly correlated with good adjustment was family solidarity.

7 FAMILY DYNAMICS AND OBJECT-RELATIONS THEORY: AN ANALYTIC, GROUP-INTERPRETIVE APPROACH TO FAMILY THERAPY

ROGER L. SHAPIRO

Psychoanalysis became an object-relations theory when Freud proposed the structural hypotheses in *The Ego and the Id* (1923). Prior to that, in psychoanalytic theory, interest in objects was limited to their role in affording need gratification through drive discharge, and identification was conceived of as a mechanism of defense. Freud's increasing recognition of the role of identification in mental life led him to propose that identification was a crucial factor in the formation of ego and superego. This was a change in his conceptualization of the role of object relations in development.

In structural theory, internalizations of object relations were crucial constituents in the formation of psychic structure (Loewald 1966). The structural theory established psychoanalysis as a developmental theory. Subsequent contributions to psychoanalytic theory in ego psychology and the work of the British school of object relations were built on the foundation of structural theory. These contributions continued the effort to comprehend the relation of the individual to reality through conceptualizing processes of internalization of object relations during development and their persistence and state of organization in both conscious and unconscious mental processes (Shapiro 1978).

This position is consistent with that of Kernberg (1976), who states: "In the broadest terms psychoanalytic object-relations theory represents the psychoanalytic study of the nature and origin of interpersonal relations, and of the nature and origin of intrapsychic structures deriving from, fixating, modifying and reactivating past internalized relations with others in the context of present interpersonal relations. Psychoanalytic object-relations theory focuses upon the internalization of interpersonal relations, their contribution to normal and pathological ego and superego developments, and the mutual influences of intrapsychic and interpersonal object-relations.''

Psychoanalysis was established as a personality theory and as a therapy before the structural theory was formulated. The methods of psychoanalysis as a therapy were based upon prior topographic theory. Although the structural theory soon led to important changes in analytic technique—specifically, the methods of defense analysis (Settlage 1974)—other modifications of technique, derived from developmental considerations and from the role of object relations in personality formation, have evolved more slowly in the years since the structural theory was formulated. These modifications have been particularly significant in the treatment of children and adolescents. The methods of child analysis are one example of such technical development.

This chapter is concerned with another technical development which addresses specific problems in the treatment of adolescent disturbances. In it I will discuss methods of analytic assessment and treatment of the family of the disturbed adolescent. I believe treatment of the family may be required because of the body of findings, predicted by structural theory, relating pathology in children and adolescents to disturbances in relationships within the family.

First, I will discuss the need for an analytic framework for the assessment of families of disturbed adolescents and indications for the application of such a framework to the group-interpretive treatment of certain of these families concurrent with the individual psychoanalytic psychotherapy of the adolescent. I will then outline an analytic theory of family functioning which conceptualizes family regression and is derived from Bion's (1961) theory of small groups. Finally, I will describe findings in families of adolescents with borderline conditions or pathological narcissism which are indications for combined individual and family treatment.

Assessment of Families of Disturbed Adolescents and Indications for Concurrent Family Therapy

In one of Freud's (1917) last discussions of theory of the therapeutic effect of psychoanalysis, he says that most of the failures of psychoanalytic treatment are due, not to unsuitable choice of patients, but to unsuitable external conditions. He notes that, while the internal resistances to therapy, the resistances of the patient, are inevitable and can be overcome, the external resistances to therapy which arise from the patient's environmental circumstances are also of great practical importance. Freud writes:

> In psychoanalytic treatment resistances due to the intervention of relatives is a positive danger, and a danger one does not know how to meet. One is armed against the patient's internal resistances, which one knows are inevitable, but how can one ward off these external resistances? No kind of explanations make any impression on the patient's relatives; they cannot be induced to keep at a distance from the whole business, and one cannot make common cause with them because of the risk of losing the confidence of the patient, who—quite rightly, moreover—expects the person in whom he has put his trust to take his side. No one who has any experience of the rifts which so often divide a family will, if he is an analyst, be surprised to find that the patient's closest relatives sometimes betray less interest in his recovering than in his remaining as he is. When, as so often, the neurosis is related to conflict between members of a family, the healthy party will not hesitate long in choosing between his own interest and the sick party's recovery.

Freud says in conclusion that he followed the rule of not taking on a patient for treatment unless the patient was not dependent on anyone else in the essential relations of his life.

Clearly, the conditions Freud recommends as optimal for psychoanalysis are by definition not possible in the treatment of adolescents. The shift from the adolescent's dependency on his primary objects (the parents) to the finding of new objects is a central aspect of personality reorganization throughout adolescence (Jacobson 1961; Shapiro 1963). Difficulty in this process is among the important causes of disturbance in the adolescent. It is therefore essential to design a therapy which helps the adolescent to manage difficulties in family relationships which interfere with the transition from preadolescent dependency on parents to a new level of autonomy in relationships inside and outside the family in late adolescence. Such a therapy requires work with the external resistances to analytic therapy described by Freud. The nature of the adolescent's dependence on his parents dictates a redefinition of the task of his treatment to include management of the external resistances. The boundaries of adolescent therapy have expanded, then, to include methods for the maintenance and repair of a working alliance with the parents.

Adequate assessment of an adolescent patient involves careful evaluation of the internal resistances, of his defensive organization, and of the causal relation between the state of ego functioning, defenses, and symptomatology (Laufer 1965). Assessment of the adolescent must also include evaluation of the external resistances, the nature of the adolescent's dependency on his parents and the nature of evidence in the family of the parents' interest in and conflict over the adolescent changing or remaining as he is. I believe this assessment is best done through interviews with the parents and adolescent together (conjoint family interviews), in addition to individual interviews with the adolescent (Shapiro 1967; Shapiro and Zinner 1976). In addition to their value for assessment of external resistances, conjoint family interviews have the goal of forming a beginning working alliance with the parents as well as with the adolescent. It is important that this alliance be established and general goals of treatment agreed upon. Family interviews establish a working situation which can be held in reserve and, in the most favorable cases, may not be needed again.

If, however, the situation is one where neurosis in the adolescent is related to conflict between members of the family, change in the adolescent may lead the parents to define the situation in a way which assumes their interests are opposed to the adolescent's; they may choose their own interests over his, and new external resistances may arise. This possibility should be anticipated in the assessment phase. A reconvening of family interviews is then indicated to attempt to manage the external resistances interpretively in a way analogous to management of internal resistances through defense analysis. In conjoint family interviews, exploration of the nature and the sources of the impasse between parents and adolescent is possible. The therapist is aided in his effort to maintain a stance of neutrality because he can orient himself to the goals of therapy the family has agreed upon. He may then proceed to examine the interferences with the accomplishment of these goals. The framework of conjoint family interviews established during the assessment phase is the foundation which authorizes the

121

therapist to work interpretively on this task. He attempts to understand and interpret unconscious assumptions activating resistances in the family to change in the adolescent, both from the side of the parents and from the side of the adolescent. The psychotherapy of adolescents with severe neurosis or higher-order character pathology may then be preserved through analysis of external resistances to treatment when they arise in the family.

The more severe disturbances of adolescence, the borderline conditions and pathological narcissism, present a specific indication for ongoing treatment of the family, concurrent with individual psychotherapy of the adolescent, because of the severe pathology in the family in the area of separation-individuation.

Interest in problems of separation-individuation in early childhood has led to new recognition of their links to processes of individuation during adolescence, which Blos (1967) has called the second individuation phase. Disturbances in separation-individuation, studied by Mahler in childhood (Mahler 1971; Mahler, Pine, and Bergman 1975), have been shown to determine borderline and narcissistic pathology in the adolescent in the work of Kernberg (1975), Masterson (1972), and my research group (Berkowitz, Shapiro, Zinner, and Shapiro 1974a, 1974b; Shapiro, Shapiro, Zinner, and Berkowitz 1977; Shapiro, Zinner, Shapiro, and Berkowitz 1975). These disturbances are seen both in the parents and in the adolescent and are treated most effectively by concurrent individual and family therapy.

The Theory of Unconscious Assumptions

Our research into the origins of adolescent disturbance has utilized evidence from direct family observations to explore the family contribution to pathologic outcome in adolescence (Berkowitz et al. 1974a, 1974b; Shapiro et al. 1975, 1977; Shapiro and Zinner 1976; Zinner and Shapiro 1972, 1974). This evidence leads us to conclude that, during the course of his development, and depending upon his particular emotional meaning to his parents, the adolescent who is disturbed has not been supported by his parents in his efforts to accomplish phase-appropriate life tasks. On the contrary, his parents have responded to his development with anxiety and repudiation of change in their relationships with him. In the face of progressive individuation in the developing child and adolescent, characteristic defensive behaviors are mobilized in these parents which distort their perceptions of the child and adolescent and dominate their responses to him. We find that the nature of disturbance in the adolescent is related to and in part determined by the characteristics of regression and the nature of defenses which dominate his parents' behaviors with him. Furthermore, our evidence suggests that these episodes of regression and related defenses in parents are activated by their unconscious fantasies regarding the child.

Our findings from observations of family interaction indicate that the nature of character pathology in the adolescent is related in specific ways to the characteristics of defenses, regression, and consequent distortions in the relationships between the parents and the developing child. In order to specify what characteristics in families are related to specific adolescent character pathology, we assess the level of regression and characteristics of defense in family transactions and the nature of unconscious fantasies which are the motives for defense. We find evidence within families for an organization of shared or complementary unconscious fantasies and related higher-level repressive defenses or lower-level defenses including denial, splitting, and projection. These shared or complementary fantasies and related defenses serve to maintain equilibrium among family members and constitute external resistances to change. The underlying assumptions of the family based upon unconscious fantasies are conceptualized as the unconscious assumptions of the family as a group. We observe repetitive behaviors in families which appear to militate against change, development, and individuation of the child and infer that shared unconscious assumptions in family members motivate and organize these repetitive behaviors. These unconscious assumptions are assumed to derive from the internalized developmental experience of both of the parents in their families of origin. An organization of motives and higher- or lower-level defenses evolves, then, in the marriage, conceptualized as the unconscious assumptions of the family. These are operative throughout the development of the adolescent. Depending upon their centrality and coerciveness as the family develops, unconscious assumptions are powerful determinants of disturbance in the maturing adolescent.

The concept of unconscious assumptions of the family group is a construct which originates in clinical observation. It derives from the small-group theory of Bion (1961) and facilitates an integration of family-systems theory and psychoanalytic concepts of individual psychology. It has proven useful both in the differentiation of families of neurotic, borderline, and narcissistic adolescents and in the clinical understanding and treatment of these families in conjoint therapy.

The small-group theory of Bion derives from psychoanalysis and is a conceptualization of both the conscious functions and tasks which define groups and the unconscious motives which are also present in group members and which may dominate group behavior. Our effort to conceptualize family behavior has been facilitated by using a similar framework, that of family functions and tasks and of a variety of unconscious motives which interfere with their accomplishment. From the point of view of adolescent development, we conceive of the family as having an important function in promoting specific developmental tasks. These include the promotion of individuation and relative ego autonomy, resulting in an integrated identity formation in adolescent family members which leads to a substantial alteration in the quality of their relationships to parents and to peers (Blos 1967; Erikson 1950, 1956; Jacobson 1964; Shapiro 1969). Adolescent development is interfered with by unconscious assumptions in the family which militate against these changes. Unconscious assumptions inimical to the task of adolescent individuation activate states of anxiety and defense in family members in response to manifestations of individuation. Regression and symptomatic behavior are then seen in the family, often most markedly in the adolescent member.

A brief review of Bion's small-group theory will help us to clarify its application to family process. Bion proposed a group theory which articulated two levels of group functioning, a mature and a regressed level. In Bion's terminology, the mature level of group functioning is called the work group, the regressed level is the basic-assumption group.

Bion brought the concepts and framework of Kleinian theory to his work with groups. The Kleinian concept of positions facilitated a conceptualization of the two levels of group functioning as being present simultaneously in all groups. Depending upon the relation of the members to leadership in the group, either the mature or the regressed level of functioning might be the chief determinant of the group's behavior. This framework is also useful in conceptualizing mature family functioning and family regression, two levels of family functioning present as potentialities in any family situation.

Through the concept of position, Klein emphasized that the

phenomena she was describing in individuals as belonging to the paranoid-schizoid position or the depressive position were not simply a passing stage or phase. Her term implies a specific configuration of object relations, anxieties, and defenses which persists throughout life. The depressive position never fully supersedes the paranoid-schizoid position; the integration achieved is never complete, and defenses against depressive conflict bring about regression to paranoid-schizoid phenomena, so that the individual at all times may oscillate between the two. Some paranoid and depressive anxieties always remain active within the individual, but, when the ego is sufficiently integrated and has established a relatively secure relation to reality during the working through of the depressive position, neurotic mechanisms gradually take over from psychotic ones (Segal 1964).

Bion applied Klein's concept of position to groups in his conception that in every group two groups are present, the work group and the basic-assumption group. The work group is the mature group, defined by its work task. But the work group is only one aspect of the functioning of the group; the other aspect is the regressive level of group functioning, the basic-assumption group. We postulate that mature and regressive aspects of family functioning are present in any family, just as both aspects of group functioning are present in any group and primitive positions of mental functioning are present along with mature functioning in the individual. Bion's capacity to effect a shift in perspective from the individual to the group as a whole was crucial to his method of working with groups and to his articulation of shared levels of regressed functioning, as well as mature functioning, within groups. This same shift in perspective from the individual to the family as a group is crucial in analytic family treatment.

In the work of Bion, a group is defined by the task it is gathered to perform. Consciously motivated behavior directly implementing this task in reality terms is called work-group functioning. The group is behaving at a mature level in that it is working at its task, its relation to reality is good, and communication among group members is logical and clear. In contrast, Bion observes that much behavior in groups appears to have some other organization and motivation. This is behavior which suggests a level of regression dominated by unconscious assumptions on the part of members that the group is gathered for quite different purposes than the realistic accomplishment of the work task. Bion postulates unconscious mechanisms in group members which are mobilized in group interrelationships and which result in behavior

unconcerned with the considerations of reality such as task implementation, logical thinking, and time. He calls these regressive states,
where group behavior appears to be determined by wishful and nonra-
tional unconscious considerations, basic assumptions. In such states a
group appears to be dominated and often united by covert assumptions based on unconscious fantasies. Bion outlines three general categories of basic assumptions which he frequently sees dominating the
regressive behavior of groups. One is the unconscious assumption that
the group exists for satisfaction of dependency needs and wishes;
another is the assumption that the group exists to promote aggression
toward or to provide the means of flight from real tasks, issues, and
objects; the third is an assumption of hope and an atmosphere of
expectation which is unrelated to reality considerations and is frequently seen in relation to pairing behavior in the group. The basic-
assumption mode of group behavior is, then, regressive behavior which
implies covert and often unconscious assumptions in group members
about the purpose for which the group is gathered. These assumptions, which have little to do with considerations of reality, have
powerful unconscious determinants and are conceptualized as expressions of shared unconscious fantasies in group members. Shifts in
direction and power of basic-assumption fantasies and behavior, and
work, are observed in groups; it is important to investigate the conditions under which these shifts occur.

Turquet (1974) has emphasized that basic-assumption group behavior is mobilized for defensive purposes having to do with the difficulties
of the work task and disturbance in relation to the work leader. The
work of the group, its functioning and task performance, is impaired
with deterioration of the ego functioning of the members. The realities
of the situation and the task are lost sight of, reality testing is poor,
secondary-process thinking deteriorates, and more primitive forms of
thinking emerge. There is a new organization of behavior which seems
to be determined by fantasies and assumptions which are unrealistic
and represent a failed struggle to cope with the current reality situation.
Thereby the group survives as such, though its essential functioning
and primary task are now altered in the service of a different task.

We derive a framework from Bion, then, an orientation to clinical
observation of the family. States of anxiety, defense, and regression in
the family are conceptualized as consequences of unconscious assumptions, in which an organization of meanings and motives is in-
ferred. These assumptions are in opposition to the developmental tasks

of the family with respect to its children and adolescents. Family-group behavior now appears dominated by assumptions that particular meanings of childhood and adolescent individuation represent a danger to family requirements, cohesiveness, and even survival. These assumptions are generally unconscious and may be denied by family members.

The family group is different in essential ways from the "stranger" small group conceptualized by Bion. In considering the family as a group, the fact that its members have a shared developmental history and have specific role relationships through development results in a differentiation and specificity of shared assumptions, motivations, and defenses which cannot exist in the randomness of the stranger group. In this sense the complexity and differentiation of family process is much closer to individual psychodynamics than it is to group process. However, the study of the family is greatly facilitated through observing the shifts from family behavior implementing reality tasks to family behavior dominated by unconscious assumptions. It is possible to characterize the level of family regression, to define shared unconscious fantasies and assumptions with precision and to describe the characteristics of shared and complementary higher-level or lower-level defensive behaviors between and among family members. In contrast, Bion's formulations about basic-assumption behavior in stranger groups are global and generalized conceptualizations of group regression and of regressive group wishes in relation to the leader.

Let us now consider the evidence in family interaction which leads us to infer that unconscious assumptions are dominating family behavior. When the family is in a situation of anxiety as a consequence of mobilization of unconscious assumptions, we find clear analogies to small-group basic-assumption behavior. Behavior showing conflicting motivations, anxiety, and higher- or lower-level defenses is seen in family members, with evidence of ego regression. Behavior in the family appears to be determined more by fantasy than by reality. Work failure is evident in the family situation, similar to basic-assumption functioning. There is emergence of confused, distorted thinking, failure of understanding and adequate communication, and breakdown in the ability of the family to work cooperatively or creatively in relation to developmental issues and tasks. It becomes impossible to maintain a progressive discussion in which family members understand each other or to respond realistically to the problems under discussion. In short, when the family is in a situation in which unconscious assumptions are

127

mobilized, associated anxiety and higher- or lower-level defensive behaviors are seen, and there is disturbance in the family's reality functioning. In contrast, in the absence of mobilization of unconscious assumptions, the family does not manifest anxiety and prominent defensive behavior, is clearly reality oriented, and relates well to tasks facilitating the maturation of children and adolescents.

Unconscious Assumptions, Defensive Delineations, and Projective Identification

In order to characterize the family contribution to adolescent disturbance we study episodes of family regression determined by unconscious assumptions carefully. We observe behaviors of the parents with the adolescent and behaviors of the adolescent with the parents in order to define the defensive meanings of their relationships to each other which are implicit in their behaviors. And we infer from these defensive behaviors unconscious meanings of the adolescent to the parents and parents to the adolescent from which we formulate unconscious assumptions of the family as a group.

We use the concept of delineation to formulate the dynamics of the parents' relationship to the adolescent and the adolescent's relationship to the parents. This is a concept closely linked to observable behavior. Delineations are behaviors through which one family member communicates explicitly or implicitly his perceptions and attitudes—in fact, his mental representation of another family member—to that other person.

Delineations may communicate a view of the other person which seems to be predominantly determined by his reality characteristics. Or delineations may communicate a view of the other person which appears to be predominantly determined by the mobilization of dynamic conflict and defense in the delineator. We call the latter defensive delineations. For example, let us consider parental defensive delineations of the adolescent. When parental delineations are observed to be distorted, stereotyped and overspecific, contradictory, or otherwise incongruent with the range of behaviors manifested by the adolescent, we make the inference that these delineations serve defensive aspects of parental personality functioning. That is, they are not simply realistic characterizations of the adolescent. Further, we find that the parents, through their defensive delineations, seek to hold the child and adolescent in relatively fixed roles throughout development, in the service of avoiding their own anxiety.

The predominant mechanism underlying parental defensive delineations is projective identification. The concept of projective identification provides a highly useful means of conceptualizing phenomena of regression and elucidating dynamics of role allocation in families. In family regression there is rapid reduction in usual ego discriminations. Dissociation and projection are increased, with confusion over the ownership of personal characteristics which are easily attributed to other family members. When one individual assumes a role compatible with the attributions of others in the family at the regressed level, he quickly becomes the recipient of projections which tend to fix him in that role. Family members project this aspect of their own personal characteristics onto him and unconsciously identify with him. The power of these projections, with their accompanying unconscious identifications, may push the individual into more extreme role behavior and into feelings which are very powerful and may be experienced as unreal and bizarre.

Bion (1961) observes that Freud's view of identification is almost entirely a process of introjection by the ego. To Bion, however, the identification of group members with the leader of the regressed group depends not on introjection alone, but on a simultaneous process of projective identification as well. The leader is as much a creature of the basic assumption as any other member of the group. Group members project onto the leader, on the basic-assumption level, those qualities required and mobilized in shared basic-assumption fantasy. This is also true in families where projective identification results in the projection onto a child or adolescent of those qualities required and mobilized by the unconscious assumptions of the family.

These parental projections have a critical effect on the individual child maturing within the framework of family-group assumptions. Developmental theory emphasizes identification processes as internalizations which are major determinants of structure formation in the child. In addition, we believe that the child internalizes through development characteristics of parental relationships with him. His dynamic meaning to his parents, attributions made to him, and attitudes toward him are delineations which modify the child's self-representation and are determinants of structure formation. Parents' delineations of the child and adolescent, where the parents' regression is at a level of impaired self-object differentiation and primitive projective identification, are particularly coercive. Behavior in the child which counters these parental delineations leads to anxiety in the parent. The child is then motivated to behave so as to mitigate this parental anxiety. Internalization by the child of the parent's defensive delineations of him moves the developing child and adolescent into a role which is complementary to parental defensive requirements. Defensive delineations are, consequently, dynamic determinants of role allocation in the family. The role allocated is necessary to maintain parental defense and mitigate parental anxiety. The dynamics of role allocation operate in a broader framework of unconscious assumptions of the family as a group. Over time, these establish a pattern of internalizations within the self-representation. Unconscious assumptions within the family, and related experience of defensive delineations, impinge upon the reorganization of internalizations required by ego-id maturation during adolescence. These influences may interfere significantly with individuation and the consolidation of identity in the adolescent.

In the families we have studied we find evidence that each family member participates in the regression we have described. It is through the participation of all family members in these regressive episodes that the level of family regression and higher- or lower-level defensive organization achieve their stability and their power.

In family assessment and family therapy we attempt to articulate the unconscious assumptions of the family as a group and to discern the participation, contribution, and collusion of each family member in the episodes of family regression, dominated by unconscious assumptions and higher- or lower-level defensive organization, which we consider to be decisive for the developmental disturbances we are discussing.

Families of Adolescents with Borderline Conditions or Pathological Narcissism

In families of adolescents who manifest borderline or narcissistic disturbances, we consistently find evidence of a powerful cluster of unconscious assumptions which equate separation-individuation with loss and abandonment. Thinking and actions of family members which are not in accord with these assumptions are then perceived and reacted to as destructive attacks (Shapiro et al. 1975; Shapiro and Zinner 1976).

There are important areas of similarity in the characteristics of regression in these two types of families. In both types of families, regression is activated by behavior in family members signaling separation-individuation and loss; in these circumstances there is clear evidence of anxiety in the family and efforts to restore the previous equilibrium. There is regression to an organization of lower-level defenses, of denial, splitting, and projection, and an active splitting of aspects of self and objects. These split self and object representations are then distributed by projective identification. There is, however, a difference in the nature of the split in the self and object representations found in these two types of families, and, consequently, there is a difference in what is projected onto the separating and individuating family member.

In families of borderline adolescents, individuation, manifested in either autonomous or needful behavior in one family member, activates unconscious assumptions in other family members about the nature of relationships containing good experiences. Such behavior is unconsciously perceived as a threat to the survival of the family as a group, leading to anxiety and projection of destructiveness onto the individuating family member.

In these families a structure of internalized object relations is found in family members in which there is splitting of all good and all bad self and object images. Family members split off those bad aspects of themselves, which are associated with painful and aggressive experiences with objects in the past. In particular, painful responses to autonomous strivings within individuals, or to needs for nurture and support, give rise to shared unconscious assumptions in the family about the dangers of such behavior. Through projective identification, they relate to the separating and individuating adolescent as they would to a repudiated part of themselves and rebuff him in episodes of aggressive turmoil and withdrawal. The result in the adolescent is an identity formation dominated by negative self and object images, a continuation of splitting of positive and negative internalized relationships, and a clinical picture of identity diffusion.

In contrast, in families of narcissistic adolescents the unconscious assumptions focus on the specific meanings of a narcissistic relationship between parent and adolescent (Berkowitz et al. 1974b). If a parent projects valued aspects of himself or herself onto a child or adolescent and utilizes him as a self-object, the narcissistic equilibrium of the parent is disturbed when, during individuation, the child or adolescent moves into a position no longer complementary to the parent's narcissistic need. This disruption of a central narcissistic relationship in the family disturbs the self-regard of other family members, whose narcissistic equilibrium depends on the parent who is now suffering an abrupt disturbance in self-esteem.

In families of narcissistic adolescents we find a structure of internalized object relationships in which there is an active splitting of grandiose and devalued self and object images. Real, ideal, or devalued images of self and object are not integrated in family members into a self-concept with stable internal regulation of self-esteem. An effort to stabilize self-esteem is seen in the activation of a narcissistic relationship within the family. In these families such a differentiated narcissistic relationship is found between a narcissistic parent (grandiose self) and the adolescent (idealized self-object). This external relationship helps maintain the split in both parent and adolescent. The adolescent, who is utilized by the parent as a self-object, also evolves a pathological narcissistic self-structure and requires the relationship to an omnipotent parental image to maintain narcissistic equilibrium. Separation-individuation produces narcissistic disequilibrium in both parents and adolescent, with episodes of narcissistic rage and projection.

Family regression militates against further differentiation of the adolescent from the family. Instead, through projective identification, boundaries between family members become even more blurred, with parents and siblings projecting onto the adolescent who is attempting to individuate those feelings of devaluation denied within themselves.

These findings lead us to combine psychoanalytic psychotherapy for the adolescent with analytic, group-interpretive family treatment in borderline conditions or pathological narcissism of adolescents. In family treatment the continuing problems of projection and loss of differentiation between parents and adolescent are interpreted, and there is an opportunity for working through the meaning and experience of separation over time. Less bound by the projections of his parents, the adolescent has a new possibility for individuation which he is able to explore more fully in his individual therapy (Berkowitz et al. 1974a; Shapiro et al. 1977).

Conclusions

In the treatment of adolescents, unconscious assumptions in the family lead to external resistances to analytic therapy. The patient's family relationships frequently interfere with therapy more than the patient's own internal resistances. This is a central problem in treatment. Methods of conjoint family interviewing have been described for the management of external resistances in the treatment of adolescents. Such interviews should be part of the initial assessment of the disturbed adolescent as they help to establish a working alliance not only with the adolescent but also with his family.

I have presented concepts and methods which we have used to study families of disturbed adolescents. An organization of shared or complementary unconscious fantasies and related higher- or lower-level defenses within family members which maintain equilibrium among them is postulated. Anxiety and intensified defensive activity are activated by behavior which challenges or contradicts the underlying assumptions determined by these unconscious fantasies. These unconscious assumptions of the family as a group are evidenced in repetitive behaviors in families which appear to militate against change, development, or individuation of children. Shared unconscious assumptions in family members which motivate and organize these repetitive behaviors derive from the internalized developmental experience of both of the parents in their families of origin. An organization of motives and higher- or lower-level defenses evolves, then, in the marriage. These are operative throughout the development of the children and adolescents and have critical effects on their personality development.

For neurotic adolescents conjoint family interviews should be resumed when the external resistances interfere seriously with treatment.

For adolescents manifesting borderline conditions or pathological narcissism, where serious disturbances over separation-individuation, found in both adolescents and parents, are profoundly interfering with adolescent development, concurrent psychoanalytic psychotherapy for the adolescent and group-interpretive family treatment is indicated.

REFERENCES

Berkowitz, D.; Shapiro, R.; Zinner, J.; and Shapiro, E. 1974a. Concurrent family treatment of narcissistic disorders in adolescence. *International Journal of Psychoanalytic Psychotherapy* 3(4): 370–396.

Berkowitz, D.; Shapiro, R.; Zinner, J.; and Shapiro, E. 1974b. Family contributions to narcissistic disturbances in adolescence. *International Review of Psychoanalysis* 1(3–4): 353–362.

Bion, W. 1961. *Experiences in Groups*. London: Tavistock.

Blos, P. 1967. The second individuation process of adolescence. *Psychoanalytic Study of the Child* 22:162–186.

Erikson, E. 1950. *Childhood and Society*. New York: Norton.

Erikson, E. 1956. The problem of ego identity. *Journal of the American Psychoanalytic Association* 4:56–121.

Freud, S. 1917. Introductory lectures on psychoanalysis. *Standard Edition* 16:448–463. London: Hogarth, 1963.

Freud, S. 1923. The ego and the id. *Standard Edition* 19:12–68. London: Hogarth, 1961.

Jacobson, E. 1961. Adolescent moods and the remodeling of psychic structure in adolescence. *Psychoanalytic Study of the Child* 16:164–183.

Jacobson, E. 1964. *The Self and the Object World*. New York: International Universities Press.

Kernberg, O. 1975. *Borderline Conditions and Pathological Narcissism*. New York: Aronson.

Kernberg, O. 1976. *Object Relations Theory and Clinical Psychoanalysis*. New York: Aronson.

Laufer, M. 1965. Assessment of adolescent disturbances: the application of Anna Freud's diagnostic profile. *Psychoanalytic Study of the Child* 20:99–123.

Loewald, H. 1966. Review of psychoanalytic concepts and the structural theory by J. Arlow and C. Brenner. *Psychoanalytic Quarterly* 35:430–436.

Mahler, M. 1971. A study of the separation-individuation process and its possible application to borderline phenomena in the psychoanalytic situation. *Psychoanalytic Study of the Child* 26:403–424.

Mahler, M.; Pine, F.; and Bergman, A. 1975. *The Psychological Birth of the Human Infant: Symbiosis and Individuation*. New York: Basic.

Masterson, J. 1972. *Treatment of the Borderline Adolescent: A Developmental Approach*. New York: Wiley.

Segal, H. 1964. *Introduction to the Work of Melanie Klein*. London: Heinemann.

Settlage, C. 1974. The technique of defense analysis in the psychoanalysis of an early adolescent. In M. Harley, ed. *The Analyst and the Adolescent at Work*. New York: Quadrangle.

Shapiro, E.; Shapiro, R.; Zinner, J.; and Berkowitz, D. 1977. The borderline ego and the working alliance: indications for family and individual treatment in adolescence. *International Journal of Psychoanalysis* 58(1): 77–89.

Shapiro, E.; Zinner, J.; Shapiro, R.; and Berkowitz, D. 1975. The influence of family experience on borderline personality development. *International Review of Psychoanalysis* 2(4): 399–411.

Shapiro, R. 1963. Adolescence and the psychology of the ego. *Psychiatry* 26(1): 77–87.

Shapiro, R. 1967. The origin of adolescent disturbances in the family: some considerations in theory and implications for therapy. In G. Zuk and I. Boszormenyi, eds. *Family Therapy and Disturbed Families*. Palo Alto, Calif.: Science & Behavior Books.

Shapiro, R. 1969. Adolescent ego autonomy and the family. In G. Caplan and S. Lebovici, eds. *Adolescence: Psychosocial Perspectives*. New York: Basic.

Shapiro, R. 1978. Ego psychology: its relation to Sullivan, Erikson, and object relations theory. In J. Quen and E. Carlson, eds. *American Psychoanalysis*. New York: Brunner/Mazel.

Shapiro, R., and Zinner, J. 1976. Family organization and adolescent development. In E. Miller, ed. *Task and Organization*. London: Wiley.

Turquet, P. 1974. Leadership: the individual and the group. In G. S. Gibbard et al., eds. *Analysis of Groups*. San Francisco: Jossey-Bass.

Zinner, J., and Shapiro, R. 1972. Projective identification as a mode of perception and behavior in families of adolescents. *International Journal of Psychoanalysis* 52(4): 523–530.

Zinner, J., and Shapiro, R. 1974. The family group as a single psychic entity: implications for acting out in adolescence. *International Review of Psychoanalysis* 1(1): 179–186.

8 DEVELOPMENTAL TASKS IN ADOLESCENCE

ALBERT BRYT

> Youth should heed the older witted
> when they say don't go too far—
> now their sins are all committed
> Lord, how virtuous they are.[1]

Adolescence is a period of increasing ability to meet critical and ever more complex demands for personality integration. Clearly marked at the start by the changes of puberty, its end is arbitrarily determined by social factors.

Adolescent tasks include the emancipation from childhood, the judicious examination of taught and learned moral and ethical values, the formation of a reliable sense of self and individuality, the clarification of vocational interests, the preparation for intimacy in interpersonal relations, the organization of genital activity, and the crystallization of a personal and social role. At least two endpoints are interrelated: the intrapsychic integration of biologic, physiologic, and psychologic processes, and their progressive and productive social integration. This chapter is concerned with an examination of the impact of social conditions on these developmental tasks.

The new capabilities of adolescence must have a social setting where they can be expressed. On the other hand, modulation of expression is necessary to avoid social disruption. These two requirements are apt to clash. They represent an element of the generation gap which is fed by the overpowering strength of the evolving adolescent potentials and by society's investment, mediated by parenting adults. A significant discordance between intrapersonal development and interpersonal, social expectations is likely to endanger the fruitful evolution of what Bettelheim (1967) referred to as the "social being."

The numerous possibilities for friction can be reduced only through compromise. Society, because of its experience in living and tried potentials for prospective planning, must take the initiative toward workable solutions. Adolescents cannot do so because of the novelty of their internal developments. There has been, however, little movement in this direction, largely because intergenerational conflict and psychopathology in adolescence are thought to be normative, at least in our Western industrialized society.

Mead's (1928) *Coming of Age in Samoa* might have led to a critical questioning of our views on adolescence, but this has not happened. Nor have Grinker and Grinker's (1962) findings on mentally healthy young males produced the deserved impact. Likewise, Offer's and Sabshin's (1976) study, despite its equally impressive documentation, has failed to be instrumental in an as yet noticeable reexamination of accepted theories. Contributions from the field of anthropology by Kardiner and his co-workers (1945), Kluckhohn and Strodtbeck (1961), Miller and Swanson (1958), and Opler (1967) or by sociologists such as Bronfenbrenner (1958), Edgerton (1971), or Merton (1957) also have been disregarded in the formulation of the psychodynamics of adolescence (Blos 1963; Giovacchini 1977).

The impact of youth on society is more difficult to overlook. Indeed, their intervention in the affairs of society has brought about significant changes in social goals and mores. Recent examples are their effective participation in the civil mobilization against the war in Southeast Asia and the dedication with which they have concerned themselves with the environmental consequences of modern life-styles and industrialization.

It has been argued that youth alleges virtue when merely expressing rebelliousness (Cohen 1968). I, among others, have disagreed with such a view (Bryt 1968). The issue of normative adolescent rebelliousness has been overplayed and constructive, emancipated behavior has received much less attention. True, protests by youth against the established order stand out in comparison with explicitly stated constructive social goals. Yet, the absence of self-seeking personal comfort and the disdain for hedonistic satisfaction are witness to humanistic motivations. The importance of the coming generation to society has often been overlooked. Its troublemaking capacities are least significant. Indeed, only the active interest of youth in social institutions can assure their preservation; passive tolerance cannot. Democracy would be in grave peril without the participation of its young people in, for instance, the electoral process. No authoritarian regime could survive long without an effective alliance between the dictatorial leaders and youth. Undeniably, nihilistic destructiveness has been perpetrated as an end in itself. This is pathological behavior and a childlike response to frustration in the face of arbitrariness by adults. In self-seeking defense, but not totally without justification, youth counters that the social fabric has been more badly damaged by the wanton self-righteous refusal by decision makers to engage in a dialogue than it has by the noncooperation (perhaps even violent actions) of those who felt shunted. A comparable argument can be extended to include family, schools, and the body politic.

Nothing denotes the adequate fulfillment of adolescent developmental tasks better than an individualized human capable of utilizing all opportunities for self-realization; those capacities existing within the person and those arising in the sociocultural setting (Sullivan 1953). Such a person will be recognized as an intelligent, dynamic, self-directing citizen capable of evaluating situations from new perspectives, defining new goals, and finding new solutions to problems.

Youth are not always compliant, but they can be malleable and accessible to reasonable compromise in a sensitive and responsive society where they can have a voice in shaping tomorrow's attitudes. Youth must have a right to recognition by society, but it must not be a privilege to be granted or withheld. When there are openings for their useful contributions to social needs, they welcome the challenge of meaningful endeavor. They do not want to be an afterthought. Modern industrialized, especially urban, society often fails to ingather its youth. This estranges them from their future and robs their present of dynamic potential.

Adolescent developmental tasks depend on the social climate. When it is unfavorable, psychosocial movement forward is vitiated, and psychological growth begun in infancy and expected to culminate in adulthood is stifled. As the number of educated, knowledgeable adolescents has increased in modern society, and because of the ease and rapidity of communication, even those who are less educated are aware when there is no place for them in the social order. They then accept and follow the leadership of more alert peers in judging social goals and social deficiencies critically. When society disregards comments by its youth, normative ability for dissent lacks a forum for expression. This creates adolescent hostility, not the revived oedipal situation. Malinowski's (1934) observations are worth recalling, not as a model, but as an illustration. In the Tobriand Islands, where matrilineal family organization prevails, the maternal uncle is the seat of autocratic familial authority. His is the task of teaching his sister's sons. The biological father, though maintaining an otherwise traditional marital relationship, exercises little or no authority over his sons beyond their early childhood. Tobriand adolescents rebel against their uncles and their power but are friendly and congenial with their fathers. This illustrates the notion that the ordering of social structures is a developmental accomplishment.

Society takes pride in its ability to integrate new ideas and to promote rapid changes. Hence, it could provide acceptable avenues for the expression of dissent instead of trying to suppress it by the imposition of discipline. This could mean not only less counterproductive interference, but actual facilitation for the pursuit of the adolescent goal of concentrating "upon socialization and preparation for and integration into the adult world" (Giovacchini 1977).

Adolescent performance is but the dress rehearsal for adult transactions. The stage for this is set earlier when the child studies a range of adult roles, leisurely and bit by bit, by validating perceptions with chums, playacting with toys, and make-believe storytelling. Adolescents enriched by intellectual maturation can then follow through, interpolating what they have learned earlier and combining it with would-be adult experimentation. There is progressive refinement of skills for later, effective adult behavior.

Experimental role acting must be allowed to have deficiencies. Social practice, in our acquisitive society, is that "nothing succeeds like success." As a consequence deficiencies or failures get special handling. Failures may be disregarded as if insignificant, losing their stimulus quality for learning, or they may be exaggerated, disqualifying its perpetrator. Neither reaction is a desirable one. Instead, deficiencies and errors could lead to correctively preventive steps. For developmental progression in this direction adolescents must have deft direction. Parents and the schools often do not see it this way. If they cannot guarantee success they may at least be able to salvage the appearance of it. To this end coercion and rote training are effective. Of course, coercion consistently applied can have the desired results. It also dulls strivings for individuality and interferes with emancipation. Ultimately, it may lead to a noncreative adaptation, that of Whyte's (1956) "well rounded man."

The value of individual emancipation cannot be overrated, nor can coercion as a most effective antidote. Modern child-rearing practices have considered this fact and have adopted permissiveness which teaches children to fend for themselves early, too early perhaps. Parents are often proud of their little tyrants who know exactly what they want. At puberty, however, as emancipation becomes a principal developmental task, abrupt changes initially restrict freedom. Later on, when adolescents demur, there may be another reversal to a laissez-faire attitude. Usually the first line of battle is the expectation of adolescents to know better. Yet, they have not been taught self-control or how to recognize and respect reasonable limits. The imposition of discipline in the schools, to which some adults object and others want more, is not a learning experience. Then, secondarily, perhaps recognizing that they have failed to set defined limits in the past, parents overcorrect and become authoritarian. True, they rationalize that they do so out of concern for their maturing child. They are, however, really driven by anxiety and are ambivalent because of their allegiance to the social ideal of personal freedom and to the contradictory social requirement of conformity. Their parental value system is on shaky foundations, as is their sense of personal independence. So, when adolescents object actively, the unavoidable clash between society's wish for restrictive modulation of behavior—denatured by the parental neurotic needs—and adolescent action proneness takes place in an impoverished atmosphere without reliable principles. Hence, everything goes. Parents are at a greater disadvantage. They realize, faintly, that their own experiences have been similarly unprincipled and that they themselves need deft direction, as do their teenage children. Society fails to provide either.

These problems, which are not new, received a big boost with the end of the First World War. There had been an early misreading of Freud's discoveries, and parents were blamed for the social unrest, dominated by youth. A more careful reading of Freud's (1930) later writings could have corrected this, but it did not happen, perhaps because Freud failed to question the authenticity of the social order while questioning the authenticity of human strivings for an ordered society. Parents at present are in a worse position. Now they are held responsible for the neurotic difficulties of the growing generation as well as its failure to respect society's values.

In the face of the assumed inability of parents, society has taken over child protection. Proprietary rights of parents over children have been abrogated. Considering the extent to which children had been exploited, there may have been a need for such measures, but they have added to the further disruption of family ties progressively weakened by the disappearance of the extended family as an institution. The progressive fragmentation of society carries into child-rearing practices that which at other times had been transmitted from generation to generation. Present-day parents must improvise in spite of uncountable rules and codifications on child care, since society does not teach skillful parenting—except for nutrition and physical needs. In addition, many children no longer have the advantage of object constancy in their early years because of damage to family bonds. Then there is the principle of personal freedom, indiscriminately applied to children, without a matching requirement for respect for others. This can destroy emotional and cognitive familiarization between members of a household and the basis for a meaningful dialogue between teenagers and parents. As a result the age-appropriate separation from parents has no boundaries.

The general awareness that early emotional privation inhibits psychological growth has led to some absurd consequences. One of these is the belief that any frustration works to the child's detriment. In the commercial exploitation of this belief new needs are artificially created, exposing parents to increased pressures. They fear adverse consequences so are loath to deny any of a child's wishes. They are no longer guided by rationally defined limits so they find themselves cornered, reacting with anger first and then with guilt. Seeking a way out of this predicament, parents turn to experts for help. Psychiatrists and educators are thus promoted to make up for the lost tradition of parenting. They, in turn, are often guided by theoretical preconceptions and may give counsel based on nothing more than their proclaimed authority.

In adolescence comparable difficulties are interwoven with developmental dilemmas, more particularly the needs for emancipation. Society has promoted would-be instant solutions to regulate the orderly progression toward adolescent maturation and adult social integration, for example, added years of compulsory education for all and the possibility for higher education for some. These do not meet pertinent developmental requirements because they do not take into account differences in personal propensities or physiological and psychological readiness. Thus sociocultural prescriptions and proscriptions have little effect or may create new developmental difficulties. In essence, adolescents are forced to work out their own solutions in an inhospitable social climate which limits options. Therefore, youth may refrain from defining their aspirations and preferences, which used to be one reliable measure of maturational progression. In some instances this hesitation has gone beyond mere postponement. More and more teenagers seek refuge in radicalism or excessive reactive conservatism (Whitehorn 1962) in order to come to terms with the extension in time of this developmental period with its socially ill-defined end.

At least one further area demands concern: the active sexuality of young people at a progressively younger age due to the combination of the earlier onset of puberty and changed mores. Current sexual practices, indulged in even by preteenagers, may correspond to their physical capabilities and may be consistent with the necessity for experimentation with would-be adult roles. Yet, in our society sexual behavior, to be legitimate, presupposes feelings of intimacy and closeness between the partners. The potentials for such feelings are sometimes inadequately developed even in adults; they certainly are in early adolescence. They depend on the building of the complex framework for individuation, including the capacity to trust and to relate acquired in childhood, and on true separation, a developmental achievement of late adolescence.

The precociously acting young adolescent, therefore, may have to escape into pretend-closeness in conformity with social standards or ostensibly reject these and opt for licentiousness. In either case the result is likely to be the untimely closure of psychosexual development, truncated self-experience, tenuous interpersonal relationships, and pseudocommitment to no cause. Licentiousness, in addition, entails the disregard of moral obligations toward the sexual partner. The social climate which dictates such nonsolutions is bound to be generative of emotional depression, a prevalent clinical symptom in present-day youth.

Precocious sexual behavior and its consequences may be placed side by side with other ephemeral pursuits to circumvent the constructive, developmental strivings for honesty, probity, and inner consistency toward idealistic goals. Irrespective of social ideals, social practice invites the neglect of cooperative interests for the benefit of rivalrous competition. Defeat over others carries more weight than feelings of belonging. Appearances have precedence over convictions; competitive winning is preferred over team effort. Reliance on devious means, including violence, has replaced competence and the rules of fair play. Respect for others has been replaced by expediency in setting the limits for what is permissible.

Puberty gives rise to a compelling wish for gregariousness. Adolescents band together in groups, obeying their own rules for social conduct. They can be compared with apprenticeship situations and can be useful. Here unresolved problems can be reconsidered and worked through. Also, new issues can become the object of collaborative examination. The peer group offers and requires the collaboration of its members for the completion of tasks which otherwise might exceed the capabilities of the single individual. The group endures because responsibilities are shared, as are the fruits of the collective endeavor. The adolescent society teaches dynamic social participation. True, the adolescent-created support system encourages self-assertive stands against parental dominance. By encouraging liberation from parental bondage it also supports emancipation from the protection of parental power. The peer group may sometimes forcibly initiate emancipation, even in the face of personal unreadiness. Increased psychological turmoil may result. This is exceptional. More often, the identification with the "social group" (Montague 1966) permits the speeding up of the normative progression toward separation in a youth who otherwise might not have succeeded in extricating himself or herself from the comfortable embeddedness of parental dependability (Schachtel 1959).

The group also demands conformity. Unfettered behavior is modulated. Conversely, inhibitions may also be lifted in response to group pressure, allowing behavior which otherwise might be morally unacceptable. Yet, the group is of great value to its members and ultimately to society. Many an adolescent can be helped out of emotional isolation. Even the peripheral association with peers offers opportunities for an exchange of views with others without the necessity for explicit side taking. Also, because the group may force participation in intragroup activities the isolated adolescent can be helped to identify dislikes, can discover and experiment with effective modes for interpersonal conflict solving and for peaceful side-by-side existence in spite of differences in opinion. Personal frailties can be exposed for critical assessment of nonthreatening others, a very difficult achievement in relation to adults. Comparisons between individual approaches become possible, giving perspective to personal crises without the threat of isolation or ostracism.

In the peer atmosphere, youth perceive themselves through the eyes of their age-mates, perhaps similarly beset by problems, without the distortions brought about by the narcissistic overlay of parental appraisal. More importantly, they experience the need and learn the means for adaptation to others. They receive training in cooperativeness toward common political, social, religious, and ethical goals. They share responsibility for the success of joint undertakings and also learn to accept failure in common with others, not at their expense. However, intergroup relations do not obey comparably high moral principles. They frequently continue to reflect less desirable social practices.

Conclusions

Personality development in adolescence is increasingly geared to interpersonal transactions. Cooperation and collaboration with others is in the service of self-realization. In spite of frequent clashes with social expectations, youth are interested in the pursuit of higher ideals and in the preservation of social institutions. Far from wanting to exclude themselves from society, their opposition to it is aimed at preventing its self-destruction.

As psychiatrists working with young people our efforts in treating maladjusted adolescents are only in partial fulfillment of our role. We also must use ourselves to facilitate the achievement of adolescent developmental tasks. We can do so by being advocates for the authenticity of the humanistic goals of young people.

NOTE

1. Wilhelm Busch, German satirical writer (1832–1908), trans. Christopher Morley.

REFERENCES

Bettelheim, B. 1967. *The Empty Fortress*. New York: Free Press.

Blos, P. 1963. *On Adolescence*. New York: Free Press.

Bronfenbrenner, U. 1958. Socialization and social class through time and space. In E. E. Maccoby, T. M. Newcomb, and E. L. Hartley, eds. *Readings in Social Psychology*. New York: Holt.

Bryt, A. 1968. Discussion of a paper by Sheldon B. Cohen. In J. Masserman, ed. *The Dynamics of Dissent, Science and Psychoanalysis*. Vol. 13. New York: Grune & Stratton.

Cohen, S. B. 1968. Rebel and reactionary, siblings under the skin? In J. Masserman, ed. *The Dynamics of Dissent, Science and Psychoanalysis*. Vol. 13. New York: Grune & Stratton.

Edgerton, R. B. 1971. In I. Galdstone, ed. *Anthropology, Psychiatry and Man's Nature*. New York: Brunner-Mazel.

Freud, S. 1930. Civilization and its discontents. *Standard Edition* 21:64–145. London: Hogarth, 1961.

Giovacchini, P. 1977. Psychoanalytic perspectives on adolescence. *Adolescent Psychiatry* 5:113–145.

Grinker, R. R., Sr., and Grinker, R. R., Jr. 1962. "Mentally healthy" young males. *Archives of General Psychiatry* 6:405–453.

Kardiner, A., with the collaboration of Linton, R.; Du Bois, C.; and West, J. 1945. *The Psychological Frontiers of Society*. New York: Columbia University Press.

Kluckhohn, F., and Strodtbeck, P. 1961. *Variations in Value Orientation*. New York: Harper.

Malinowski, B. K. 1934. *The Sexual Life of Savages in Northwestern Melanesia*, New York: Harcourt Brace.

Mead, M. 1928. *Coming of Age in Samoa*. New York: Morrow.

Merton, R. K. 1957. *Social Theory and Social Structure*. New York: Free Press.

Miller, D. R., and Swanson, G. E. 1958. *The Changing American Parent*. New York: Wiley.

Montague, A. 1966. *On Being Human*. New York: Hawthorne.

Offer, D., and Sabshin, M. 1976. *Normality*. New York: Basic.

Opler, M. K. 1967. *Culture and Social Psychiatry*. New York: Atherton.

Schachtel, E. G. 1959. *Metamorphosis*. New York: Basic.

Sullivan, H. S. 1953. In H. S. Perry and M. L. Gawell, eds. *Interpersonal Theory of Psychiatry*. New York: Norton.

Whitehorn, J. C. 1962. A working concept of maturity of personality. *American Journal of Psychiatry* 119:197–202.

Whyte, W. H. 1956. *The Organization Man*. Garden City, N.Y.: Anchor.

9 CURRENT SEXUAL ATTITUDES, SOCIETAL PRESSURE, AND THE MIDDLE-CLASS ADOLESCENT GIRL

CLARICE J. KESTENBAUM

With evidence that there has been considerable change in societal attitudes toward sex during the last decade, it becomes important to examine how current shifts are affecting the fourteen- to sixteen-year-old, midadolescent girl. Certain changes, however, are more apparent than real. The sexual revolution may in some instances have provided greater openness about behavior which was formerly carried on in secrecy. Today, young men and women openly share an apartment in experimental marriage. Previously, the double standard was rigidly applied, heterosexual exploration for adolescent boys took place with an older woman, and for girls there was no such thing as open or admitted adolescent sex.

Other changes are more genuine. The average age of the first sexual intercourse does appear to have lowered from eighteen to seventeen years for middle-class girls in the current generation. Puberty itself, as Seiden (1975) has recently noted, is occurring at a younger age. Menarche tends to be at age eleven or twelve years where a generation ago thirteen or fourteen was a more typical age, and in the nineteenth century it was as late as fifteen or sixteen. Marriage for a woman and the assumption of adult roles occurred earlier than today, when attainment of educational goals is often not completed until the mid or late twenties.

The length and quality of adolescence has strong cultural determinants. If we define adolescence as the period between puberty (with its inherent physiological changes) and the assumption of adult roles (including work that permits financial independence and the formation of an intimate love relationship), this period extends several years beyond legal majority. Moreover, class differences can be marked. Masturbation is becoming more acceptable as a normal activity among middle-class youngsters (Mussen, Conger, and Kagan 1969) while among lower-class youth the act is still stigmatized as shameful or sinful, a view held by Western society in general from the eighteenth century (Aries 1960). Young, lower-class boys have been more ready to engage in sexual intercourse and prove their manhood. Intercourse, then, becomes an antidote to masturbation, given the pressure of their post-pubescent sexual drives and their value system—which may seem to a middle-class adult overly harsh and antiquated.

Adolescence as a Developmental Phase

Adolescence, as many authors have observed (Freud 1958; Laufer 1965), is an important developmental phase with its own timetable for completion of developmental tasks. Character formation during adolescence will proceed optimally, according to Blos (1968), only if the following conditions are met.

1. *Loosening of parental ties.* The adolescent must increasingly seek new models (via teachers, counselors, friends, and heroes) with whom he can identify and by whose example he shapes his own efforts at individuation and independence. The movement is toward autonomy; away from a dependent role within the family and toward relationships outside the family matrix. Ordinarily, ego-ideals become more realistic, and goals are revised so as to be more in line with what is attainable. As a result, the adolescent's value system (superego) undergoes considerable modification and becomes less punitive.

2. *Resolution of earlier traumas.* The adolescent must come to terms with certain traumatic events of his childhood, whether these involve only early disappointment with one or another parent or something as severe as the death of a parent.

3. *Establishment of continuity.* Here the adolescent seeks to establish a sense of continuity both with respect to his own previous feeling states and remembered experiences and to the history of his own family. One cannot have a future without having had a past.

4. *Solidification of a sexual identity.* Adolescence is characterized by solidification of one's sense of gender identity (an aspect of self-awareness with preoedipal roots) and a growing capacity to make a heterosexual object choice.

By late adolescence, if development has proceeded optimally, the individual will have achieved the sense of a unique personal identity, firmly established work goals, and a well-developed capacity for heterosexual intimacy. By late adolescence one expects that the healthy individual has enough judgment, self-esteem, and sense of personal integrity to withstand the external pressures of a complicated society so that he will not succumb to the preachings of false prophets or the cultural fads of the day.

The Midadolescent

The young and midadolescent girl, still in the process of development, is in a vulnerable position regarding her self-concept and her role in society. Early adolescence is a period of reactivation and reorganization of sexual and aggressive drives. The push toward maturity comes about, of course, from the hormonal changes that accompany this period of life as well as from societal expectations.

The young adolescent will often experience considerable difficulty coping with the host of physical changes occurring in her body. The onset of menstruation has far more significance than just that of a simple physiological phenomenon. Menarche is a symbol of sexual maturity and forces her to contemplate more intensely her future role as wife and mother. Even among so-called enlightened girls of today the first menstrual period can be a traumatic event if preparation has been faulty or distorted. Her attitude will be greatly influenced by her mother's own attitude toward menstruation and toward sex in general. The girl is sensitive not only to what her mother conveys in words but, more importantly, to what she conveys in her gestures, in her relationship with her husband and other men, and in what she chooses not to say to her daughter. If the mother's own feminine identification is unsatisfactory, she may convey to her daughter negative feelings about all that is uniquely female and, along with it, all that pertains to the menses.

The girl's reaction will also be shaped by the attitudes and reactions of significant others. The timing of the menarche is of particular importance. If a girl is the first or last among her friends to have her period, she may suffer the humiliation of being different from her peers. Still, in the long run, it is chiefly the mother who determines whether the girl will regard menstruation as a milestone—or a millstone. Breast development is one of the more prized achievements of female puberty. Girls will compare breast size, order training bras, and in general derive great pleasure from the comments of classmates about the new protuberances in their T-shirts.

By now, masturbation will have become a central concern to young adolescents of both sexes. Although it is an essential part of growing up, in spite of more permissive societal attitudes adolescents continue to generate many false and frightening ideas on the subject. Girls have less difficulty as a rule than boys, since they can deny that the pleasurable sensations derived from pressure on the inner thigh is a masturbatory act while boys with their obvious erections cannot. Guilt feelings, especially in relation to incestuous fantasies, can act as powerful deterrents to otherwise natural urges. Actually, masturbation constitutes a way of controlling and integrating the new urges. It can be viewed as a method of experimenting with one's physiological capacities. Certainly, before intimacy with another can be achieved (at a later stage of development), the young individual must learn the functioning of his own body; he must learn to recognize and to accept the rhythms of sexual tension and the experience of orgasm.

In early adolescence the sense of self is weakened by powerful drives not yet under control. Sexual urges are as often disruptive as exciting. There will be a phase of heightened curiosity about one's own body as well as about that of the opposite sex. Peer relations are still apt to be with the same sex, particularly with one or two best friends. For these young girls, heterosexual exploration at this early stage has less the function of establishing an intimate tie than of helping them explore and understand new sensations developing within themselves. Hence this activity is still largely directed at problems relating to the self (the narcissistic path of development) rather than toward others (the object-libidinal path of development).

The behavior of parents may be such as to intensify the conflicts with which the young adolescent is struggling. The father who used to kiss and fondle his little girl unembarrassedly suddenly finds a nubile young woman in his lap, capable of arousing him to a degree too great for comfort. Both become ill at ease, awkward, and tend to give up this kind of playfulness. It is no longer just play. To make matters worse, the mother finds herself furious, fighting valiantly to keep down her envy of the young woman's firm breasts and shapely waist while her beautiful, blossoming daughter runs around the house in bra and panties.

How does the young adolescent handle the powerful drives that threaten to make life unbearably turbulent? A generation ago the prevailing social mores made the sexual initiation rites somewhat easier. Dating was accompanied by more rules and rigid structure and therefore, in most cases, less anxiety. A boy would expect a girl's parents to be waiting up for her at the prescribed hour. All he could expect was a kiss on the cheek—but since this would often be all either of them could handle comfortably there was a great sense of relief (for both), despite the boy's complaint to his buddies that he couldn't "get more." Boys and girls would exchange endless phone calls (as they still do), notes in class, and torrid sonnets, all in the security of knowing that nothing more than verbal activity of this sort was expected or even allowed.

Now that we have moved into the era of the permissive society or newer freedoms this kind of safeguard through distance does not always operate. According to Planned Parenthood,[1] 30 percent of teenage girls fifteen to nineteen have had their first sexual intercourse (in San Francisco, the rate was noted as high as 60 percent). Boys and girls are immersed in an atmosphere of swinging singles, open marriage, high divorce rates, and loosened restrictions on their parents as well as themselves. Many single again, middle-aged parents compete with their adolescent offspring quite openly, bringing home weekend sex partners in relationships often of brief duration. Perhaps the parents can cope with such situations, but the children are frequently made quite anxious.

Parties for adolescents are often unchaperoned. Alcohol, marijuana, and sex are freely available. Some parents have come to believe that early sexuality of this sort will be a liberating experience—one that will minimize the kind of sexual conflicts suffered by the parents as a result of their own more repressive childhood experiences.

The effects of this early and, I feel, premature sexual activity will differ somewhat depending on the sex of the child. Despite all attempts to liberate women, the double standard still exists, rooted in inescapable biological differences. Only the girl can become pregnant. Only for her is abortion an experience of bodily invasion and poignant loss. The experience is not one to be considered a simple event, a brief interference with life, but a sad and humiliating occurrence which can lead to negative feelings about sex and men in general. Moreover, the new freedom has not shed light on the appalling degree of ignorance the adolescent usually brings to the matters of sexual function, conception, and birth, despite the best efforts of modern sex education, school lectures, and the popular press. Testimonials to these unpleasant realities are the increased (in middle class) early adolescent pregnancy and abortion rates (Shaffer, Pettigrew, Wolkind, and Zajicek 1978). The rate of illegitimate pregnancies among fifteen- to seventeen-year-old white girls has increased by 6 percent in a decade (Zelnick and Kantner 1978). It would seem that widespread availability of the pill is no match for the impulsivity of many adolescents or the rather meager sense of responsibility many of them have for their own bodies. Moreover, judgment is sadly lacking. If, indeed, in some cases pregnancy is a status symbol,[2] little thought has been given to planning for the new baby, who is in any case seen more as a doll than an independent human being.

Throughout adolescence the difference between the sexes in level of psychosexual maturity is profound. Girls are usually two or three years ahead of boys in this respect. Sex for the fourteen-year-old boy is still a proving ground for genital competence or a defense against homosexual concerns. The girl is already further ahead in the business of separating herself from parents and is beginning to seek a new person who will supply love, warmth, nurturance, and devotion.

Sex still has primarily narcissistic meanings for the boy; a masturbatory act in the company of another. The girl, on the other hand, is moving in the direction of object relationships, if only, at this early stage, to fulfill unmet dependency needs.

Many young adolescents now feel pressure from peers to experiment (details to be shared by all) as well as from their parents to be sexually free. Catapulted into relationships that mimic heterosexual intimacy long before they are ready, these adolescents become involved in romances that are necessarily quite superficial. The disappointment suffered at the all but inevitable dissolution may be much keener, owing to the immaturity of the participants. Girls may feel abandoned after a sexual encounter and may experience a lowering of self-esteem.

Clinical Examples

1. Susan was a fourteen-year-old honor student from a liberated home. Her mother assumed she was a responsible and intelligent girl, gave her a "facts of life" lecture with her first menstrual pad, and told her she could now handle her own private life, "no questions asked." She came for consultation after two months of difficulty studying, sleeping, and concentrating. She told me she had missed two periods and was sure she was pregnant. Since she had had intercourse with three boys during that time span, she did not even know who the father might be. Susan at first indicated that she was the active member in search of sexual partners. She did not mind not being loved or not loving, because the peaceful feeling after orgasm was "satisfying enough." She shared the details of her conquests with her two best friends and felt they envied her for "being like the boys." Later, however, she admitted she always felt terribly hurt when the boy did not call back, was secretly ashamed of her reputation, and felt used and manipulated by her classmates. As it turned out, she was not pregnant. She began psychotherapy but had still a way to go before working out her contempt of men and of herself as well.

2. Mary was another fourteen-year-old, middle-class girl whose parents had divorced two years before. Taller than most of her classmates and beset with braces and acne, she gave no inkling of the beautiful girl she would become in several years. She felt insecure, because boys "are only interested in me because I help them with their homework." She was determined to be popular at all costs. At an unchaperoned party one night she engaged in a transient sexual relationship with a boy who was clearly interested only in another conquest. He immediately spread the word to all his buddies about having "scored" with her; she felt humiliated and ashamed.

Discussion

The cautionary statements I am making are derived from clinical experiences with girls designated as patients. Presumably they had other problems which led to their behavior in the first place. We cannot really generalize from clinical vignettes about the millions of healthy adolescents who do not appear in our offices. The dire warnings about the youth of the sixties ended in congratulatory statements about the children of the seventies. Many adolescents do not succumb to the pressures to do things before they are ready.

I am thinking of one seventeen-year-old in particular who found that the permissive house rule in her college dorm (boys and girls living on the same floor with a unisex bathroom etc.) was "too hot to handle." She, along with her roommates, presented a list of rules to the dean asking for more structure, that is, men and women on different floors, no opposite-sexed roommates "sleeping over" ("hard to do homework with sexual noises emanating from the next bed"). The rules were approved by an overwhelming majority of students.

There is no absolute timetable regarding readiness for intimacy. Many seventeen-year-olds have such relationships (and they do not share details of their sexual activities with their best friends, either), while some twenty-two-year-olds are still immature. We can, however, speculate about the toll societal pressures take on some vulnerable adolescents. Some adolescents, unable to separate from parents successfully, become thrust prematurely into structureless sexual situations and employ extremely maladaptive defensive maneuvers. Defense by displacement to parental substitutes is not uncommon. The numbers of youngsters who follow fringe religious cult leaders testify to this. One patient, a sixteen-year-old upper-class girl from an extremely permissive family, "adopted" the Baptist parents of the seventeen-year-old boy next door "because they go to church, are very very strict (sexually), and I feel safe with him and them."

Some young adolescents, having great difficulty separating themselves from their primary objects—the parents—attach themselves to a partner in an intense fashion, each clinging to the other in a way that precludes the formation of more appropriate intimate relationships at a later time. They become frozen into a togetherness from which neither seems able to extricate himself. Occasionally such liaisons do end up in successful relationships. More often they are a burden not easily borne by the participants, who in the process lose valuable time that might otherwise have been spent in more profitable interaction with a wider variety of other age-mates. Sex is a powerful force binding people together, but where boys and girls of thirteen and fourteen are concerned for this very reason it can impede growth. Here I refer to growth in self-awareness and in the formation of identity, both of which are ordinarily fostered by the freedom to move in and out of briefer and less intense friendships with the opposite sex.

Other maladaptive solutions encountered with certain adolescent girls include narcissistic defenses, asceticism, hypochondriasis, and self-starvation as ways of controlling burgeoning sexual and aggressive drives. Obviously those girls would have had difficulty coping with pubertal changes in any generation, but current societal pressure is for them an additional stress.

Finally, a word about homosexuality. The girls with identity problems, in particular those who have had great difficulties identifying with their mothers, are easy prey for lesbian seductions (Kestenbaum 1978). While in former years the same problems confronted these girls and caused great internal conflict, there was little group pressure then to act on them. Once sexual behavioral patterns are established, it is more difficult to return to heterosexual behavior. I have seen a number of young girls when confronting their homosexual identification become greatly conflicted, depressed, and trapped between two worlds: gay and straight.

Conclusions

Now that the culture surrounding the young adolescent girl is providing her with so few limits, she often feels torn between desire and prudence in a manner seldom encountered in her mother's generation. A girl of thirteen or fourteen may feel pushed in the direction of intimacy, lacking guidelines either from within herself or from the environment. She may be led to ask her mother, "Is it all right to go all the way?" In the vast majority of such instances the very act of asking permission is a clear message that she is not emotionally ready. She wants her mother to say no.

When an adolescent girl has reached the point of genuine readiness for sexual intimacy she no longer feels the need of expressed parental permission. This development, however, is itself a hallmark of late adolescence and lies well beyond the phase we have just been discussing. It is a characteristic of middle-class adolescence today that many young people try to crowd the kinds of exploration and the intimacy associated with later stages into the earliest stages of adolescence.

Here it is wise to keep in mind that just as every gardener knows there is a minimum time necessary to grow a rose there is a minimum time for growing a person. Even modern technology cannot accelerate these processes.

NOTES

1. *New York Times* (April 11, 1977).
2. Ibid., "Many teenage girls feel it is very much a status symbol to be four to seven months pregnant and wearing maternity clothes"—spokesman for planned parenthood, Santa Clara County, Calif.

REFERENCES

Aries, P. 1960. *Centuries of Childhood*. New York: Knopf.
Blos, P. 1968. Character formation in adolescence. *Psychoanalytic Study of the Child* 23:245–263.
Freud, A. 1958. Adolescence. *Psychoanalytic Study of the Child* 23:245–263.
Kestenbaum, C. 1978. Some practical considerations in the assessment and treatment of adolescent girls with separation problems. *Journal of the American Academy of Psychoanalysis* 6:353–368.
Mussen, P.; Conger, J. J.; and Kagan, J. 1969. *Child Development and Personality*. New York: Harper & Row.
Shaffer, D.; Pettigrew, A.; Wolkind, S.; and Zajicek, E. 1978. Psychiatric aspects of pregnancy in schoolgirls: a review. *Psychological Medicine* 8:119–130.
Seiden, A. 1975. Sex roles, sexuality, and the adolescent peer group. *Adolescent Psychiatry* 4:211–225.
Zelnik, M., and Kantner, J. F. 1978. Contraceptive patterns and premarital pregnancy among women aged 15–19 in 1976. *Family Planning Perspectives* 10(3): 135–142.

10 ADOLESCENT GIRLS AND MENSTRUATION

LYNN WHISNANT, ELIZABETH BRETT, AND LEONARD ZEGANS

Puberty is a time when girls begin to take a particular interest in their bodily structure and function. Not only is their attention drawn to changes in external body size and shape, but questions also arise concerning the mysteries and workings of their inner anatomy. During puberty a girl must actively address issues about her changing body and the meaning and control of new bodily functions. She must also find new roles for herself in her family and peer group. A girl's approach to menstrual hygiene may reflect and be important in dealing with these diverse issues.

Menarche and menstruation have been treated as taboo and have remained relatively undiscussed in our culture. Menstrual hygiene as a somewhat isolated topic has been more widely acknowledged, in part because of the efforts of commercial manufacturers of sanitary supplies to market their products through educating girls in their use (Whisnant, Brett, and Zegans 1975). However, little systematic attention in the literature on development has been paid to the role of education about, and choice of, sanitary protection in a young girl's experience of menstruation even though this choice represents an area in which she can exercise discretion in coping with a new bodily function.

The devices most widely used for menstrual hygiene—the napkin and the tampon—are significantly different. A napkin can be worn with only the most rudimentary understanding of the anatomical relations of the external genitalia and vaginal canal and without direct manual contact with the genitalia. Insertion of a tampon not only necessitates contact with the genitalia but also requires some sense of anatomical relations.

First marketed about thirty years ago, tampons are now widely used.

When tampons were first made available, numerous articles in the medical literature discussed the physiological and anatomical aspects of tampon use in an attempt to allay fears (e.g., tampon use in unmarried females might have unfavorable moral implications with regard to masturbation and virginity) (Dickenson 1945; Diddle and Boulware 1942; Gosling 1960; Karnaky 1956; Thornton 1943).

Few reports of their experiences of the biological changes of puberty have been based on interviews with the adolescent girls themselves. This study presents one aspect of a girl's perceptions and way of coping with beginning menstruation and examines how her relationship with her family and peers may influence her style of perceiving and dealing with her own body.[1]

Method

Data were obtained during August 1973 and August 1974 from interviews with white middle-class campers and counselors at an overnight nondenominational girls' camp in New England. Girls who had received parental permission for participation in this study were selected for interviews by age groups in the order they were listed on the camp roster. There was no preselection in regard to menstrual status. The girls were interviewed by one of two women clinicians. Only one girl refused to be interviewed. Seventy girls were interviewed: twenty-six premenarcheal campers, thirty-two postmenarcheal campers, and twelve postmenarcheal counselors (table 1).

The interviews were semistructured and without forced answers. The number of replies represents spontaneous answers to general questions; the girls who did not comment on a particular aspect of tampon use may or may not have shared the feelings of those who did. Since this study is an exploratory hypothesis developing understanding rather than a hypothesis testing procedure, the application of statistical tests to the data would not be appropriate. The advantage of this open form of information gathering is that it may render the instances when the majority of girls answered and agreed more interesting.

In addition to the interviews, written questionnaires—administered to subjects drawn from the same population—elicited answers to specific questions about demography, education, menstrual history,

TABLE 1

THE POPULATION

	N	Mean Age
Interview subjects:		
Premenarcheal campers	26	11.3
Postmenarcheal campers	32	12.8
Postmenarcheal counselors	12	19.0
Total	70	...
Questionnaire subjects:		
Premenarcheal campers	101	11.0
Postmenarcheal campers	51	12.4
Postmenarcheal counselors	19	16.5
Total	171	...

and menstrual hygiene practices. This sample included 171 girls: 101 premenarcheal campers, 51 postmenarcheal campers, and 19 postmenarcheal counselors (table 1).

In examining the data the population was first partitioned into three main groupings: (1) premenarcheal campers, (2) postmenarcheal campers, and (3) counselors. Second, the two postmenarcheal samples were grouped by their choice of product used for menstrual hygiene: (a) girls who used only napkins, (b) girls who had tried tampons and used them occasionally, and (c) girls who used only tampons.

Results

Girls reported learning about tampons from a variety of sources including mothers, friends, school educational programs, and pamphlets or instruction sheets prepared by the manufacturers of tampons (see table 2). Age and menstrual status were important in determining the source of a girl's information about tampons and their use. Almost all the girls had talked with their mothers about menstruation and menstrual hygiene before or at menarche. The majority of girls (95 percent of those interviewed, and 86 percent of those responding to the questionnaire) were given napkins for sanitary protection by their mothers at the time of their first period (see table 3). (The girl who used tampons the first day was seventeen years old at her menarche).

159

TABLE 2

WHERE GIRLS LEARNED ABOUT TAMPONS

Subjects	Mother	Sister	Friend	School Nurse	Commercial Pamphlets	Total*
Interview	4	0	9	0	17	30
	(.13)	(0)	(.30)	(0)	(.56)	...
Questionnaire ...	11	1	8	0	31	46
	(.23)	(.02)	(.17)	(0)	(.67)	...

NOTE.—Percentage shown in parentheses.
*Girls who replied to this question from both premenarcheal and postmenarcheal girls.

In contrast to the number of girls who remembered their mothers giving them napkins when they talked about menstruation, only 57 percent said their mothers specifically mentioned tampons. Of those, all but three talked about tampons before or at menarche. One girl's mother discussed tampons in response to her daughter's questions and another on discovering that her daughter was using them. Girls who recalled the mother offering advice and instruction about the tampon, found her quite influential. None of the girls who used only tampons reported the mother saying "no" or "wait," whereas 42 percent of the girls who used only napkins said their mother advised them, "no" or "wait." Only 21 percent of the girls who used napkins

TABLE 3

SOURCE OF PRODUCTS FOR MENSTRUAL HYGIENE

Subjects	Mother	Sister	Friend	School Nurse	Self	Total*
Postmenarcheal interview:						
Received napkin from	41	1	1	0	0	43
	(.95)	(.02)	(.02)	(0)	(0)	...
Received tampon from	10	0	7	0	13	30
	(.33)	(0)	(.23)	(0)	(.43)	...
Postmenarcheal questionnaire:						
Received napkin from	59	4	3	2	0	68
	(.86)	(.05)	(.04)	(.02)	(0)	...

NOTE.—Percentage shown in parentheses.
*Number of girls who replied to this question.

exclusively felt their mothers gave permission to use tampons. In girls who use tampons exclusively, twice as many (40 percent) of the girls who used tampons exclusively believed that their mothers were in favor of tampons. Girls reported that their mothers had told them to "wait" but did not specify why or how long. Some remembered their mothers vaguely suggesting they should wait until their periods would be "regular" or their bodies "more mature." In all of these interviews there were only one or two explicit references to the issues of masturbation or virginity in discussions about tampons. One of the girls who expressed this most directly said, "I was afraid to use tampons at first—I thought I'd do it wrong and it would hurt me. My stepmother said I should use it only after I've gone to bed with someone. She said something could break inside. I used it anyway. I didn't tell her." The group of girls who used both napkins and tampons restricted tampon use for specific occasions such as swimming. The mothers in this group were least likely (12 percent) to give permission for tampon use (see table 4).

The girls seem to be influenced by their perceptions of the mothers' attitude with regard both to initiating the use of tampons and to using them exclusively. But regardless of what they reported their mothers said, girls in this group began to use tampons within a year or two after menarche. In the group of twelve counselors interviewed (ages 15–21)

TABLE 4

GIRLS' PERCEPTIONS OF THEIR MOTHERS'
ATTITUDES TOWARD TAMPON USE

| | | Mothers' Attitude | | |
Interview Subjects	N of Girls Interviewed	Yes	No or Wait	Not Mentioned
Premenarcheal campers	26	2	6	15
	...	(.07)	(.23)	(.57)
Postmenarcheal campers:				
Who used napkins	14	3	6	5
	...	(.21)	(.42)	(.36)
Who used napkins				
and tampons	8	1	4	3
	...	(.12)	(.50)	(.37)
Who used tampons	11	4	0	6
	...	(.36)	(0)	...

NOTE.—Percentages shown in parentheses.

only one did not use tampons. (This counselor expressed concern that she must be abnormal because she did not.)

Girls, who either did not discuss tampons with their mothers or felt that their mothers took a negative attitude, turned to peers for support and information. "I didn't discuss when to use tampons with my mother. The only source of information was my friends. I accepted their statements." Girls often talked about tampon use, encouraged each other to try tampons, and frequently taught one another (a favorite method is for one girl to stand outside the bathroom door and to read instructions to her friend inside). This is in marked contrast to girls' reticence with friends at the time of menarche. Some girls independently decided to use tampons and taught themselves how using the instructions in the tampon package. While 43 percent of the girls secured tampons for themselves, none of the girls provided their own napkins. Ninety-five percent of the girls who used napkins obtained them from their mothers—only 33 percent of the girls who used tampons obtained them from their mothers.

The girls were asked what advantages they perceived in the choice of tampons rather than napkins (see table 5). Their reasons were predominantly social. First, they could be more active and engage in sports, especially swimming. Second, the girls considered tampons a more "adult" mode of menstrual hygiene. Third, they could hide the evidence of menstruation (they referred to their dislike of wearing

TABLE 5

PERCEIVED ADVANTAGES OF TAMPON USE

Interview Subjects	N of Girls Interviewed	Advantages		
		Increased Activity	Excretory Control	Maturity
Premenarcheal campers	26	13	7	8
	...	(.50)	(.26)	(.30)
Postmenarcheal campers:				
Who used napkins	14	9	3	3
	...	(.64)	(.21)	(.21)
Who used tampons	18	11	10	7
	...	(.61)	(.58)	(.41)
Postmenarcheal counselors who used tampons	11	4	10	9
	...	(.36)	(.90)	(.81)

NOTE.—Percentages shown in parentheses.

sanitary napkins which they described as uncomfortable, bulky, smelly, dirty, and diaper-like). The girls who already used tampons were likely to volunteer that tampons offered control over messiness or odor. "They said a lot of blood comes out and you can't stop it—but with tampons it was controllable." These girls were graphic in descriptions of their disgust: "Napkins leak and stain—you sit on dried blood"; "Using napkins—you feel like a baby." The tampon users offered emotional, vivid descriptions concerning napkin use, worries about tampons, and the experience of menstruation. The girls who used only napkins were more restrained in their comments. Several girls asserted that their attitude toward menstruation changed about the time they started using tampons (e.g., "when I use it I feel normal; when I don't, I don't").

The girls were also asked about the disadvantages of tampon use (see table 6). Those who did not use them regularly expressed their current fears or doubts. Regular tampon users asserted that there were no disadvantages but recalled those they had before beginning to use tampons. The disadvantages can be placed in three categories. First, girls should be "mature" before using tampons (this factor was mentioned most often by the postmenarcheal girls who still used napkins, least by those who used tampons). Second, tampons were potentially damaging (they might fall out, get stuck, or damage something inside). Girls narrated stories about this concern—"One of my friend's sisters

TABLE 6

PERCEIVED DISADVANTAGES OF TAMPON USE

Interview Subjects	N of Girls Interviewed	Disadvantages		
		Ignorance	Damage	Maturity
Premenarcheal campers	26	10	16	11
	...	(.38)	(.61)	(.42)
Postmenarcheal campers:				
Who used napkins	14	8	9	10
	...	(.57)	(.64)	(.71)
Who used tampons	18	5	13	2
	...	(.29)	(.76)	(.11)
Postmenarcheal counselors				
who used tampons	11	8	5	7
	...	(.72)	(.45)	(.63)

NOTE.—Percentages shown in parentheses.

put one up. It would not come down. Her brother had to go in with pliers to get it." This perceived disadvantage—potential damage—was emphasized equally by all groups.

The third disadvantage was that girls feel unsure about the correct way to use tampons. Girls' doubts were related to their lack of knowledge about their external genital anatomy, which they expressed in comments like "I wouldn't know where to find the vagina" and even "the vagina, it's where you urinate—same place." Ignorance about the body and the technique of tampon use seemed to act as a strong deterrent to girls who were making a decision concerning their use. This factor was discussed most fully in retrospect by the older girls who had by this time been using tampons for a while.[2]

The importance of this lack of information was endorsed in the girls' descriptions of their first use of tampons. The girls interviewed often described themselves as never having systematically, either manually or visually, explored their genitalia; most attempted to insert the tampon by blind poking. "I practically killed myself getting it in—no idea where to put it. I never realized until then that I had two holes." Even the girls who tried using mirrors as aids felt unable to identify the structures they saw and found this method was more confusing. Girls preferred to try to learn to insert the tampon alone, with their mother (in the case of younger girls) or friends verbally encouraging them. One girl's mother inserted the tampon. The first experience in inserting the tampon was often characterized as extremely difficult and painful. Many girls made several attempts before succeeding. Girls described themselves as having been preoccupied with the "ordeal" of "getting it in" the first time. Some, in retrospect, described their success with a sense of pride—"It was a big thing at camp, the "older and wiser" club. The toilets were all lined up, and you'd go in there and learn to use tampons. It was a rite of passage." Girls who mastered the use of tampons were proud of their competence and often encouraged their friends to try tampons.

Discussion

Adolescent girls' use of a tampon rather than a sanitary napkin for menstrual hygiene may serve as an important, hitherto unrecognized, role in female psychosexual development. Several important tasks may be aided or impeded: coming to terms with the maturing body, loosening childhood ties to mother, developing a positive body image, and making a positive identification as a mature female beginning heterosexual experiences. While this study includes data collected from healthy subjects, clinical vignettes from patients are used to call attention to the role that menstrual hygiene may play in pathological sexual development and to illustrate the relevance of this topic in clinical work.

COMING TO TERMS WITH A MATURING BODY

Menarche ushers in a developmental epoch in which numerous pregenital conflicts are reawakened (Blos 1970). The mother and child struggles with issues of independence in establishing control over excretory functions during toilet training may be recalled at menarche when this new excretory-like function begins (Lewin 1930). The spontaneous flow of menstrual blood revives earlier experiences involving incomplete sphincter control and associated fears of soiling. An extreme example of this conflict and the role of menstrual hygienic practices is that of a formerly anorectic girl who responded to the resumption of her menstrual periods with great anxiety. She attempted to override the involuntary cramping and "soiling" by overdosing on laxatives thereby inducing "voluntary" cramping and loss of sphincter control with fecal soiling. After a time she began to insert tampons days and even weeks before her period was due in an effort to insure control over the flow. An example of the exhibitionistic quality displayed by a small child offering a fecal gift is that of a hospitalized sixteen-year-old psychotic girl who insisted on using no sanitary protection and wearing her stained jeans for several days so that everyone could see that she had begun to menstruate.

A sanitary napkin given by the mother to the daughter on the first day of the first period may heighten the regressive pull. The napkin is reminiscent of the infantile diaper that provided both a covering for the genitals and a means of absorbing bodily excretions. The healthy adolescent subjects in this study described the menstrual flow as dirty, messy, uncontrolled, and the sanitary napkin as "diaper-like" and public. They evidenced a fastidious modesty in which they appreciated the cleanness, control, and privacy offered by tampons.

The influence of an adolescent girl's peer group in loosening ties with mother is highly important. However, during the pubertal years relationships with her girl friends often undergo several viscissitudes. Although prepubertal girls discussed their curiosities about menstruation freely with each other (Whisnant and Zegans 1975), they became more secretive near the time of their first menstrual period and turned to their mothers for advice. A conflict situation is created in early puberty when the daughter has a need for separateness and individuation with a simultaneous opposing need for increased closeness with her mother. The mutuality is intensified at menarche by the female adolescent's tendency to rely on her mother as a source of information and guidance in managing new bodily functions.

The onset of menstruation enables the young girl to perceive her genitalia as more defined and specific (Deutsch 1944, Kesterberg 1961). Mother-daughter discussions, which before menarche may have seemed unreal and abstract to the girl, are perceived as more directly personal and intimate after menstrual flow has been experienced. The mother's interest in directing the adolescent's menstrual hygiene practices was perceived by some of the subjects in this study as excessive curiosity about the genitalia. Their mothers were seen as being intrusive and seductive. Communication about the tampon, an object which must be inserted into the vagina, is more explicitly personal and can occasion more anxiety and embarrassment than talk about the sanitary napkin which is used externally to cover a large, amorphous area.

Interaction between the mother and daughter regarding the use of the tampon may reactivate issues of infantalization and intrusive fusion with the mother. In several clinical cases, the mother's insertion of the tampon into her daughter at the first period created a traumatic event for the girl. One such girl who came for treatment at fourteen refused to insert tampons herself but had repeatedly required her mother's aid. Another refused to use tampons after the initial insertion by her mother. At twenty-one she still rejected self-use of the tampon and any contact with her own genitalia.

Interaction between mother and daughter regarding the use of the tampons, however, may assist in the detachment of the daughter from the mother and increase the girl's awareness of her own body and her individual responsibility for self-control. The mother's permissive attitude to the use of tampons can be interpreted as a way of acknowledging directly the daughter's vagina and indirectly the daughter's potential for adult sexuality. The girl's perception of her mother's acceptance of her autonomy and sexuality is reinforced and hence construed as approval of the girl's growing identification toward competent, independent adult womanhood. The mother's approval of tampon use implicitly assists the task of female adolescence in reworking the oedipal conflict.

The younger girls in this study, when interested in tampons, did not turn to their peers for instruction as readily as did the older subjects. One might speculate that this early reticence relates to the psychosexual stage of development in which their homosexual urges and acting out are much closer to conscious recognition (Lewis 1971). Containment of homosexual urges may no longer be of such imminent concern to the older girls who are thus able to turn to peers for help in mastering tampon use. The older girls who had learned to use tampons were eager to help and encourage others to do likewise.

Insertion of a tampon requires manual dexterity and a knowledge of spatial relations. It is a procedure that can be taught most easily by example and by direct assistance. However this kind of teaching among peers was quite unusual. Girls were reluctant to have their genital looked at or touched by their friends. The commonly used method of teaching evidenced in this study—one or more girls standing outside the closed bathroom door, reading instructions from the tampon insert, and offering suggestions—provides intimacy and support without seeing and touching. Certainly, relatively little new factual information seems to be transmitted by this method of instruction. Rather the presence of friends may serve to provide permission and to reduce anxiety and guilt about use of the tampons. Learning to use tampons with the help of a peer group may foster autonomy and individuation and so aid in the process of establishing independence from the mother.

MAKING A POSITIVE IDENTIFICATION AS A MATURE FEMALE BEGINNING ADULT HETEROSEXUAL EXPERIENCE

When tampons were first marketed, questions were raised about their use by young girls. The concern was primarily regarding the

167

physical rather than the psychological aspects of tampon use. A vigorous advertising campaign has sought to reassure mothers and doctors that the use of tampons does not affect virginity. Persistence of vague fears of damage because of the size of the hymeneal opening and widespread feeling or belief by the girls in this study that they should be older or that their bodies should be larger or more mature before starting to use tampons suggests that concerns about virginity and defloration are active in the girls' psychic reality.

It seems reasonable to expect that the penetration taboo (Lederer 1968) would be affected by the use of the tampon and that the psychological experience of the first intercourse might well be different for both partners when the penis is not the first object to have entered the vagina. Many of the sensations ascribed to the first use of tampons such as pain, anxiety, and a sense of rite of passage are similar to those of the interpersonal experience of defloration. One girl in this study had been urged by her boyfriend to practice using tampons before intercourse so the first time would be easier. This idea is reminiscent of the use of a ritual object for defloration in some primitive cultures and may be one way of addressing the "fear of virginity" in our culture. Use of the tampon may alleviate some of the anxiety of adult heterosexual experience.

DEVELOPING A POSITIVE BODY IMAGE

The insertion of the tampon, a neutral and nonsexual object, provides a socially sanctioned opportunity for the girl to touch and explore her external genitalia. If she has not previously done so, she can begin to form a conscious mental representation of the vagina and to connect internal and external sensations. This new perception, which will become part of the entire body image, may be as rudimentary as the notion that a space exists within her body where something may be placed safely and then retrieved, or it may be a more complex and complete concept of anatomical relations and sensations. In any case, insertion of the tampon allows or encourages a gradual self-regulated exploration.

The girl's independence in managing the insertion of the tampon permits her to begin, at her own pace, a repetitive series of experiences which facilitate a gradual familiarity with her genitalia. This can influence a girl's perception of herself as either active or passive in relation to her developing body image and her experience of her invisible internal genitalia. It is a step in discovering the vagina as part of her body which can be explored and entered without damage and thus may have an important effect on a girl's experience of her sexuality. It is possible that the mastery of the use of tampons which requires a girl to place an object in the vagina may also have important practical implications for a girl's or woman's later choice of contraceptive method and her ultimate willingness and ease of acceptance of an intravaginal method of contraception such as the diaphragm.

Conclusions

Adolescence is a vital epoch when integration of bodily and emotional experiences shape subsequent attitudes and behavior. During adolescence a girl must confront several tasks including: undoing childhood ties to mother, forming a positive identification as a woman, and coming to terms with her maturing body. This study is concerned with the effect that beginning use of tampons has upon a girl's view of herself; her body, especially her genitalia; and on her relationships with her mother and peers. Data were obtained from interviews and questionnaire survey of normal adolescent girls in a naturalistic, nonclinical setting. Results indicate that for many girls the use of tampons rather than napkins marked acquisition of an "adult" way of dealing with menstruation. Menstruation was initially described as a sickness which limits activity. Napkins were regarded as infantile, diaper-like, and dirty. Mastery of the use of tampons may repeat the earlier triumph of sphincter control and undo the confusion of menstruation with excretory function. Many girls anticipated waiting several years before attempting to use tampons, yet, the majority of these girls experimented with tampons as early as during the first year after menarche. This experience then becomes a stage in the girl's increasing awareness both of her genitalia as familiar and defined and of her developing sexuality. This learning experience may be dealt with by the girl either alone or in the peer group, in contrast to coping with the first menstrual period when girls turned to their mothers for advice. A girl's opportunity for discussion with peers reduces the regressive pull to the mother; assists her in arriving at a more conscious, differentiated sense of herself; and helps her to achieve greater autonomy. Clearly, from the perspective of the adolescent girl, the experience of learning to deal with menstruation extends beyond hygiene, and the mastery of hygienic practices may involve issues of growth and independence which are basic to the formation of a female identity.

NOTES

1. It is acknowledged that the girls' reports may be at variance with what the mothers' attitudes or behaviors actually were. However this study deals with the perceptions of the adolescent girls regarding their mothers communication. If a future study should indicate that the mothers were, in fact, more positive in their actual statements, the present data would be more significant in that it would demonstrate that the adolescent girls' psychic reality had distorted the actual situation in a predictable way.

2. A more complete description of the education of this population and in the misconceptions, in spite of exposure to educational materials, may be found in Whisnant, Brett, and Zegans (1975).

REFERENCES

Blos, P. 1970. *The Young Adolescent.* New York: Macmillan.

Deutsch, H. 1944. *Psychology of Women.* Vol. 1. New York: Grune & Stratton.

Dickenson, R. L. 1945. Tampons as menstrual guards. *Journal of the American Medical Association* 128:490–494.

Diddle, A. W., and Boulware, L. 1942. Vaginal tampons for menstrual hygiene. *Journal of the Iowa Medical Society* 32:256–257.

Gosling, P. H. 1960. Internal tampons. *British Medical Journal* 1:879.

Karnaky, K. T. 1956. Vaginal tampons for menstrual hygiene: second report—eighteen-year study. *Clinical Medicine* 3:545–548.

Kestenberg, J. S. 1961. Menarche. In S. Lorand and S. Schneer, eds. *Adolescents: Psychoanalytic Approach to Problems and Therapy.* New York: Hôeber.

Lederer, W. 1968. *The Fear of Women.* New York: Harcourt Brace Jovanovich.

Lewin, K. 1930. Kotschmieren, Menses und Weibliches über-Ich. *International Journal Psychoanalysis* 16:43–56.

Lewis, M. 1971. *Clinical Aspects of Child Development.* Philadelphia: Lea & Febiger.

Thornton, M. J. 1943. Use of vaginal tampons for absorption of menstrual discharge. *American Journal of Obstetrics and Gynecology* 46:259–265.

Whisnant, L.; Brett, E.; and Zegans, L. 1975. Implicit messages concerning menstruation in commercial educational materials prepared for young adolescent girls. *American Journal of Psychiatry* 132(8):815–820.

Whisnant, L., and Zegans, L. 1975. A study of attitudes toward menarche in white middle-class American adolescent girls. *American Journal of Psychiatry* 132(8):809–814.

PERSPECTIVES ON THE EFFECTS OF SOCIAL AND CULTURAL CHANGE

11   INTRODUCTION: THE EFFECT OF GEOGRAPHIC MOBILITY ON ADOLESCENTS

SIDNEY L. WERKMAN

Anyone who has moved to a new residence knows that, as Matthew Arnold wrote, "Change doth unknit the tranquil brow of man." Yet there has been very little scientific study of the psychological effects of moving on adults, and even less on the effects of moving on children and adolescents. Since geographic mobility is one of the major defining qualities of the contemporary world—the average American moves fourteen times in the course of life—it is worthwhile to examine the unique stresses and challenges that relate moving to psychological development and functioning.

The chapters in this section are addressed to extreme aspects of the phenomena of moving in the hope that these special situations might illuminate general principles embedded in ordinary life changes. One chapter chronicles the effects of the involuntary move of Vietnamese adolescent refugees who came to the United States following the close of the Vietnam war; another compares aspects of self-image, family relationships, and views of intimacy of teenagers in a highly mobile military community with those of military teenagers who have undergone fewer moves; and one examines the peculiar problems of American teenagers returning to the United States as adults after having lived abroad for a considerable part of their lives. In each case the moves were involuntary rather than made by choice, such as to go to college, initiate a career, or travel for recreation. Thus the teenagers described in this section are in effect chattels to the moving process and have experienced at least one more developmental stress than adolescents who did not need to move.

A move to a new home, especially one at a great distance from home or origin, carries with it a number of special stresses. Friendships, athletic activities, hobbies, and club involvements are disrupted. Mobile adolescents typically must live without any regular contact with grandparents and other relatives. Parental relationships become distorted in varying ways. Typically, fathers are away from home a good deal of the time and find their careers unusually compelling; this leaves their children to be reared almost exclusively by mothers who themselves may feel uprooted and in need of more support than is available. Thus it becomes difficult to develop and maintain intimate nurturant relationships.

Mobile adolescents are faced with novel customs and school requirements and must develop flexible coping strategies in order to be accepted in widely varying community situations. They are torn from friendships repeatedly yet must have the energy to invest in new ones. A definite experience of mourning becomes necessary, as does a recognition that it is impossible to return to the life known before. Many of the difficulties involved in geographic mobility relate to an inability to recognize these stresses, to master them, and to give up living in the past.

One of the most fascinating questions surrounding geographic mobility has to do with how much change is optimal and how such change can be managed most effectively by families and their teenagers. A number of observations suggest that highly mobile adolescents are at high risk for developing problems involving self-image, views of the future, and their ability to make new, intimate relationships with others. These concerns are among those discussed in the chapters.

As yet, we do not possess adequate data to document the hypothesis that mobility typically results in psychological dysfunction. In fact, some studies conclude that there is no psychopathology inherent in moving. Such a view would suggest that we have invented a cure for which there is no known disease. However, the following chapters do indicate that there is a definite psychopathology related to geographic mobility. It may well be that psychological difficulties related to geographic mobility become visible not in short-term observations of adaptation but in long-term studies of character structure and attitudes. This position coincides with the conclusions developed from the study of parent loss and, indeed, fits with the whole genetic point of view in dynamic psychological development. Therefore, it seems apparent that further studies of the phenomena surrounding geographic mobility will be fascinating in themselves and potentially useful in defining a new and important dimension of adolescent developmental stress and variation in our highly mobile society.

12   COMING HOME: ADJUSTMENT PROBLEMS OF ADOLESCENTS WHO HAVE LIVED OVERSEAS

SIDNEY L. WERKMAN

American children who live overseas for extended periods of time encounter unusual developmental challenges. They face repeated experiences of separation and loss, the hazards of transitions, and confrontations with novel patterns of culture and behavior. These children comprise an ongoing experiment in an alternate style of growth and differentiation that may be of considerable importance to our understanding of events and stresses that mold normal character development.

Many aspects of their lives are similar to a much larger group of people from other native lands. In this historical period of extensive geographic mobility and increasing international travel, the total group constitutes a new category of people of a "third culture" (Useem, Useem, and Donoghue 1963)—an international population which has loosened its ties to a home country, yet has not become totally integrated into the host country. These internationalists, more knowledgeable about each other than either the countries in which they live or their lands of origin, share attitudes, interests, concerns, and intrapsychic processes which may well be distinctive and enduring. Some unique aspects of growing up within this population followed by a return to life in the United States will be examined in this chapter.

For many, the task of readapting to the United States is the most difficult hurdle in the entire cycle of international life. People uniformly report that it is far less stressful to leave the United States and find a place in a new country than it is to experience the unexpected jolt of coming back home. As a twenty-year-old woman recalled: "People pushed and shoved you in New York subways or they treated you as if you simply didn't exist. I hated everyone and everything I saw here and had to tell myself over and over again, Whoa, this is your country, it is what you are part of."

Very little attention has been paid either in the research literature or in clinical work to the issues involved in return and readjustment to the United States or of the stress of geographic mobility in general (Bower 1967; David and Elkind 1966; Kantor 1965; Werkman 1972, 1977). Yet clinical experience and the anecdotal reports of returnees, expatriates, or internationals—in the United States we do not even have such a sanctioned term as "colonials" to describe these people—indicates that the stress of fitting into a new geographic situation can have serious and long-lasting effects.

My own involvement with this population has included work with the Peace Corps here and in Asia, with the Department of State, and in consultation positions with the Business Council for International Understanding and American schools overseas. The population from which these observations were made consist of four groups: (1) adolescents and adults interviewed during consultation trips to international schools overseas; (2) extensive tape-recorded interviews with thirty university students (average age: twenty) who had lived overseas at least one year and were attending the University of Colorado at Boulder; (3) patients from my clinical practice whose problems began in relationship to living overseas; and (4) a research sample to be described.

Approximately 1,700,000 Americans live overseas, of whom 230,000 are children attending international schools. The nonmilitary population is predominately a highly selected group of professionals and college-educated administrative personnel, largely with intact families, who probably represent a more than usually stable, psychologically resilient, competent group of people.

Any comparisons of mental health between overseas Americans and the general population of the United States are complicated by the unusually high socioeconomic status, level of ambition and achievement, education orientation, and intactness of families in overseas communities. Though a search for psychopathology is implicit in work of this kind, the further such investigation is pursued, the more the focus turns to an examination of styles of adaptation, character, and attitude studies rather than the attempt to diagnose psychiatric dys-

179

function. That is, the major differences, some positive and others negative, in such conditions as schooling, language, community supports, cultural advantages, novelty, sense of purpose, and even availability of mental health facilities greatly impede the attempt to assess levels of psychological health.

Psychocultural Conflicts

The following short examples from interviews and writings of people who have lived overseas describe aspects of the special qualities of such lives and highlight significant issues to be faced on returning to the United States:

Several things make an overseas childhood difficult. It is hard to reestablish roots and find new friends after each uprooting, especially when "home" can be such different places in just a few years. The family stays intact when it moves, but it is usually maids who take care of young children, and they have to be left behind. The culture, the language, the faces, and the scenery surrounding a child change much more drastically when moving between continents than moving around within the United States. The resulting discontinuity in hobbies and life style leaves you feeling scattered and confused.

For a child who has been a foreigner most of her life, being different from the surrounding society gets to be a habit, and when she moves to the United States she still feels like a foreigner. Even though children may have been to American schools, they do not know much about the United States if they cannot remember having lived there. It is frightening to go back; crime and violence in the United States seem even worse from outside the country. The usual problems of fitting into a new place are compounded by the problems of trying to conceive of an adult future in a society barely experienced. Sensitive children pick up characteristics in the countries they live in that may not fit smoothly into American life.

A young woman in college raised overseas described her plight in this way in an open letter to her parents:

A particular aspect of my "heritage" is that unlike most, it's not a shared one. I don't have anyone to "swap notes with," if you know what I mean. Even you and Daddy experience things in a radically different way—you were adults and already formed, while I was a child, malleable, susceptible, and unmolded. The uniqueness, while precious, is also very lonely at times. Being a child, I had a child's ability to adjust. I learned to assume that things were only temporary, that upheavals were always around the corner. This enabled me to survive, of course, but in the process I learned not to trust in "security," not to invest too much of myself in any one place for fear of losing it—in short, I learned to cultivate a sort of inner distance from the world around me. These are things I must unlearn today for they are handicaps to me as an adult trying to send down roots. But the habit and conviction of uninvolvement are very hard to break.

Intimate friendships develop quickly and with great intensity, in part to fill the vacuum left by the loss of the extended network of social, recreational, and athletic activities available to youngsters in the United States. These friendships, almost like shipboard romances, have built-in self-destruct qualities. "Never once did I have to break up with a girlfriend," a young veteran of such brief encounters reminisced.

My love affairs were always beautifully, romantically severed in first flush. Either I was transferred or she was. You could stand at the airport or shipside and wave the relationship away—just like that. When I was in high school, I found a girlfriend in February, knowing she was going to leave in June. I took her for what she was on the surface, and she did the same with me. Knowing that, we didn't have time to change each other or get to know each other very well. There was no sense of history in what we were doing. Even now I still tend to assume in some place deep inside of me that there is no need to confront problems or adjust to them, because I feel they will just sail away when my tour is up.

Another observer described his experience as follows: "There was a separate reality in my mind, a part of me held back. You didn't learn to be tentative or cautious. Instead, you developed an ability to throw yourself totally into a situation, expecting that you were also going to pull yourself out totally at a later date. It was sort of like the total commitment of early childhood, continued forever."

A move overseas with its intoxicating immersion in a foreign language and culture often frees a person to try experiences he would not seek out in his usual home. Impressionable young people may find themselves recurrently drawn to the vividness of new experiences and intense friendships out of the very intensity of their loneliness and isolation. As one philosophic returnee recalled, "I am forever pursuing experiences as intense, exotic, and elemental as the ones I encountered in my youth abroad. I have developed a kind of fearlessness, a kind of survivor's euphoria and optimism." One youngster recalled his difficult readjustment to the United States in this way: "I had lots of friends and played on the school soccer team in Pakistan. When I got back nobody noticed me and nobody was going to go out of his way to be nice to me in that big school. My marks slipped and I was miserable for two years."

On return to the United States, a significant part of the experience of an overseas person is left behind. Unfinished tasks and unfulfilled dreams must be dropped or forgotten. The need to abandon intense friendships and cultural supports frequently results in disturbing feelings characteristic of a grieving process. Though most returning Americans seem to make a good surface adjustment to this country, that adjustment may, at times, cover over a host of barely contained feelings of uncertainty, alienation, anger, and disappointment, as in the following report:

I felt out of everything when I came back. I didn't know about the music, what to wear, or how to get into the tight cliques that have formed from people who have been together all their lives. My junior high school graduating class in Saudi Arabia had just fifteen other kids. This high school has 2,000 kids, and it is unbelievable. You even have to get a pass to go to the john. The school is filled with cliques, the kids who do dope, the cheerleaders, the sports kids. I just couldn't get in with any of them. I didn't like them, and they didn't like me. I felt I was more mature than the other kids, and the things they thought were important seemed trivial to me. What am I going to wear at school today? Who am I going to walk home with? Those are just not big things in my life. I was afraid of these kids because, even though I felt mature, they knew a lot more about living in America than I did.

Issues that grip people in the United States lose their urgency, and the person overseas frequently develops a new group of interests based on an entirely different premise, that of being an observer and guest. As a visitor, his attention tends to be drawn to the grand, proud expressions of a host country's culture—art, music, architecture, theatre, holidays—rather than the mundane, daily ones. He loses contact with the anchoring points of daily life both in the United States and overseas.

Such conditions foster the development of a rich fantasy life that may be difficult for others to comprehend. An adolescent girl told me that, when she was in Paris, she had lived out a vision of herself as a turn of the century beauty, strolling through museums and stopping along the Champs-Elysées for a glass of wine. No one questioned the role she was playing out, least of all herself. On return to the United States little support can be found to nurture international fantasies, and, in addition, the returnee has lost track of the current events in this country. Bafflement and frustration may ensue on all sides.

Much of our experience is primarily nonverbal. It is difficult to translate into words certain of our touch, taste, smell, or visual perceptions, even though these perceptions may exert a potent influence on one's consciousness and self-definition. "You simply can't describe the feel of the hot wind on your skin in Sicily or the noise and commotion of traffic in Rome," a youngster lamented. "It just can't be reproduced in conversation. When I try to tell people what it was like, it probably sounds like I just want them to envy me. But, it's not that. I just want them to know what I felt, who I am." This large component of experience, nonverbal and unshared, creates a painful barrier to effective communication, so that the person who has returned from overseas may feel isolated and become prey to all kinds of distorted perceptions and disturbing fantasies.

Symptomatic Problems of the Returnee

Many returnees describe feelings of discomfort and vague dissatisfaction with their lives, though they cannot pinpoint the basis of their difficulty. They are able to adjust to the United States but are not comfortable with that adjustment. Most of the problems I have encountered fit the category of vague adjustment reactions rather than the more traditional psychiatric diagnoses. Long-lasting feelings of restlessness and rootlessness are typically recalled, even by those who are overtly well adjusted to their return from overseas.

A DIFFERENT SELF-CONCEPT

Attitudes of teenagers overseas about themselves and others were examined in a recent research study (Werkman and Johnson 1976). Differences in attitudes and values between teenagers raised overseas and those raised exclusively in the United States were studied by comparing 172 teenagers who lived overseas with 163 teenagers matched for age, sex, and socioeconomic status who had lived exclusively in the United States. Using the semantic differential technique, the subjects' reactions to certain concepts were rated on the dimensions of evaluation, activity, potency, and sensitivity. The groups were separated at statistically significant levels in rating the following concepts: Teenagers who lived overseas rated "themselves" as less strong, good, or happy than those in the United States; "the future" was not as strong, colorful, stable, or close to them; "friends" were less important, close, strong, and colorful; "loneliness" was more interesting, close, stable, and comfortable for them; and "restlessness" was more interesting, good, and happy for them.

The results suggest that overseas teenagers are unusually searching and open about themselves and especially capable of acknowledging potentially disturbing affects. They appear to be less secure and optimistic than adolescents who live exclusively in the United States, but in many ways they are more psychologically sensitive. The self-concepts of overseas teenagers appear to be less positive, and they seem to show less of a feeling of security and optimism about life in general. These results do not suggest that teenagers who have been raised overseas are less psychologically healthy than those in the United States but, rather, that overseas experience does have a significant effect on their values and attitudes.

Discussion

Because of the attitudes described, it well may be that overseas teenagers are candidates for becoming restless, possibly rootless people who have a constant need to be on the move. Indeed, it is a general clinical impression that the majority of people who have grown up overseas do not want to settle down in one place during their adult lives. Approximately two-thirds of the people seen in the Boulder sample as well as in my clinical practice hope to return overseas and expect to live geographically mobile lives.

Some children develop what can best be called a fixation on a stage in their growth and experience, often of a romantic nature, that may result in prolonged grieving or depression when they return to the United States. A wise teacher in Italy summarized the passionate nature of such encounters in this way: "American teenagers who come to our school develop strong attachments and sometimes intense crushes with Italian youngsters. They become inseparable, for each sees in the other, at a time when both are bursting with vitality, an opportunity to fulfill all of life's wishes. The breaking off of these friendships when the American goes home can be devastating for the visitor and the Italian child alike. Both suffer the effects of separation, as I know from conversation and letters, for such a long time."

Children who develop this syndrome have idealized every aspect of life overseas and have repressed the ordinary, boring, or anxiety-provoking components. They dismiss everything in the United States as uninteresting, worthless, or harmful. They are unwilling to integrate themselves into a new school, the pleasure of American sports, or the challenges of making friends when they return to the United States.

Instead, there is a desperate clinging to memories that are exquisitely pleasing precisely because they do not need to be tested against the reality of what actually happened. The dynamics of children with such problems bear considerable resemblance to those of cases conceptualized by Fleming (1972) as "parent loss" situations, in which a deeply experienced loss results in a kind of freezing of psychological maturation, an inability to engage in new experiences, and a distorted sense of time.

IDENTITY PROBLEMS

A child growing up in the United States incorporates a considerable part of his identity from the youth culture that surrounds him. Only in stressful circumstances does he need to ponder the question, Who am I? On the other hand, the child from overseas must integrate a heritage of externally prescribed behavior, which may hinder his own personal exploration and differentiation, with a uniqueness of experience that makes it necessary for him to seek out his own selfhood in the spotlight of bewildered isolation. For example, he may be told repeatedly that "You are a little ambassador," cautioned against chewing gum in public, and warned never to utter any negative statements about the host country. (A teenager confided to me that "my dying fear will be that a fight I had with a Pakistani boy would ruin American relations with the subcontinent.")

A polyglot background may add to the complications involved in developing a coherent sense of self. "My first language was Dutch, my second Greek, and I believe my youngest brother spoke Armenian when he was small," a young returnee told me, and added, "I developed certain ways of thinking in Dutch and Greek that remain today more vivid and accessible to me than English." Another said: "I'm two people. The one who uses English is quiet and precise; the Portuguese one gestures and is poetic and free."

The forging of an American identity is made difficult by the lack of authentic role models in adolescence. One youngster remembers his groping concerns in this way:

We were this whole group of Americans desperate to be Americans, but we were in India. So we would sit around and talk about hamburgers. Really! We would talk about hamburgers, and about half of us wouldn't remember what a hamburger tasted like, but we pretended we did. And I remember we read movie magazines and at one point even decided that our school should have cheerleaders. Our school didn't even have any teams, but we decided we had to have cheerleaders. So there we were having tryouts and learning cheers. In India! Someone who had been a cheerleader in America had just come, and she taught us all the cheers. We made these little skirts out of Indian material. It was weird.

In order for a firm sense of identity to develop, the adolescent depends upon the support of a stable society to confirm the value of his growing sense of inner coherence. The youngster growing up overseas often must move during adolescence—the very time when stability of behavioral expectation and easy availability of role models and ego ideal figures are most needed. As a result, he must make many individual, often lonely decisions that define his being. He cannot fall back upon parental experience for guidance, as his parents have grown up in a different societal situation, typically that of the United States. Because a premium is placed on conforming behavior overseas, the adolescent is both under pressure to adhere to generally rigid American community standards, while at the same time he is bombarded with the standards and values of the host country. (In some Southeast Asian countries, for example, there may be rigid rules about dating within one's peer group, at the same time that sexual experience with prostitutes is quite acceptable within the community.)

A teenager described another aspect of this complexity this way:

You end up with a double concept of yourself. There is this sense that you have an extra talent, your knowledge of another language and another culture, that has no value except in planning your life. I think where people get into trouble is that they tend to come back and know they have this asset, but think that everybody else should know about it and feel "you should respect me because I've got this extra experience," but it doesn't apply. What you gain from experience abroad is going to be maintained, but it's better to tuck it away. What you have learned not only doesn't get you anywhere, but it tends to threaten or irritate people.

A young adult offered these observations on the same theme: "When I came back to college, I kept observing and adapting my behavior to suit my country, all along feeling something like those transsexuals we hear about who adjust the best way they can to the fact that they seem to have been born into the wrong body. What they have is called gender dysphoria syndrome. What I have might be called culture dysphoria syndrome." A part of the culture dysphoria syndrome was described as a legacy of "fitting myself into many strange situations and places where I was an outsider but trying somehow to be part of it. It gives you a minority group empathy, being always yourself a foreigner. You are more sensitive to outsiders' needs than most people."

The sense of self developed from overseas experience can be one of great strength and resilience but, as described by a particularly gifted American who grew up overseas, it must be worked at and won with pain and effort. He wrote: "Once you realize you can never penetrate the hermetically sealed, parochial xenophobia of the natives here in the United States, you breathe a sigh of despair mixed with relief and set out toward a native country you know you must create for yourself, inside."

The paradigm of separation-individuation defined by Mahler (1968) usefully places these observations in context. It is as if the overseas-reared youngster retains a symbiotic attachment to his international experiences or returns symbolically to that attachment under the stress of the demands for individuation made by his return to the United States. If the attachment to overseas life was too intense or too gratifying, the returnee may find it exceedingly difficult to venture into the anxiety-fraught area of new experiences, particularly if the adults involved are, themselves, unable to give up the fantasied gratifications of their overseas past. Conversely, too headlong a rush into new experiences, without having mourned the loss of previous attachments, may leave the returnee with a heritage of concerns with desertion, rejection, and devaluation. A significant portion of life experience may remain isolated and become a hindrance to the development of autonomy and a firm American identity.

Faced with a bewildering group of what a patient of mine once called "cultural orders," it may be difficult to define a sense of self that is more than a series of changing masks. A youngster who returned from an overseas life to boarding school in the United States called the process one of "adopting of expressive masks, hoping to find a core from the various disguises we chose in incestuous emulation of one another."

Conclusions

The splitting highlighted by several of the examples described may be the result of an adaptive need to suppress significant portions of one's developmental experiences. An important part of the self remains foreign, hidden, split off, except when brought into consciousness through the mediation of someone who has shared a similar experience. The American who has grown up overseas typically finds it necessary to create in himself a complex identity, one that includes an ability to withhold significant experiences without developing feelings of guilt or anxiety, while retaining them in readiness for expression when the opportunity for a shared relationship becomes available.

Though we possess a time-honored tradition of farewell parties to send people overseas, and a considerable literature of adventure and self-discovery to guide them, we are endowed with very little ritual and writing to help them on their return. We are in need of a body of writing that can interpret America to returning Americans and, at the same time, explain them to those who have remained at home. Similarly, we need to devise societally recognized events that will reintroduce travelers to the people of their home country and guide them to a recognized place in their community.

The task of readapting to the United States or to any significant geographical change is an important one. Useful strategies for dealing with the stresses of mobility are emerging and can be modified for inclusion in individual therapy, group process situations, and classrooms. Geographical relocations occur frequently in our society, and we might hope that "rites of passage" related to such relocations will become part of our culture.

REFERENCES

Bower, E. M. 1967. American children and families in overseas communities. *American Journal of Orthopsychiatry* 37:787–796.

David, H. O., and Elkind, D. 1966. Family adaptation overseas: some mental health considerations. *Journal of Mental Hygiene* 50:92.

Fleming, J. 1972. Early object deprivation and transference phenomena: the working alliance. *Psychoanalytic Quarterly* 41:23–49.

Kantor, M. B. 1965. *Mobility and Mental Health.* Springfield, Ill.: Thomas.

Mahler, M. S. 1968. *On Human Symbiosis and the Vicissitudes of Individuation.* New York: International Universities Press.

Useem, F.; Useem, R.; and Donoghue, J. 1963. Men in the middle of the third culture: the roles of American and nonwestern people in cross-cultural administration. *Human Organization* 22(3): 169–179.

Werkman, S. L. 1972. Hazards of rearing children in foreign countries. *American Journal of Psychiatry* 128:992–997.

Werkman, S. L. 1977. *Bringing Up Children Overseas: A Guide for Families.* New York: Basic.

Werkman, S. L., and Johnson, R. 1976. The effect of geographic mobility on adolescent character structure. Unpublished data available from the authors, University of Colorado School of Medicine, Denver, Colorado.

13 ADOLESCENTS IN THE MOBILE MILITARY COMMUNITY

JON A. SHAW

It is estimated that there are over 2,100,000 children in the military community (Bennett 1974). While these children experience the same developmental and maturational processes as other children, the voluminous literature on the military family has tended to elaborate upon those social and facilitating processes which are unique to the military way of life. The critical pressures associated with frequent family moves, intermittent experiences in strange and foreign countries, and transient father absence have all been described. Most of these studies, however, have necessarily preferred to perceive the stresses inherent in the military way of life within the framework of social systems theory, with little attention to developmental perspective.

The child in the military community is a member of a social system in which there is a high expectation of mobility. Studies of these children have, however, rather consistently failed to find any predictable relationship between emotional and behavioral problems and the frequency of family moves (Shaw and Pangman 1975). As Pedersen and Sullivan (1964) have noted, the predominant factors determining the child's adaptation to frequent family moves are the family and parental processes and, most important, the parental attitudes, assimilation, and identification with the military way of life.

A study of military children from a high school in Germany revealed that the average high school graduate had attended nine schools prior to graduation (Strickland 1970). In one of the few studies of the adolescent experience in the military family, Darnauer (1976) interviewed separately and in structured formats sixty adolescents, ranging in age from sixteen to eighteen years, and their parents from a large military training installation. He noted that the average adolescent had moved 5.8 times. Sixty-seven percent had experienced at least one family move since the ninth grade. While they stressed the importance of travel and cultural experiences, they indicated that frequent family moves were the predominant negative factor in military life. Although 75 percent had experienced a period of father absence during adolescence, this was rarely mentioned.

While observers have recognized the momentous significance of physical and psychological dimensions of puberty, there has been little effort to view the problems of geographic mobility from the perspective of phase-specific tasks of adolescence. The essence of adolescence is the withdrawal of childhood yearnings from the object representations of youth and the modification of self- and object representations through increased cognitive development, maturational processes, and a new exploring of interpersonal and intimate relationships. This process of separating from infantile ties to parental objects represents an intrapsychic shift or discontinuity in development. The adolescent has to give up forever his youthful dependency and passive longings for the parental images of his childhood if he is to secure his own independence and autonomy. The family move represents a discontinuity in his social relationships with its loss of friends and others and interferes with the consensual validation of his emerging identity and capacity for intimacy. It has been speculated that the imposition of a social discontinuity in the form of a family move may resonate with the intrapsychic discontinuity in development characteristic of the adolescent process and may render him peculiarly vulnerable to a failure to progress normally in the resolution of his adolescence (Shaw 1978). Inbar (1976) has indicated the profound vulnerability of the mid-adolescent to crisis in his environment.

How does the adolescent in the military family experience the constant uprooting intrinsic to military life, with its loss of friends, young loves, and the continuity of a stable social milieu? Does he respond like Alice, who asks the Cheshire cat in her search for the enchanted garden: " 'Would you tell me, please, which way I ought to go from here?' 'That depends a great deal on where you want to get to,' said the Cat. 'I don't much care where' said Alice. 'Then it doesn't matter which way you go,' said the Cat. 'So long as I get somewhere,' Alice added as an explanation'' (Carroll 1960, p. 88). Or is he like Thomas Wolfe, who asked about man's tormented wandering in his writings: "Where shall the weary rest? Where shall the lonely of heart come home? What doors are open for the wanderer? . . . Where the weary of heart can abide forever, where the weary of wandering can find peace, where the tumult, the fever and the fret shall be stilled" (1935, "The Proem," p. 2).

This study will attempt to explore the adolescent's self-perception relative to a number of personality variables and attitudes toward interpersonal relationships, frequency of moves, and life in the military family. Particular attention will be given to his description of himself vis-à-vis an adjective checklist with the intent of determining if this is influenced by the frequency of moves. It is hypothesized that increasing frequency of family moves interferes with the adolescent process with its movement toward consolidation of an ego identity and capacity for intimate relationships.

Method

Adolescents consecutively attending the Adolescent Medicine Clinic for a wide range of general medical problems were tested on a modified Werkman Family Move questionnaire, as well as on a checklist of sixty-five descriptive adjectives. They were asked to answer a number of open-ended questions requiring sentence completion, to itemize the history of family moves during their life, and to make discriminative judgments relative to dichotomous descriptive adjectives on a six-point scale to ten primary questions: (1) I am ———; (2) Loneliness is ———; (3) A close (intimate) friend is ———; (4) Restlessness is ———; (5) Intimacy is ———; (6) My feelings (spirits) generally are ———; (7) My mother is ———; (8) My father is ———; (9) Moving is ———; and (10) Living in the military family is ———.

There were sixty-six forced choice discriminative response selections among the ten primary questions, such as important-unimportant, strong-weak, secure-insecure, stable-unstable, interesting-uninteresting, intimate-distant, good-bad, happy-unhappy, friendly-unfriendly, outgoing-withdrawn, available-unavailable, colorful-colorless, possible-impossible, safe-dangerous, optimistic-pessimistic, high-low, exciting-dull, and easy-difficult. The adjective checklist required the subjects to circle twenty of the following words "which you feel most describes you as you usually are."

Subjects were excluded from the study if they had not lived in a military family or failed to complete the questionnaire. Ages ranged from thirteen to seventeen years. The subjects were divided into five groups for the purpose of statistical analysis: (1) an all-adolescent group, (2) a male group, (3) a female group, (4) a group of subjects experiencing four or less family moves, and (5) a group of subjects experiencing five or more family moves.

Results

This report is necessarily limited in that it represents a pilot study in which an attempt is being made to explore various instruments and to establish clearer paradigms of investigation. Certain trends appear to be evident in the ongoing research, and they will be reported as they presently stand at this level of investigation and statistical analysis of the data.

There were no significant differences noted between the groups in the distribution of rank and the mean ages of the groups. Table 1 indicates the various sample sizes, the distribution of males and females, and the mean age of adolescents, as well as the mean of the number of family moves for each group. For the purpose of this chapter, the data will be explored relative to the adolescent population with specific attention to the high-move and low-move groups.

In response to the question, I am ———, several trends were noted. The high-move group rather consistently perceived themselves in a less positive way than the low-move group. This was clearly evident in their propensity to see themselves as more changeable, boring, and distant, as well as somewhat more withdrawn and unhappy.

The high-move group perceived loneliness as less distant and more

TABLE 1
ADOLESCENT GEOGRAPHIC MOVES

Group	N	Male	Female	Mean Age	Mean N of Moves
Adolescent......................	45	18	27	15.4	4.7
Adolescent (male)	18	18	...	15.2	3.7
Adolescent (female)	27	...	27	15.5	5.0
Adolescent: low move	30	15	15	15.5	2.1
Adolescent: high move	26	19	7	15.4	9.5

intimate than the low-move group. Restlessness was perceived in a clearly more negative profile by the high-move group, as compared with the low-move group across all the dimensions of strong-weak, colorful-colorless, interesting-uninteresting, good-bad, and happy-unhappy dichotomies. Intimacy was perceived by the high-move group as being less stable and more important and dangerous than the low-move group. The high-move group tended to perceive their feelings in a more negative profile than the low-move group. They saw themselves as more unimportant, colorless, changeable, boring, pessimistic, and low.

There was no clear distinction between the manner in which all groups perceived their mother and father. Mothers were perceived by all groups as being more available than the father. Family moves were perceived as clearly more important, easy, and exciting to males than females, who described them as unimportant and difficult but, paradoxically, more exciting. The high-move group saw moving as more important, interesting, and exciting than the low-move group. Life in the military family was perceived as more secure, interesting, and close to the high-move group. Females clearly perceived life in the military family as more secure, yet also more difficult.

On the adjective checklist in which the adolescent described how he usually perceives himself, there were significant statistical differences across a number of variables. The high-move group consistently perceived themselves in a more negative manner than the low-move group. This difference was found to be statistically significant in that subjects in the high-move group consistently checked a greater frequency of negative rather than positive adjectives, compared with the low-move group. Several adjectives were statistically more commonly checked in the high-move group. Thus, the high-move group was found to perceive themselves significantly ($P \leq .05$), more insecure, more complaining, less intimate, more inconsistent, and more critical than the low-move group. While not statistically significant ($P \leq .10$), adolescents in the high-move group more frequently described themselves as less predictable, more gloomy, and less reliable.

Discussion

Various observers of human behavior have commented on the psychological effects of family moves. The Joint Commission on Mental Health of Children Report (1969) indicates that there is conflicting evidence as to whether geographic mobility has adverse effects on children and their families. Tooley (1970) has written that "moving seems to improve family adjustment or individual adjustment almost as often as it disturbs it." Studies of the effects of geographic mobility have been characterized by a variety of findings that frequently are contradictory. The predominant finding is that the effects of mobility may be positive or negative, depending on how the individual defines the situation and, most important, how the individual in the military family has identified with the military community (Gabower 1960; McKain 1973; Pedersen and Sullivan 1964).

Nevertheless, it is apparent that every change of residence requires some degree of adjustment to the changing environmental conditions. From this viewpoint, the adolescent's adaptation to the family move can be interpreted within the context of crisis theory as representing an "emotionally hazardous situation temporarily upsetting, not always in an unpleasant sense, yet constantly requiring reorganization and mobilization of the individual's personality resources" (Caplan 1965). In this context, it is an experience which implies neither good nor ill.

The results of this study suggests that frequent family moves in the history of the adolescent leave him with a rather negative self-descriptive profile. He perceives himself as changeable, boring, distant, less intimate, more insecure, inconsistent, critical, and more complaining than his comparable peers in the low-move group. He is less predictable and reliable and more gloomy. He tends to see intimacy as something that is important but also as less stable and more dangerous. Restlessness is perceived as a less desirable trait across all dimensions, while loneliness is construed as intimate, suggesting a positive experience.

The vulnerability of the adolescent to frequent moves in his history may be related to the task of adolescence itself. The process of separating from the infantile ties to the parental objects is comparable with the process of mourning after the loss of a loved one. The child who has had so many of his initial relationships terminated by translocations, his attempts at intimacy thwarted by loss, is left with a sense of loneliness. He yearns for intimacy but is frightened by the danger of becoming too intimate with another. There is the fear that he will once again inevitably experience the loss of a loved relationship with the too commonly experienced anguish and grief.

The lack of stability in the continuity of interpersonal relationships, as well as discontinuity in social-cultural experiences, may interfere with the consolidation of an identity that has continuity and sameness through time. The adolescent with a sense of insecurity and lack of trust in intimate relationships will have difficulty disengaging from the infantile object representations. He will be less able to use his social group as an ego support system through which his individuation is to be realized. The group provides the opportunity for social role experimentation. It is through relationships with his peers that the individual guilt that accompanies his emancipation from childhood dependencies, prohibitions, and loyalties is alleviated. It is through peer relationships that one's social, personal, and sexual identity evolves and is confirmed by others. A family move occurring at the time the adolescent is frantically turning to the peer group as a substitute for family and parental objects is an undue stress. The added stress of a family move imposed on the adolescent process may tip the balance in the direction of the regressive forces. It may interrupt the process of disengagement from the infantile objects and force him momentarily into a dependent, passive position in the family. In some instances the adolescent will defend himself from the regressive pull by a pseudo-independence which may be manifested by truancy, running away, delinquency, pseudoheterosexuality, promiscuity, negativism, and poor school performance.

Conclusions

The adolescent's response to a geographic move is determined by a complex layering of systemic influences. Among those factors which have to be explored when trying to understand the adolescent's response to the family move is the individual's struggle with the second individuation process, the character of which is multidetermined by a whole complex of epigenetic, familial, and biosocial-cultural variables. It is suggested that in some instances frequent family moves leave the adolescent with an impoverished sense of self-esteem and trust in his capacity for autonomy and self-direction. There may be a failure to progress normally in the resolution of his adolescence, with impairment of his capacity to consolidate a sense of self, as well as in his capacity and readiness for intimate relationships.

REFERENCES

Bennett, W. M. 1974. *Army Families*. Published group research project. Carlisle Barracks, Penn.: U.S. Army War College.

Caplan, C. 1965. Opportunities for school psychologists in the primary prevention of mental disorders in children. In *Protection and Promotion of Mental Health in Schools*. Public Health Service, Mental Health Monograph 5, Publication no. 1226 (Washington, D.C.).

Carroll, L. 1960. *The Annotated Alice: Alice's Adventure in Wonderland*. New York: Potter.

Darnauer, P. 1976. The adolescent experience in career Army families. In H. McCubbin, B. Dahl, and E. Hunter, eds. *Families in the Military System*. Beverly Hills, Calif., and London: Sage.

Gabower, G. 1960. Behavior problems of children in Navy officers' families. *Social Casework* 41:177–184.

Inbar, M. 1976. *The Vulnerable Age Phenomenon*. Beverly Hills, Calif., and London: Sage.

Joint Commission on Mental Health of Children, Inc. 1969. *Crisis in Child Mental Health: Challenge for the 1970s*. New York: Harper & Row.

McKain, J. 1973. Relocation in the military: alienation and family problems. *Journal of Marriage and the Family* 35:205–209.

Pedersen, F. A., and Sullivan, E. J. 1964. Relationship among geographic mobility, parental attitudes and emotional disturbances in children. *American Journal of Orthopsychiatry* 34:575–580.

Shaw, J. A. 1978. The adolescent experience and the military family. In E. Hunter and S. D. Nice, eds. *Children of Military Families Apart and Yet Apart*. Washington, D.C.: Government Printing Office.

Shaw, J., and Pangman, J. 1975. Geographic mobility and the military child. *Military Medicine* 140(6): 416–446.

Strickland, R. C. 1970. Mobility and achievement of selected dependent junior high school pupils in Germany. Doctoral dissertation, Miami University.

Tooley, K. 1970. The role of geographic mobility in some adjustment problems of children and families. *Journal of the American Academy of Child Psychiatry* 9:366–378.

Wolfe, T. 1935. *Of Time and the River*. New York: Scribner's.

14 ADOLESCENTS AS REFUGEES

JOHN G. LOONEY

When adolescents move it is usually the result of an elective decision by their parents. In this chapter I would like to describe my involvement with adolescents who were forced to move in an involuntary and precipitous manner. I plan to describe the responses of Vietnamese adolescents to the stress of forced immigration into this country.

In the spring of 1975, the fall of the South Vietnamese political regime was imminent. The United States Department of State hastily formulated a plan to relocate over 150,000 South Vietnamese citizens in this country. These citizens were usually those who had assisted the American government in the war effort, and they consequently feared severe reprisals from the Communists. Their exodus from Vietnam was sudden and chaotic. After short stays at preliminary camps in the Philippines, Wake Island, or Guam, these refugees arrived at one of several refugee relocation centers within military establishments in the United States. The refugee facilities were hastily built tent communities, and living in these crowded tent communities was a distressing experience. In many instances family members were separated. Some members arrived at a refugee camp in Arkansas while others arrived at a similar camp in Pennsylvania. Compounding the distress was the long wait for relocation in America. In order to leave a refugee camp a Vietnamese family had to find an American sponsor to provide them clothing, housing, employment, and other basic essentials.

Being a refugee unfortunately has become a common experience for many. A United Nations report (1969) estimates that between 1945 and 1969, 45 million people have been denied residence in their homelands. Numerous publications have documented that emotional problems are increased when people must migrate, and even voluntary migration has been shown to result in an increasing prevalence of mental illness

(Malzberg and Lee 1956; Ødegard 1932). Refugees, those who migrate involuntarily, have been shown by many authors to have a markedly increased prevalence of mental disorders (Burvill 1973; Edwards 1956; Eitinger 1959, 1960; Eitinger and Grunfeld 1966; Kino 1951; Krupinski, Stoller, and Wallace 1973; Kuepper, Lackey, and Swinerton 1974; Meszaros 1961; Mezey 1960a, 1960b; Murphy 1974; Pederson 1949; Pfister-Ammenda 1955; Rumbaut and Rumbaut 1976; Strotzka 1961). Particularly relevant to the plight of the Vietnamese refugees is the finding that psychological problems are increased when the period between immigration and final resettlement is prolonged (Pfister-Ammenda 1955). Also relevant is the finding that problems increase when group or family cohesiveness is interrupted (Kino 1951; Strotzka 1961). It also has been noted that mental health problems increase when refugees move into a markedly dissimilar culture (Kuepper et al. 1974). In all these accounts children and adolescents appear to be passive participants whose special problems have not been addressed. There are no published reports documenting the particular effects on adolescents of being a refugee.

As noted, the purpose of this presentation is to (1) describe, in brief, a consultation experience in which I was responsible for meeting the mental health needs of refugee children and adolescents; and (2) to note something of the responses of the adolescents to this particularly stressful experience (Caplan 1964).

The Consultation: Findings, Recommendations, and Results

The commanding general of Camp Pendleton Marine Base was called from Washington and asked to establish living facilities for Vietnamese refugees. Incredibly, within twenty-four hours tent communities were built for approximately 20,000 individuals. These communities contained complete dining, plumbing, electrical, and health facilities. During ensuing months over 60,000 individuals moved through this refugee facility. The medical corps of the navy was responsible for health care. Regional clinics were located throughout the tent communities. Because of concern that the refugees might be suffering significant depression, a team of mental health consultants was obtained.[1]

The consultation team's initial activity was that of gathering information. Team members visited the tent city and, through interpreters, talked to many of the Vietnamese people, including indigenous leaders. As a child and adolescent psychiatrist, I spent my time interviewing children and adolescents and discussing the plight of these youths with their parents (Harding and Looney 1977).

It was apparent that meeting the mental health needs of the young people in the camp would be a problem of massive proportions. Children and adolescents made up approximately 70 percent of the refugee population. I was struck by differences between Vietnamese and American youth, particularly with regard to adolescents. The differences were manifested by the Vietnamese adolescents' intense sense of family loyalty. Large multigenerational families were common, and teenagers were quite busy helping with the care of their younger siblings or aged relatives. It was common to note teenagers and small children happily playing the same games, and they expressed a sense of being important and useful to their families. This sense of commitment and importance for the teenagers seemed to mitigate against the development of boredom and its possible sequelae—antisocial behavior. The younger children seemed to be unusually outgoing and happy and, although the camp was full of babies, there was little crying. I felt that a great deal of the positive adjustment of these children could be attributed to the attention they received by their adolescent siblings. In general, I was impressed with how well the adolescents fared under the pressures of their situation. The positive findings were as follows:

1. The adolescents appeared to be well nourished and well developed.

2. There was little evidence of serious acute illness.

3. The adolescents took pride in their appearance. Although in many cases their donated clothing did not fit, it was kept in good condition and often was decorated with gayly colored patches or other insignia.

4. The adolescents were vivacious and outgoing, and interacted freely with the consultants and their Marine Corp hosts.

5. The teenagers appeared to be optimistic about entering American society. Their optimism was demonstrated by their keen interest in learning American teenage customs and slang.

6. Many spontaneous social activities among adolescents occurred throughout the camps.

7. The teenagers appeared eager to learn or improve their English.

8. A high degree of family support through several generations was noted.

9. There was no interest in intoxicants.

Despite the fact that these youngsters appeared to be making an adequate initial adjustment, a number of things caused concern. Although during the early phases of camp life young people were full of the intense excitement of a great adventure, I feared that in time this excitement would abate and deleterious environmental factors would have an increasingly negative impact.

There were the following negative impressions:

1. The adults within the camp often masked considerable anxiety, a sense of serious loss, and fear of the unknown with great bravado. It was feared that in time their covert concerns would become more manifest and have a correspondingly deleterious effect on the young people.

2. Because of the change from a tropical to a temperate climate, the adolescents suffered from the cold. They had been given heavy combat jackets, but their legs and feet were bare. The situation limited their activities to the interior of their tents and restricted their interactions with other youngsters.

3. There was an absence of educational devices or athletic facilities within the camps.

4. There were no organized activities such as schools or athletic teams.

5. There were small groups of adolescent boys who appeared to be bored, depressed, and ready to cause trouble; and there were a few teenage girls dressed in a sexually provocative manner.

6. Families were broken up in the process of leaving the camp. Since some of these families were very large (as many as thirty members), American sponsors were reluctant to take on such an overwhelming responsibility. The Vietnamese families, sensing this difficulty, began splitting themselves up into smaller groups, hoping they might be reunited later. However, there was no assurance that these different groups would find sponsors in the same community or the same state.

7. There were adolescents within the camp who were not attached to families. In some cases these were teenagers whose families had been sent to another refugee camp. In some cases they were those whose

families had contracted with another family to take them to America to a "better life." Once inside the camp, however, these teenagers sensed their unofficial families' anxiety about sponsorship. They understood that chances of being sponsored decreased with increased family size. As a result they acted out their anxiety by running away and reporting to Red Cross nurses that the families had rejected them. Instead of responding to the meaning of such behavior by attempting a negotiation between the children and their unofficial families, the nurses placed these children in a compound for "unaccompanied youth." Other adolescents in the camp simply had no group attachments at all. In the chaos of leaving Vietnam, groups of people might have jumped from one boat to another. Sometimes only the adolescents were able to make the jump, and the rest of the family was left behind. These youngsters also were placed in the compound for unaccompanied youth. The adolescents in the compound exacerbated each other's misery. Severe psychiatric symptoms, including depression (with attempted suicide) and transient psychotic episodes, emerged.

Since I had the responsibility for making recommendations accentuating positive factors and offsetting potentially deleterious ones, the crucial task was to translate knowledge of the developmental needs of adolescents and the functioning of teenagers within the context of the family into recommendations that seemed reasonable and feasible to the camp administrators, officials who had little experience dealing with the emotional needs of young people. It is beyond the scope of this presentation to outline the recommendations which addressed the problems within the community, but a list of the consultation recommendations (and the generally positive results) are outlined in a separate report (Looney, Rahe, Harding, Ward, and Liu 1978).

These adolescents suffered a moving experience much more cataclysmic than is likely to be experienced in the modal American family. These families were separated from their country, their friends, a familiar culture, and, in many cases, from their previously accumulated wealth. They came to this country with little more than optimistic fantasies about what life in this society might be. Living in the crowded tent communities rapidly brought a harsh reality into conflict with these hopeful fantasies. Eventually, reports of many problems encountered by those families who had been sponsored out of the refugee camps filtered back and made the refugees aware that they indeed would be facing many trials in their new land.

Although the range of responses manifested by adolescents to this stress was from that of optimistic enthusiasm to psychotic decompensation, the usual response was one of determination, cautious optimism, stable mood, and unusual cooperativeness with other adolescents and family members. It should also be noted that this good level of adjustment did not significantly deteriorate during the four and a half months the refugee camp was in operation. Many factors might have accounted for this perhaps unexpectedly good adjustment of the teenagers—for example, many had previous experiences with adversity. It was my clinical impression, however, that the factor most highly correlated with good adjustment was family solidarity. In those large families in which leadership was shared by the elders of several generations, and in which the family itself was an effective support system, children and adolescents fared well. The stabilizing influence of grandparents, great-grandparents, aunts, and uncles was apparent. Although Vietnamese adolescents' affiliation with peers was clearly apparent and important, their continuing affiliation with their own families would seem unusual in contrasting these teenagers to American youth.

Although what I previously described have been clinical data, I have a few research data which merit brief mention. The consultation team used several standardized questionnaire instruments to try to measure the degree of stress incurred by the refugees. One of these was the *Recent Life Change Questionnaire*, an inventory of representative life-change events, high scores on which have been shown to correlate with illness vulnerability. The second instrument was the *Cornell Medical Index*, an instrument used since the early 1950s as an aide in reviewing body-system symptomatology. This index consists of 195 yes or no questions that measure the presence or absence of somatic and psychological symptoms. The third instrument was the *Self Anchoring Scale*, which was previously developed to document an individual's perception of his or her position on a one- to ten-step scale. This placement represents how close or how far an individual is from his or her best or worst possible world. These instruments were administered to a randomly selected sample of families in the refugee camp. The results of these surveys have been presented in detail in a previous report (Rahe, Looney, Ward, Tung, and Liu 1978). The results show that refugees of all ages documented scores on the severely stressed end of the scales of these instruments. The point to be made is that, whereas these people were highly stressed and viewed their circumstances as quite unsatisfactory, they adapted well. To explain this finding we have to take into account coping strategies used. As I have suggested from a clinical perspective, the maintenance of family solidarity was the most impressive probable factor. At the present time I am working with colleagues to correlate individual differences between degrees of stress as measured by these instruments and independently derived measures of family competence. My hypothesis is that the strongest families will contain adolescent members whose stress scores are relatively lower. The highest stress scores would be expected in those adolescents who had no family attachments at all.

Conclusions

The Vietnamese adolescents described in this report were studied during an extremely stressful period in their lives. They had lost all anchoring in their previous culture. Despite the stress, these adolescents generally adapted well, although, as I have mentioned, the range of responses was from extremely competent functioning to extreme manifestations of psychopathology. Why was the modal adolescent in this setting doing well? A number of explanations might be offered. As I suggested, these people might have been conditioned to adversity by events in South Vietnam. It should be noted, however, that most of these families were of middle-class status or above and had enjoyed relatively secure lives in Saigon or other urban centers. They had been little affected by the horrors of the war itself. Another possible explanation for the good response is that these young people were sustained by visions of an exciting life in an affluent new country. However, as I have noted, these people routinely did receive reports from refugees who had established lives in America that they could expect multiple and severe problems. They were told they would not readily be accepted by a people with a history of prejudice toward minorities—a people who wanted no reminders of the embarrassment of South Vietnam. Another possible factor contributing to the good adjustment was that of peer-group support. These youngsters were all in the same predicament, and they openly shared their feelings about their plight. Peer-group solidarity was apparent. As I have also noted, the most powerful explanation for the adequate adjustment of these youngsters was the sustenance they received by being members of strong family groups. They had a sense of being needed by their families. I had fantasied reflections of what it must have been like for American adolescents in rural settings years ago in this country when the labor of the teenagers was actually needed for the survival of the family.

One major unanswered question is that of how these people are faring now. Unfortunately, only anecdotal data exist, and these are contradictory. Following the relocation of the refugees I was asked to be a member of the Vietnamese Resettlement Advisory Committee, an ad hoc committee which was asked to make recommendations to the Congress about how to assist these people. One of the major recommendations was that HEW be commissioned to carry out a systematic follow-up study. No such study has been carried out. I still hope that one can be completed because I think it is possible we will learn a great deal about the adjustment of these people which would be helpful in assisting others in our culture who are faced with the necessity of relocation.

NOTE

1. The team was headed by Dr. Richard Rahe, a psychiatrist with extensive experience in responses to stress. Also on the team were Dr. Looney, a child psychiatrist, Dr. Harold Ward, a psychiatrist with advanced training in public health (M.P.H.), and Dr. Hamilton McCubbin, who held a doctorate in social work.

REFERENCES

Burvill, P. W. 1973. Immigration and mental disease. *Australia–New Zealand Journal of Psychiatry* 7:155–162.

Caplan, G. 1964. *Principals of Preventive Psychiatry.* New York: Basic.

Edwards, A. T. 1956. Paranoid reactions. *Medical Journal of Australia* 1:778–779.

Eitinger, L. 1959. The incidence of mental disease among refugees in Norway. *Journal of Mental Science* 105:326–338.

Eitinger, L. 1960. The symptomatology of mental disease among refugees in Norway. *Journal of Mental Science* 106:447–966.

Eitinger, L., and Grunfeld, B. 1966. Psychoses among refugees in Norway. *Acta Psychiatrica Scandinavicas* 42:315–328.

Harding, R. K., and Looney, J. G. 1977. Problems of Southeast Asian children in a refugee camp. *American Journal of Psychiatry* 134:407–411.

Kino, F. F. 1951. Aliens' paranoid reaction. *Journal of Mental Science* 97:589–594.

Krupinski, J.; Stoller, A.; and Wallace, L. 1973. Psychiatric disorders in East European refugees now in Australia. *Society of Science and Medicine* 7:31–49.

Kuepper, W. G.; Lackey, G. L.; and Swinerton, N. 1974. Ugandan Asians in Great Britain: forced migration and social absorption. Unpublished manuscript.

Looney, J. G.; Rahe, R. H.; Harding, R.; Ward, H. W.; and Liu, W. T. 1978. Consulting to children in crisis. Unpublished manuscript.

Malzberg, B., and Lee, E. S. 1956. *Migration and Mental Health*. New York: Social Science Research Council.

Meszaros, A. F. 1961. Types of displacement reactions among the post-revolution Hungarian immigrants. *Canada Psychiatric Association Journal* 6:9–19.

Mezey, A. C. 1960a. Personal background, immigration, and mental disorder in Hungarian refugees. *Journal of Mental Science* 106:618–627.

Mezey, A. C. 1960b. Psychiatric illness in Hungarian refugees. *Journal of Mental Science* 106:628–637.

Murphy, J. M. 1974. Psychological responses to stress. In G. P. Murphy, N. L. Murfin, and Jamieson, eds. *Beliefs, Attitudes, and Behavior of Lowland Vietnamese, Part B: The Effects of Herbicides in South Vietnam*. Washington, D.C.: National Academy of Sciences.

Ødegard, O. 1932. Emigration and insanity. *Acta Psychiatric Neurology* 4:Suppl. 4.

Pederson, S. 1949. Psychopathological reactions to extreme social displacements (refugee neuroses). *Psychoanalytic Revue* 36:344–354.

Pfister-Ammenda, M. 1955. The symptomatology, treatment, and prognosis in mentally ill refugees and repatriates in Switzerland. In *Flight and Resettlement*. New York: United Nations.

Rahe, R. H.; Looney, J. G.; Ward, H. W.; Tung, T. M.; and Liu, W. T. 1978. Psychiatric consultation in a refugee camp. *American Journal of Psychiatry* 135:185–190.

Rumbaut, R. D., and Rumbaut, R. G. 1976. The family in exile: Cuban expatriates in the United States. *American Journal of Psychiatry* 133:395–399.

Strotzka, H. 1961. Action for mental health in refugee camps. In E. Thornton, ed. *Planning and Action for Mental Health*. New York: World Federation for Mental Health.

United Nations. 1969. *Refugee Report*. New York: United Nations.

PART III

PSYCHOPATHOLOGY AND ADOLESCENCE

EDITORS' INTRODUCTION

The psychiatrist's chief concern is with the mental processes characteristic of psychopathology. Adolescent patients present us with many interesting challenges. First, they have to be understood, and they can be understood, in various ways. Developmental background and behavioral constellations provide us with valuable information that will enable the clinician to listen empathically and to respond to his patients with intuitive resonance. This response may be particularly alien to adolescent patients since they have usually felt completely misunderstood.

The chapters in this part focus on the impact both of the infantile traumatic environment and of the trauma associated with faulty adaptation due to ego defects as well as constitutional handicaps. This constitutes a wide spectrum, but it is interesting that all the authors choose to discuss patients that can best be understood in terms of structural defects. Psychopathology is viewed as the outcome of primitive fixations and correspondingly primitive defensive and adaptive mechanisms. This approach seems to be inevitable because of the types of patients that enter our consultation rooms. However, in spite of early developmental fixations, these chapters do not share the patient's despair. On the contrary, they indicate optimism and hope perhaps as a reflection of the resiliency of the adolescent's mind and the striving for the achievement of a world that will incorporate enthusiasm and idealism.

Peter L. Giovacchini emphasizes how parental psychopathology specifically influences the formation of defective early ego states which

211

determine the course of later development during adolescence. He discusses serious psychic defects found in the borderline patient: inability to maintain a mental representation without the reinforcement of an external stimulus, primal confusion between frustration and gratification, and lack of adaptive mechanisms to bind potentially painful tensions. Giovacchini traces these ego distortions to defective mothering, an absence of the soothing mother modality during feeding resulting in an ineffective nurturing modality which becomes manifest in the transference-countertransference relationship during therapy.

Pauline F. Kernberg examines normal developmental paradigms in order to construct a profile of borderline adolescent function. Symptoms of borderline function (persistence of primitive defense mechanisms, lack of a stable sense of self, and identity diffusion) are compared with normal developmental tasks and highlight deficits in the areas of object relations, reality testing, affects, impulse control, frustration, anxiety, and depression tolerance. Kernberg concludes that the lack of integration of self and object structures results in chronic ego disability.

Alexander Deutsch and Michael J. Miller present a case study of a young female who had joined a religious cult several years previously. Still a member of the group, she underwent extensive interviews and psychological testing. They found her repressed and inhibited, and characterized her defensive style as one of benevolent transformation. The authors believe that some of her psychological conflicts and character trends appeared to influence her conversion to a religious cult.

Ake Mattsson and David P. Agle review the dynamics of psychosomatic disorders and state that psychophysiologic disorders include those physical illnesses where emotional factors significantly contribute to the onset or course of the illness and where adolescence, as a developmental phase, serves as a vulnerability factor. The authors describe some hemic disorders to illustrate how the biopsychological stage of adolescence may influence the expression of physical disorders.

Raphael Greenberg examines the impact on the family of chronic disability. He believes that cooperation between the patient's family and the rehabilitation team is more important than in any other medical situation because of the extensive use of denial by these patients. Greenberg emphasizes the importance of mourning the loss of function and the role of the physician in facilitating this working through.

15 THE SINS OF THE PARENTS: THE BORDERLINE ADOLESCENT AND PRIMAL CONFUSION

PETER L. GIOVACCHINI

The psychoanalytic approach emphasizes developmental continuity. The early environment assumes central importance, although its specific attributes were not particularly stressed by Freud as he was studying the psychoneuroses. At first, he differentiated the different effects of childhood sexual trauma on the basis of whether they were passively or actively experienced (Freud 1896). When he abandoned the traumatic theory of the etiology of neuroses (Freud 1905), he retained the role of sexuality, but he needed to concentrate on intrapsychic processes apart from their connections with factors in the external world.

Freud has been criticized by the Neo-Freudians for ignoring interpersonal relationships. Here, I wish to introduce an interpersonal approach in that I want to include the influence of the external world on the developing psyche or its influence on the occurrence of psychopathology. However, I propose to maintain Freud's intrapsychic orientation and to extend it to studying the intrapsychic effects of the external world, that is, the infantile environment with its significant external objects.

The title of this chapter now becomes relevant. I mean to emphasize how parental psychopathology will specifically influence the formation of early ego stages and later determine the course of developmental process and consolidation of the identity sense that occurs during adolescence. I do not mean, however, that anything sinful in a *moral* sense is involved.

In their enthusiasm for a strictly deterministic viewpoint, many young therapists tend to be somewhat critical of parents, even to the point of being judgmental, when dealing with children's psychopathology. Over the course of years, however, especially when they have children of their own, their attitude mellows. Rather than being critical, they develop a more understanding attitude. Once involved with the dynamics and structure of the parent-child interaction, value judgments recede into the background.

The reader will also note that I have paraphrased the expression, "the sins of the father." The mother's role is usually emphasized, but I do not want to be accused of discriminating. I prefer to think in terms of a function, the nurturing or parental function. What we are really interested in is a process.

What occurs during childhood is recapitulated in psychoanalytic treatment. Consequently, the transference relationship supplies us with an opportunity to reconstruct the events of early childhood. These are also reexperienced in a more complex fashion during adolescence. The analyst becomes the servant of a process, as Masud Khan (personal communication, 1973) once felicitously stated. Our unobtrusive presence will teach us a great deal about the subtle parental relationships that lead to the formation of psychic structure, defective or otherwise.

Definition of Borderline

The diagnosis "borderline state" is a statement about phenomenology. The term refers to a clinical condition that hovers between a psychosis and neurosis. Kernberg (1978) believes that such patients have a well-structured psychic organization that can, under stress, decompensate into a transient psychosis. They reconstitute relatively quickly and maintain some kind of adjustment with the external world. The latter may be quite effective. According to Kernberg, and Masterson (1978) agrees, these patients suffer developmentally from fixations at the separation-individuation stage described by Mahler (1972).

I too believe that the phenomenological implication of the diagnosis is important and agree that these patients can easily regress and recover from a psychotic state. Unlike some earlier writers, however, I do not see the borderline patient as being on a continuum between a neurosis and a psychosis. Rather, the borderline patient hovers on the edge of a psychosis, but he has not regressed from a neurotic state (Giovacchini 1979).

This brings us to another meaning of borderline that supplements phenomenology. I am referring to the significant ego defect that is characteristic of this entity. The borderline patient makes a borderline adjustment to the external world. He barely has the ego executive techniques that enable him to master the exigencies of the external world and to meet inner needs.

External reality may be inordinately complicated for borderlines. They feel lost and inadequate when facing situations that other persons find pedestrian. Thus, these patients are borderline in two senses, which I feel is a good reason for reserving the term for this group.

The patients described by Kernberg and Masterson have achieved stable defenses that permit them to relate to their environment with some security. Some of their patients, especially those that have been called narcissistic personality disorders (Kohut 1971) can be eminently successful. I prefer the label "character neurosis," since the clinician is clearly dealing with characterological defects that lead to conflicts with the outer world, but these conflicts have been handled by a defensive superstructure. These are primitive defenses, such as overcompensatory narcissism and splitting mechanisms, but they have sufficient organization to enable the patient to achieve psychic equilibrium.

By contrast, the patients I prefer to call borderline are usually overwhelmed by their pervasive sense of inadequacy and helplessness. These developmental fixations are extremely primitive, involving symbiotic and even presymbiotic stages. I propose to explore the parent-child interaction in order to illuminate the psychic processes that lead to the acquisition of psychic structures that determine the course of character development. The impact of the mother's character structure in particular, but also the father's view and adjustment to the external world, determine how various ego subsystems are constructed. The parents' psychopathology causes specific structural defects in the child that become manifest in the adolescent and adult as a borderline syndrome.

Clinical Perspective

The emergence of early ego states during the transference regression gives the analyst clues as to how the neonate and the infantile environment interacted. Patients will reveal the impact of the nurturing relationship upon their developing ego. In turn, their current characterological adaptations will also help us learn how they influence their children's psyche and either promote or disrupt the course of emotional development. The material to be presented will demonstrate the effects of symbiotic and presymbiotic fixations as well as later defensive adaptations or failures of adaptations as seen in the character neuroses and borderline states. Fortunately, I have material from the analyses of both parents and adolescents. Occasionally a patient will reveal that a son or daughter is having severe problems. I have often succeeded in referring the child to a colleague for analysis. Later we have been able to compare notes, and the relevance of the parent's needs to the child's ego defects becomes strikingly clear. These conclusions have implications about the course of emotional development, especially during the early phases of psychic structuralization.

I will begin with a vignette about a woman in her late forties, the mother of three children all of whom eventually became engaged in an analytic relationship. My patient fit the criteria of the borderline state that I have enumerated. She periodically regressed into a state of psychotic helplessness and she was inadequate to meet the exigencies of daily life. She had made a minimal adjustment to reality.

A colleague referred the patient to me. He frankly told me on the telephone that he could not stand her, and neither could her husband and children. The patient supposedly was a hopeless alcoholic who made everyone miserable. I recall my immediate response. I felt a profound sense of sorrow for this woman whom I had never seen. Nevertheless, I formed an image of a helpless, misunderstood person who was exploited by a sadistic husband and selfish children. I was partially right—that is, about the husband, but not about the children.

It was obvious during the first interview that the patient was very pleased to be there. She had an aristocratic but soft manner, revealed herself as an example of good breeding and gentility, and spoke with pride of her social-register background. She did so to such a degree that I might have formed the impression that there was something saccharin about what seemed to be retrospective reconstructions of the infallibility and largesse of her immediate and remote ancestors, a lineage she could easily trace back to the *Mayflower*. She spoke in reverent tones of her father, a ruthless tycoon. Perhaps I might have felt appropriately irritated inasmuch as she could have been lording it over me, a mere tradesman, a psychoanalyst, who was not included in the rosters of the privileged gentry. Thinking back on this initial session, I am surprised I had none of these feelings. Later I could only wonder why I did not, since they would have been an expected response to this woman's espousal of standards and values that did not belong to my world. To look at her attitudes as the products of defensive adaptations would mitigate any reactive resentment, but I was not trying to make formulations about her psychopathology. I was not trying to do anything. All I know is that the profound sorrow I felt with the referring colleague was still with me; in fact, it was intensified.

I know now that I was reaching out to her fundamental helplessness. Her clinging to her noble origins represented a weak and pathetic attempt to cling to some vestige of dignity and integrity. She basically loathed herself, but not with the misery and agitation of the typically depressed patient. Underneath her porcelain-like veneer of worldly sophistication, she felt totally helpless and vulnerable, unable to handle even the simplest tasks of everyday living. She jokingly rationalized her physical clumsiness and the fact that she had never worked a day in her life by reminding me that she was raised in a setting where servants took care of all her needs. She boasted that she had never worked, nor would she ever. However, it became apparent how frightened she was of a world that was moderately complex for her, one where she did not have the adaptive techniques (represented as work) to cope with internal needs and external problems. She bordered on panic and sought relief by drinking herself into a state of perpetual insensibility.

I became aware of her drinking when I had to change a morning appointment to late afternoon. Up until then I had almost forgotten that one of the reasons for consultation was a drinking problem. She was unsteady as she lay on the couch and her speech was slurred. She fairly reeked of alcohol. To my amazement, she began lecturing on temperance and telling me how unladylike it was to overdrink. Perhaps an occasional aperitif or a little vintage wine would be decorous, but no more. I was further astonished because I had the conviction that she really believed what she said.

She did not drink in the morning. Every day she would have lunch with one of several lady friends at a local restaurant. By 4:00 P.M., she would be moderately inebriated, and by late evening she had become dead drunk as she drank continuously. In spite of this obvious behavior, she insisted that she did not drink. I gradually realized that she could not distinguish between drinking and not drinking since, for all practical purposes, she was drinking all the time.

For many years, the patient needed to present herself to me as a paragon of purity and self-sufficient gentility. In the external world, I later discovered she continued in the same regressive alcoholic fashion. She was on a morning schedule and would not accept any afternoon appointments. Around eleven o'clock one evening her husband rang my front doorbell and presented his wife to me. She was obviously drunk and humiliated. She mumbled incoherently and cried loudly, plaintively calling my name. I did not let her or her husband in. I simply suggested that she be taken home and that I would see her the next morning.

After this episode, her demeanor changed remarkably. She was no longer a fashion plate. She was usually dishevelled and openly revealed how helpless, vulnerable, and miserably inadequate she felt. She continued regressing and drinking more, but instead of liquor having a calming effect, as it usually did, she became increasingly agitated. She was repeating a pattern that had brought her into treatment in the first place.

At the beginning of treatment, she felt similarly inadequate, but it was directed toward the overwhelming problems her children were causing her. They were acting out in a variety of ways, some of which I will describe later, and the patient felt confused, not knowing how to deal with them. Her agitation mounted, but she still was able to exert a modicum of control. Now her loss of psychic equilibrium was considerably more intense. In both instances, her usual defenses failed and her underlying vulnerability surfaced. When she saw the referring psychiatrist, she was facing the quandary of not having sufficient adaptive techniques to master her children's problems. In our recent sessions, she indicated that her husband, because of his sadistic needs, had succeeded in toppling her defense of social superiority.

The patient and I were able to survive the regression. During this stormy period, she exposed various features of the primitive aspects of her psyche. These qualities, I believe, are responsible for the transmission of the borderline factor which starting with the defect in the ego executive system is also manifested by other distortions of psychic structure.

During this regressive episode, the patient exposed how inadequate and inept she was in dealing with the simplest facets of reality. She was helpless and almost totally paralyzed, indicating the lack of executive ego techniques. This lack was especially noticeable when she had to care for her children during their infancy. She was required to mother them, but she could not handle such a complex task. She could not autonomously gratify her own needs. How could she possibly minister to her children? I surmise that they would not have survived if she did not have constant help.

In spite of the omnipresent nursemaid, the children also had poorly developed executive systems. All three have problems in adapting to the external world, and this became especially evident during adolescence when they had a miserable time getting through high school. One of them had to be tutored and attend special classes, but none managed to complete the first year of college. To this day, neither of her sons has ever been able to hold a job. For all practical purposes, they and her daughter have never worked—although they do not brag about it as their mother does when she states that she will not work—and are alcoholic. Furthermore, my patient is inconsistent in that she is not proud of her children's inability to work, whereas she takes pride in her own refusal to do so. Quite clearly, she is as incapacitated as her children, a defect that they have acquired from her. The children could not introject the mother's skills for mastering external problems, because she had none.

A person can be defined by what he does. To submit to hyperbole, if a person does nothing, he is nothing. My patient's ego defects caused her to have a vague, amorphous identity sense, an attribute which is commonly found in borderline patients. Her children also had no concept of who and what they were. An unformed identity sense is characteristic of adolescence, but in them it had achieved psychopathological proportions.

The primitive organization of the patient's self-representation, as might be expected, was part of an ego state in which object representations are also amorphously constructed and the boundaries between the psyche and the outer world are correspondingly blurred. In turn, the ambiguity and lack of distinction of the inner world and external reality were accompanied by an inability to identify and discriminate inner needs. I was surprised to learn that the patient had difficulty in recognizing various biological tension states. For instance, she literally did not know whether the visceral sensations she experienced meant that she had to urinate, defecate, or that she was hungry. She could only decide by physically locating her feelings. I have noted this lack of drive development and discrimination to be fairly typical of the borderline syndrome. It was startling that all of her children were similarly handicapped.

This lack of discrimination also extended to sensory impressions from the external world. She had absolutely no taste for food or drink. Everything tasted alike. Her insistence that she did not drink was, in part, the consequence of her indifferent sensations. Whatever she drank tasted like water, so outside of its soothing effects, alcohol really had no meaning for her. I wondered how she was able to nurture her children, since she could not identify her needs and had such little capacity to view external objects as separate from herself. This blurring of boundaries, in addition to her lack of adaptive techniques, would make the task of mothering inordinately difficult.

Perhaps her children survived because of the nursemaid, who, incidentally, still works for the patient. Still, in her own clumsy way, she attempted to care for them. I asked her to tell me how she fed the children. I knew I was abandoning for the moment the analytic viewpoint that does not interrupt the spontaneous flow of material, but I was immensely curious. She did not mind my intrusion and went on uninhibitedly and naively to describe what she did both by words and gestures. I was horrified by what I heard, although I do not believe she knew it. She was too absorbed in reliving these experiences of many years ago. Apparently she picked up her babies by the waist and then swung them in a wide arc. This was her idea of rocking. Then she placed (in her imitation of the motion, it seemed to be a shove) the bottle into the infant's mouth. At the same time she hummed, but to me it sounded as if she were keening. She also stroked the child. Her fingers, however, made pinching motions.

My patient was in treatment seven years, and I still see her occasionally on an irregular basis. Inasmuch as I wish to concentrate upon the effects of the mothering experience on the formation of early psychic states, I will emphasize her relationship to her children, about whom I have considerable data, rather than her early childhood as it was reconstructed during the transference regression. Briefly, concerning the latter, there was a remarkable but not unanticipated similarity between the way she was treated as a child and the way she treated her children. The most outstanding characteristic of her early relationships was how frustration and gratification become confused.

As mentioned, all of the children are alcoholic. Excessive drinking upset their lives to the point that they were expelled from school and are unable to stay employed or to sustain stable object relationships. All three are living from the income of a trust fund, but in spite of its sizable amount, they are constantly in debt and are unable to manage their lives. I will report the clinical material relating to the treatment of the youngest child. She was fourteen when I referred her to a colleague. She often missed or cancelled sessions, evidently being too frightened to become involved in a psychotherapeutic relationship. Nevertheless, a transference was established and the therapist was able to gain considerable insight about her intrapsychic processes. She remained with him for two years. At the age of nineteen, I saw her six or seven times for consultation.

When she started treatment, the patient had just managed to get her elementary school diploma. She had already been drinking heavily. She often attended classes drunk. Like her mother, she denied drinking when she was obviously intoxicated.

The principal believed that her drinking was a reaction to her scholastic inadequacy. She seemed unable either to learn or to retain what was being taught, although she had average scores on psychometric examinations. In spite of these scores, some of her teachers believed that she had organic brain damage. The psychologist disagreed and strongly recommended therapy. Her mother turned to me helplessly pleading to tell her what to do.

Reluctantly, the daughter agreed to see a psychiatrist. As seemed to be typical of her reactions, she did not actively protest becoming involved in psychotherapy, but she passively resisted by being late or not coming to her appointments. She never offered any excuses for her behavior.

The therapist learned that his patient had lived a life of perpetual confusion. She perceived the world as harsh and ungiving and did not believe she had any place in it. She described herself as an "alien from another planet." What caused others joy made her feel sad and tense. In fact, she always felt some degree of inner agitation. She found life joyless and was not able to find pleasure in anything. However, she was not depressed; she just could not understand how her friends learned how to enjoy themselves. If anything, she was bitter about her lack of capacity to engage herself in something that would give her satisfaction. She also considered herself totally unable to give or to be sensitive to someone else's needs. Drinking somehow helped in that when she drank, she felt "numb," although as mentioned, she never admitted drinking directly.

Her fantasy life was meager, but she had a fantasy or daydream that was nearly always with her. She saw herself "sitting in a locked car illegally parked on the ice of a frozen lake." Since she should not be there, policemen are hovering around the automobile, but it is locked so they cannot get in. She sits there, more or less complacently, smoking cigarettes. The daydream characterized her treatment. She sat in the therapist's office for two years smoking cigarettes and remaining impervious to all of his interventions and interpretations.

Interestingly enough, the therapist confessed to me that he was unable to remain nonintrusive. She stirred something within him that made it necessary to "do something." He felt frustrated in that he did not know what that something should be. He understood that most likely he was reacting to the patient's projection of her helplessness into him. What disturbed him was that in spite of his insight he continued feeling both helpless and obliged to help her. He was dismayed because he did not have the adaptive techniques to deal with her therapeutically and found that his professional identity was threatened.

I have chosen to discuss this particular adolescent, but I could just as easily have written about the clinical material of her siblings. In essence, their histories and courses of treatment are practically identical. Briefly, they sustain themselves by drinking, they cannot support themselves or remain engaged in meaningful employment, and they find the world confusing. They cannot adapt to the exigencies of everyday life and have never formed any lasting commitments. They have all married, but the three of them have also been divorced or separated. None has been hospitalized, and there have been no delusional or overt psychotic indications. They started therapy as adolescents, but because of their failure to become involved, treatment has been discontinued. Usually the patient has left, but much to the relief of the therapist. I have seen all three on occasion, the sons once or twice, the youngest daughter six or seven times. Therefore, I will rely upon the data derived from what I learned from her first therapist (she saw four or five more) and from her consultations with me to draw inferences about her structural fixations and the effects of the early maternal relationship.

I can make such inferences from clinical material which, in a sense, runs parallel to what I observed in the transference regression of the mother. To begin, the daughter's learning difficulties were related to her inability to maintain a mental representation without the reinforcement of an external stimulus. This was a serious deficit that made it difficult for her to internalize what was being taught. Concerning her mother, I can recall many sessions when she would feel her image of me receded further and further into the background until it completely disappeared. Then she might become panicky. I, in turn, had the vision of the couch and chair moving away from each other, making me want to reach out my arm and pull the couch back where it belonged. When I saw the daughter, she presented me with a considerable amount of evidence that she still had problems in holding a mental representation but not to the same extent as previously.

This type of ego defect must be related to early processes of perceptual organization that may date back to presymbiotic phases. I will describe a presymbiotic disturbance associated with the inability to sustain a mental representation, something which probably develops later as the infant emerges from symbiotic fusion (Giovacchini 1978b). I am referring to the confusion between frustration and gratification which was so clear in the mother and which the daughter also prominently demonstrated. This early, perhaps primal, confusion would determine the developmental course of the registration and organization of perceptions, the formation of memory traces and introjects, and the assimilation of adaptive techniques. Inasmuch as the identity is, in part, defined by this structural sequence, such an initial developmental disturbance will also result in a confused identity.

The daughter jokingly complained to me that she must be a mental defective because she was never able to remember anything. She especially could not recall names. On the whole, however, her memory seemed to be adequate. She had special difficulties in forming mental images of significant persons who had some responsibility in looking after her. She meant her parents and the nursemaid. This heightened her insecurity and sense of helpless inadequacy because she had to turn perpetually to others to meet basic needs. She could not rely on the internalized representation of a nurturing source, and as a consequence, she had not developed the ego executive techniques to care for herself in a fashion approaching autonomy. She experienced a constant tension that bordered on panic, and alcohol was the only relief she could recognize.

I purposely use the word "recognize" because, as I already mentioned, she did not know what gratification or release of tension meant. I am again pointing out her primal confusion. Whereas the ordinary adoles-

223

cent has the task of consolidating characterological adaptations in order to be able to attain goals that will lead to satisfaction, she had neither the techniques for such goals nor the perceptual discrimination to recognize satisfaction. The latter would, of course, make the former impossible. I remembered the mother's description of her techniques of nurturing her children, and now the daughter was telling me that she could not be soothed. For example, soft music and lights, a quiet room, would make her feel unbearably agitated, whereas a frenetic tempo, a noisy discotheque, a jarring sound, all created a sensation, if not exactly of well-being, at least of a relative equilibrium. Still, she never really felt calm or tranquil. At the most, she was toxic, as in a drunken stupor, and the peace of mental harmony was as alien to her as were most facets of the external world.

Primal confusion is also a determinant in the construction of the recurrent fantasy of the locked automobile parked on the icy lake. Whereas most people prefer warm open spaces, she chose a cold closed space. She often stated that she felt frozen inside, but paradoxically, the frozen state was the only one in which she found a degree of comfort. She believed that if she exposed herself to warm air, she would disintegrate.

Since then, I have encountered some similar material in a young adult patient who could regress to a state of catatonic immobility. Her adolescence had been particularly stormy and similar to the patients described. She had enormous problems because of an amorphous identity dominated by helplessness and self-hatred. She had the following quasi-delusional episode when seeing me. I call it "quasi-delusional" because, even though she lived the experience with great intensity and realism, she did not seem to be consumed by it. She still had considerable judgment and reality testing. She told me about her feelings as if they were a fantasy, and yet they went beyond fantasy but not entirely to the point of a fixed delusion. She suddenly told me she was pregnant. The next day she spent the whole session having labor pains, and the following session she announced that she had delivered a baby. This baby, a boy, had no facial features so she had to punch a hole in him with a can opener in order to be able to feed him. He had leprosy, and the only way he could survive was by being kept in the refrigerator. If he were put on the windowsill in the sunlight, parts of him would break off. Besides having an amorphous face, his arms were the stretching, curled-up type of telephone cord. The patient kept her son for two weeks and then she caused him to disintegrate by putting him out in the sun.

As the patient's associations confirmed, the baby represented the deteriorating, diseased aspect of her self-representation. I direct attention to the two outstanding features of this fantasy or delusional child that are similar to the ego defects being discussed. First, the child had no mouth. He was born without the equipment by which he could be fed. Initially there was no way by which he could obtain gratification of inner needs. In order to feed him, mother had to punch a hole in his amorphous face, a reflection of the amorphous nature of her self-representation. He had no arms. The telephone cords could not wrap themselves around the mother, therefore he could not cling or hug. In addition to being unable to be nourished, this baby could not reach out to be loved and soothed. Lacking these elements, it would be impossible to reduce tension, so any ministration would be experienced as disruptive. Next, this grotesque creature could not survive in warmth, only in a cold environment. The fantasy of my patient's daughter involved an automobile parked on ice. This was her refrigerator. Again, what is ordinarily satisfying and soothing cannot be tolerated and the opposite is also true, that is, what would ordinarily be disruptive is vital for survival.

On the surface, this reversal and confusion might seem to be similar to, although more primitive than, Bateson's (1960) concept of the double bind. This similarity is only superficial. Bateson was describing communication patterns where the mother would send out a certain message at one level and convey the opposite meaning at another level, often a somatic level, as by gesture or facial expression. The patterns I have described for borderline and other primitively fixated patients relate to an inability to develop the capacity to organize perceptions even to the extent that they can be subjected to double-bind messages. Because of faulty structure, interactions with the outer world lead to paradoxical effects. The interactions themselves are not internally inconsistent. The mother's attempts at soothing, which are, in fact, disruptive, cannot be equated with contradictory messages. The mother was attempting to soothe. For a variety of reasons, she did not know how.

The leprous baby lacked the fundamental equipment that would enable him to be gratified. Inasmuch as this child represented the diseased parts of the mother, she believed that she also lacked such equipment. From this it follows that she would not be able to soothe her child's inner disruption. A caress could be murderous choking.

Those primitive vital relationships can be viewed in terms of two components, not to be confused with the two messages of the double bind. The interaction has both background and foreground elements. The fantasy baby emphasized defects in both areas in that he lacked all receptive access. Ordinarily a mother feeds and soothes the child at the same time. She holds her infant affectionately as she is supplying nurture. The background is soothing and the foreground reestablishes homeostasis by replenishing. Disturbances of these early modalities can have devastating effects.

The patients I have described here did not have a soothing background to achieve a tranquil feeding experience. Recall the mother's description of how she held and fed her children. Primal confusion can best be understood in terms of the lack of synthesis between background and foreground. My patient, the alcoholic mother, and her daughter were not achieving inner harmony because of the inability to effect such an integration during early childhood. Thus, they had to use various defensive devices to control their inner disruption, such as withdrawal and alcohol. From a structural viewpoint, they had been unable to internalize an adaptive mechanism designed to bind potentially painful tension. They have not been able to form a soothing introject, although I am using the word introject in a very loose sense. These processes occur before the psyche has the structural capacity to form and hold introjects, but it is still able to make endopsychic registrations that are important determinants for the formation of later ego structures.

Theoretical Perspective

I have discussed the course of emotional development elsewhere, outlining the hierarchical elaboration from an internalized modality to an introject, a mental representation, a memory trace, and finally the assimilation of an adaptive technique as it becomes integrated into the self-representation (Giovacchini 1978a). Here, I simply wish to emphasize one factor that will have deleterious effects upon this sequence. The absence of the soothing modality has profound effects upon the feeding experience, which will then lead to specific vicissitudes that determine how the psyche will be able to respond to inner needs.

This relationship of maternal jarring is disturbing from the very beginning. As soon as the child develops beyond a physiological reflexive state, such early object relationships determine how mentational elements are structured. The initial psychological level is presymbiotic, and we can only think in terms of modalities and primitive endopsychic registrations during these first few months of life. During the next stage, the symbiotic stage, there is more organization of intrapsychic factors even though the boundaries between inside and outside have not yet been established. The fact that there are no boundaries makes it possible for such boundaries to be constructed. Disturbances in the acquisition of the soothing modality interferes with the achievement of the blurring between inside and outside that is characteristic of symbiosis.

Once again Winnicott's (1953) work becomes significant. I am referring to his concept of the transitional phenomenon. I have described in detail how the transitional phenomenon and later the formation of the transitional object can be conceptualized in terms of modalities (Giovacchini 1978b). Briefly, Winnicott described an infantile condition in which the child believes he is the source of his own nurture. This occurs because the mother is so empathically in tune with her child's needs that her instantaneous response creates the illusion that gratification is coming from within. In this optimal state of fusion there is no distinction between the inner and outer world. Boundaries are blurred, a precondition for the emergence of symbiosis and the formation of boundaries.

Winnicott is, of course, indulging in metaphor. The neonate is incapable of believing anything, and he knows nothing about sources or the inner and outer world. However, his psyche undergoes structural changes and further organization because of a satisfactory maternal relationship characterized by a soothing background and a nurturing modality.

The primal confusion caused by disruptive mothering interferes with the structuring of an effective nurturing modality. This would then determine how well introjects are formed and mental representations are retained (Giovacchini 1978a). All the patients discussed here could not maintain a mental representation without reinforcement from the external world. They had difficulties in organizing and holding percepts, the latter often being experienced as faulty memory.

Patients suffering from ego defects have been subjected to many varieties of pathological nurturing. The type described here is different and distinct, a characteristic of the borderline state as it has been defined. It can be contrasted to other relationships, especially those that primarily involve abandonment. As is to be expected, there is considerable overlapping between various maternal constellations, as there is with clinical syndromes. A frequently encountered mothering pattern concerns the projections of hated parts of the mother into the infant. The child is used as a narcissistic appendage; he is made into an extension of her psyche.

The relationship between the mother and daughter could be mistaken for narcissistic projection. Still, projection is not involved to any significant extent. Neither the mother nor the infant had the structural integrity to support even such a primitive mechanism as projection. The mother is behaving ineptly. Within herself she lacks a soothing mechanism as part of her background. Therefore, she is unable to function as a calming influence for her child. This is quite different from projection, which is tendentious. The infant does not introject the mother's inadequate self-representation. He fails to register a soothing experience, and instead associates the lack of soothing, the disruption, with the foreground of nurture. Inasmuch as these events occur during the presymbiotic stages, introjection and projection are not yet possible, since these mechanisms require some distinction beyond the dissolution of the symbiotic phase.

Borderline patients, however, may use projective mechanisms even to the extent of some paranoid ideation. These are not predominant elements of the clinical picture, but they are not incompatible with the developmental arrests that have been postulated. To repeat, presymbiotic structural defects will determine the course of later development. When the child becomes capable of forming introjects, the inadequate, hateful parts of the nurturing environment become part of the emerging self-representation. The mother also obtains relief from her self-hatred by projecting, but there are both qualitative and quantitative differences between these, what might be called secondary, projections and those relationships in which projection is the primary psychic mechanism. These latter interactions involved fixations on symbiotic fusion and early postsymbiotic formations of part-object relations.

Therapeutic Perspective

Although projection is minimal in these borderline patients, the clinician can still think in terms of transference and countertransference. Again this is a matter of definition. If only the projection of feelings or parts of the self determine whether a phenomenon can be classified as transference, then the patients I am describing have only minimal transference reactions. Nevertheless, they recapitulate the infantile environment during treatment and cause the analyst to have feelings toward them similar to those felt by significant figures of the past.

Borderline patients, because of their lack of adjustive techniques, often form intense dependent relationships. They tend to idealize their therapists. Their helplessness and clinging can cause many therapists to feel frustrated. Still, in spite of the oppressive and frenetic atmosphere the patient may create, he is trying to achieve some kind of stability and equilibrium. However, the therapeutic relationship can become so intense that therapeutic goals are lost sight of and the patient and analyst may resort to blaming each other. The patient is bitterly disappointed because the analyst does not fulfill magical rescuing expectations and the therapist reproaches the patient for his dependency by accusing him of resisting and not otherwise working hard enough in treatment. Adolescents and their therapists are especially prone to become involved in a struggle against each other rather than in an experience of mutual interest and sometimes sharing intrapsychic events.

The adolescent daughter of my patient showed me an interesting side of herself; either she had hidden it or it had remained submerged with my colleague, her first therapist. Before I saw her I expected a resentful young lady who would triumphantly withdraw from me. On the contrary, she seemed eager to be there and revealed that she needed me to comfort her. I knew I was having a soothing effect upon her and I was glad to be fulfilling that function.

I only consented to see her because her mother literally pleaded with me to do so. Her daughter lived in another city and would not see anyone else but me. Since she was not to be my primary patient and I thought that, at the most, I would be seeing her only two or three times, I set up an appointment. I felt my most relaxed, as I often do when I am seeing someone toward whom I will not have the responsibility of being their therapist on a long-term basis. I felt tranquil as she sat in front of me and quite evidently she did too. The second time I saw her some weeks later, she told me how well she had slept since her first session. In fact, she had been dozing in my waiting room the ten minutes she arrived before her appointment time. I note this reaction because it emphasizes how she was able to achieve a soothing background with me whereas with my colleague the atmosphere was turbulent and confused. I believe that she could have returned to him and worked out her inner chaos, which can be conceptualized as primal confusion, now that she had been able to have a soothing experience.

I believe that the first therapist was not able to work with her because of a particular type of countertransference. This conjecture is based upon my experience with the mother, toward whom I felt the disruptive impact of disorganizing countertransference reactions. Various episodes of her treatment were characterized by an almost indefinable urgency which enveloped us. She would describe certain tasks that she had laboriously and with an incredible expenditure of energy tried to perform and failed to do so with a predictable and inevitable frequency. She lamented her failures with such agony and anguish that I felt literally jarred. I reflexively gritted my teeth and had an immense urge to shake some competence into her. I was surprised how my response was one of being forcefully shaken up. Certainly, my reactions had no soothing potential whatsoever.

After a particularly intense episode, my patient reported that she became especially clumsy. She was always clumsy, but now she frequently stumbled. She never fell or hurt herself, but she was afraid she would because she would come very close to falling down. Clearly, my feeling jarred by her anguish did nothing to help her achieve equilibrium.

To use Winnicott's (1960) expression, I failed to provide a holding environment. I make this assumption because I could feel myself becoming a replica of her jarring infantile environment, not as a projection, but as an externalization of a turbulent inner space. After many upsetting sessions, she was able to derive some soothing and later even considerable soothing from our relationship. With her adolescent daughter, on the other hand, I apparently was able to provide a holding environment, but I do not know whether this would have been possible if her first therapist had not absorbed her disruption.

I have often discussed the daughter with her first therapist and learned from him that her subsequent therapists, especially younger ones, found it difficult to contain their excitement. They found the patient sexually disturbing. I believe that the jarring elements of the infantile environment would become erotized, the therapists then felt very uncomfortable with her, and finally therapy would be terminated much to everyone's relief.

Thus, the countertransference may become the chief obstacle to treatment. During these early stages of psychic development, the background assumes a greater importance than during more structured ego states. The analyst finds himself immersed and surrounded by the disruptive elements of the infantile ambience. Consequently, he is unable to create a holding environment, a secure, calm setting in which the therapist can effectively function analytically. Analytic activity represents the foregound which the patient may accept as satisfying nurture. Failure in achieving a harmonious blend between background and foreground causes a fixation on the regressed ego state which recapitulates primal confusion. As happened with the adolescent patient, the treatment may be prematurely terminated or there may be a therapeutic impasse in which the patient fails to progress.

To repeat, the regressed ego state represents a presymbiotic developmental phase. In the next phase, the symbiotic phase, the mother, the nurturing source, and the infant become fused. Distinctions between background and foreground are blurred. If the two are discordant, the fusion is imperfectly formed. This will seriously affect the transitional phenomenon, the acquisition of the nurturing modality, and the consolidation of ego boundaries. Treatment as it reenacts defective early development reveals the vulnerability of the symbiotic phase. If the therapist's countertransference recapitulates the discordance between background and foreground, then the transference will not achieve the symbiotic unity that is a necessary intermediate pathway to the establishment of object relationships and autonomy.

Conclusions

Early object relationships—that is, the qualities of presymbiotic nurturing—are responsible for certain character disturbances that define the borderline syndrome. The early maternal relationship can be divided into two components, background and foreground. When these elements clash, the child experiences a particular disruption that can be conceptualized as primal confusion.

The clinical examples cited here indicate the difficulties in treating the borderline adult and adolescent. Therapeutic impasses can be explained on the basis of specific countertransference reactions which repeat the jarring qualities and the discordance between foreground and background elements of maternal nurturing. The therapist must create a holding environment, one in which the outer world can be beneficially internalized so as to promote structure and development. These clinical experiences indicate that there is a resiliency and plasticity to the psyche, both the patient's and therapist's, that enable us to approach human misery and elemental confusion with some hope that the effects of early traumas can be overcome in the moving, sometimes painful, therapeutic interaction.

REFERENCES

Bateson, G. 1960. Minimal requirements for a theory of schizophrenia. *Archives of General Psychiatry* 2:447–491.

Freud, S. 1896. Further remarks on the neuro-psychoses of defence. *Standard Edition* 3:157–187. London: Hogarth, 1962.

Freud, S. 1905. My views on the part played by sexuality in the etiology of the neuroses. *Standard Edition* 7:269–281. London: Hogarth, 1953.

Giovacchini, P. 1978a. The analytic introject and psychic development. *International Journal of Psychoanalytic Psychotherapy* 7:62–87.

Giovacchini, P. 1978b. The impact of delusion and the delusion of impact: ego development and the transitional phenomenon. In S. Gralnick and L. Barkin, eds. *Between Reality and Fantasy*. New York: Aronson.

Giovacchini, P. 1979. *The Treatment of Primitive Mental States*. New York: Aronson.

Kernberg, O. F. 1978. The diagnosis of borderline conditions in adolescence. *Adolescent Psychiatry* 6:298–319.

Kohut, H. 1971. *The Analysis of the Self*. New York: International Universities Press.

Mahler, M. 1972. On the first three phases of separation individuation. *International Journal of Psycho-Analysis* 53:333–338.

Masterson, J. 1978. *New Perspectives on the Psychotherapy of the Borderline Adult*. New York: Brunner/Mazel.

Winnicott, D. W. 1953. Transitional objects and transitional phenomena. *International Journal of Psycho-Analysis* 32:89–97.

Winnicott, D. W. 1960. The theory of the parent-infant relationship. *International Journal of Psycho-Analysis* 4:585–596.

16 PSYCHOANALYTIC PROFILE OF THE BORDERLINE ADOLESCENT

PAULINA F. KERNBERG

The descriptive symptomatology of borderline personality organization in adolescence, as well as in other age groups, does not alone suffice for the understanding of this syndrome. Symptoms, in fact, may occur across diagnostic categories; thus, patient studies that take only this dimension into account often result in heterogeneous groupings. It is therefore necessary to develop multiple criteria within the psychoanalytic framework to conceptualize more thoroughly the borderline syndrome.

The authors who have contributed to the further elaboration of the borderline syndrome (Frijling-Schreuder 1969; Geleerd 1958; Grinker, Werble, and Drye 1968; Kernberg 1975; Knight 1953; Masterson 1967, 1972, 1975) in adults as well as in children and adolescents, have had a common matrix of experience: (*a*) psychoanalysis as a theoretical framework, (*b*) work with severely regressed young or adult patients, and (*c*) an intense interest in or research commitment to child development. Perhaps many of the barriers to understanding the developmental issues, the psychopathology, and, most important, the principles of psychotherapeutic technique in borderline cases originate in lack of experience in one of these areas.

The importance of the precise delineation of borderline adolescent functioning lies in the assumption that borderline adult patients represent chronologically older adolescents. The adult borderline does not differ substantially from the adolescent except in the accrual of secondary complications in the course of living (marriage, children, career vicissitudes) which do not essentially modify the borderline personality organization in these patients. For example, a forty-five-year-old patient acknowledged to me quite candidly that she just did not feel her age; she felt she was either a little girl or at most a budding adolescent. Her three marriages, four children, college education, and multiple travels throughout the world had not left much of an imprint on her. Due to the persistence of primitive defense mechanisms (such as splitting and its related defenses, early forms of projection, denial, primitive idealization, omnipotence, and devaluation), with their ongoing ego-weakening effects, the patient is unable to integrate his experience because of incomplete, distorted relations with external objects. The chronic instability of unintegrated superego components deprives the patient of guidelines for self and other evaluation and hence of a stable sense of identity. The borderline patient is thus not basically affected by positive life circumstances, for he cannot learn from experience. Time has stopped for him.

Normal Developmental Paradigm

In constructing a borderline profile, it is useful to examine normal developmental paradigms. Table 1 presents the achievements expected of the preschool child, the latency-age child, and the adolescent (modified from Senn and Solnit 1968). This outline will serve as a reference point in the discussion of borderline functioning that follows. By comparing the borderline adolescent's development with normal developmental tasks, we will gain a better understanding of the significance of the borderline patient's symptoms.

The Borderline Adolescent Profile

OBJECT CONSTANCY

The borderline adolescent has not acquired a sense of autonomy or secure independent functioning. In part this deficiency is due to the lack of object constancy, which a normal preschool child has already begun to establish. Object constancy implies the capacity to establish a whole object representation, integrating the aggressive and libidinal

TABLE 1

NORMAL DEVELOPMENTAL PARADIGMS

Developmental tasks for preschool children:
1. Increased dexterity in motoric functions.
2. Mastery of body functions, including sphincter control, eating, and sleeping.
3. Differentiation from mother; development of secure sense of autonomy (implying history of normal transitional object).
*4. Tolerance for separation from mother, despite ambivalence toward dependency or independence (on the way to the establishment of object constancy).
*5. Establishment of standards of bad and good with the beginning of reality testing.
6. Acquisition of social skills; signs of acculturation in handling of aggression, relation to peers, and activities.
*7. Ability to express feelings, such as shame, guilt, joy, love, and desire to please (implying the establishment of the superego).
*8. Learning of sexual distinctions; broadening of sexual curiosity as the Oedipus complex is repressed with the capacity for object constancy and superego formation.
9. Use of repression and related mechanisms (reaction formation, isolation, identification, and others).

Developmental tasks for latency-age children:
1. Progression in cognitive functions from intuitive thinking toward concrete operations.
2. Development of greater physical prowess.
*3. Acquisition of sense of identity of sex and role through play, fantasy, learning tasks and roles.
*4. Improved impulse control with predictable ego states.
5. Enhanced self-confidence and pride.
*6. Increased independence from parents, with a relative increase in importance of peers.
*7. Enjoyment of peer interaction and competitiveness in well-organized games.
*8. Awareness of world at large and issues of birth and death; tolerance for depression.
*9. Sense of belonging to an extended collective community.
*10. Well-established peer relationships.
*11. Oedipus complex expressed in derivative forms and resolved primarily through sublimatory channels.

Developmental tasks for adolescents:
1. Mastery of physical power and coordination in coming to terms with bodily changes and anchoring the various aspects of the sense of identity.
*2. Acquisition of sense of identity in the process of exploration of and experimentation with self and the world.
*3. Struggles for emancipation and independence from the family; ability to contain anxiety.
*4. Development of abstract thinking and incorporation of learning into a gestalt of living; development of sublimatory channels.
5. Acquisition of moral and ethical standards, as well as critical functions toward self and others.
6. Establishment of sex role, with capacity for intimacy and heterosexual adjustment.

236

  *7. Realistic perception of the family. Enhanced tolerance for siblings; conflicts with parental authority mainly concerned with increasing struggle for independence around everyday practical matters.

  *8. Masturbatory fantasies; fantasies connected to sexual relations with inaccessible women, including voyeuristic, exhibitionistic, and sadomasochistic components in the service of sexual relations with the opposite sex.

  9. Absence of psychotic states in the average, expectable environment.

  10. Lastly although not a developmental task but developmentally expected is the presence of transient symptoms and traits (depression, identity crisis, neurotic conflicts with authority, even activation of primitive defense mechanisms in the normal identity crisis, including occasional antisocial behavior and infantile narcissistic object relations).

SOURCE.—Modified from Senn (1968).
*These tasks are of particular relevance in a comparison with borderline functioning.

affective ties to the object. With the attainment of object constancy the representation of the object is in congruence with its characteristics in the external world. The object representation persists in the actual absence of the object and thus can be used for identification as well as to monitor, support, and approve the individual's functioning in the absence of the object.

Object constancy also implies a capacity for differentiation and integration into currently real, remembered, potential, and imaginary positive and negative object and self-images. Object constancy acquisition is concomitant with the integration of the self-representation into the self-concept: the child progresses from object representations to object constancy, from self-representations to self-constancy. In borderline patients this complex patterning has not been completed. The external object is needed. Without its presence, the connection to a world now recognized as separate from self is lost, resulting in feelings of alienation or self-dissolution (this can be seen, for example, in the borderline's panic states and marked regressions during periods of separation from the parents or therapist).

REALITY TESTING

In terms of reality testing, the borderline adolescent is at a stage similar to that of the preschool child. He has contact with reality but, as with the preschool child, the reality span is brief and the ability to test reality has to be borrowed from the parent or therapist (Geleerd 1958).

237

The ability to test reality in the here and now has been assessed by Kernberg (1977). The patient is asked to evaluate his own behavior and the behavior of the interviewer, or to empathize with the different perception that the interviewer may have about the patient's productions. If the patient is able to empathize with the interviewer's perspective and with some social norms, which he may not comply with but that he at least can recognize, he shows an important capacity which differentiates borderline conditions (where this capacity exists) from schizophrenia (where it is not present). This capacity to test reality through empathizing with another person can thus be used for diagnostic purposes.

A young adolescent described by Geleerd (1958), for instance, used her mother to integrate her reality testing. During a visit, the mother expressed grief over her daughter's ideas of reference; the girl corrected these ideas when she noticed her mother's sadness in relation to her. Thus, the borderline adolescent, like the preschool child, borrows from the examiner's or the parent's ego the necessary support to test reality or, in other words, to test the congruence between object representations and external objects.

AFFECTS

In terms of affects, the borderline adolescent is less advanced than the preschool child, conveying a chronic lack of gratification or anticipation of gratification. His affects are mostly fear, distrust, and rage, and usually there is a lack of modulation of affects. Anger, demandingness (as an expression of coercion), exploitative behavior, and lack of social tact are described by authors such as Geleerd (1958) and Grinker et al. (1968).

The quality of affective expression is reminiscent of the intense anxiety and disruptive rage characteristic of the first and second year of life. Similarly, the all-or-nothing quality of affective discharges is reminiscent of the wide mood swings characteristic of the separation-individuation process (eight to thirty-six months). The elation present in the practicing subphases and depressive moods alternates with a sense of omnipotence in the rapprochement-phase crisis. The angry, coercive attitude and hypomanic elation can thus be considered as the affective counterpart to the main fixation point of this psychopathology, namely, the separation-individuation subphase, especially the rapprochement crisis.

Affects follow the structural integration of self- and object images. The less integrated these images are—the more splitting is in operation—the more likely it is that extreme all-bad and all-good object images will be present. Because in borderline patients the complex patterning of integration of self- and object images, with the widening variety of self-other relationships, is missing, the affective derivatives linking self- and object representations also lack modulation.

EGO FUNCTIONING

The borderline adolescent's lack of impulse control and the unpredictability of his ego states contrast with the expected achievement of the latency years. The changing levels of ego organization indicate an underlying failure to establish a solid hierarchy of ego states and function. The synthetic function of the ego is inoperative. In a way, splitting has a reciprocal relation to the synthetic function of the ego, which involves the synthesis of self- and object images as well as the integration and depersonification of the superego.

Nonspecific ego deficits are present in functions negatively affecting the degree of impulse control, that is, low frustration tolerance, low anxiety tolerance, and low depression tolerance. The deficits in these functions are common to borderline conditions. What is important, however, is that the lack of impulse control may not necessarily represent an ego defect, in the sense of lack of capacity to control, but may be used defensively to bring about different ego states for the purpose of controlling anxiety.

The lack of anxiety tolerance indicates the inadequate development of anxiety used as a signal—an indirect indication of deficits in the structuralization of the psychic apparatus. In regard to his low frustration tolerance, the patient may defensively withdraw into fantasy life, have severe temper outbursts, or lose contact with reality to ward off what he experiences as an attack.

Tolerance for depression is an important indicator of ego strength and predictability of ego states. Depression may reflect the capacity for guilt, for concern for the loss of an object; it thus implies an ability to grieve, to mourn, and to accept the reality of human limitations. This capacity to tolerate depression is missing in the borderline adolescent, who instead may experience emptiness, pseudoeuphoria, or apathy.

SUPEREGO FUNCTIONING

The lack of integration of the superego because of the splitting and deficient synthetic function of the ego allows for negative representations remaining at the level of introjects, which are easily projected onto external objects. This explains both the paranoid potential of these patients and their relative lack of guilt and concern for others (Kernberg 1975).

EXPERIENCE OF SELF

In contrast to the normal adolescent identity crisis, the borderline adolescent suffers from identity diffusion, defined as the lack of integration of the concept of self, and the concept of significant others. Here I would like to elaborate on the pathology of the self-experience in connection with the separation-individuation process. The adolescent may have any or all of the following experiences of self (in my formulations I have attempted to verbalize the predominant fantasy):

1. "I am hooked to my mother and therefore she cannot survive without me or I cannot survive without her." This fantasy corresponds to Mahler's stage of differentiation. It contrasts to the true symbiotic relation characteristic of psychosis where there is fusion of self- and object representation with no boundaries between them—where, to put it into words, "I and mother are one."

2. "I carry mother all around and I don't need her." This formulation relates to the experience of self in the early practicing subphase.

3. "Mother is inside and part of me for a while. If she is not around I may cease to exist—lose her inside of me—and therefore I need her around to refuel." This verbalization corresponds to the experience of self in the practicing phase proper.

4. "Mother is not part of me or I am not part of mother, but instead she is under my control or I am under her control." This is the experience of self in the rapprochement phase.

In my opinion, what appears descriptively as fear of merging may have a variety of structural implications different from those of the truly symbiotic psychosis, where self and object dissolve into each other and feel like one. In borderline cases fears and wishes of merging preserve the distinction between self- and object images, primitive as these may be. I would like to propose that borderline conditions may stem not only from the rapprochement crisis, but also from fixations or regressions to the earlier differentiation or practicing phases of the separation-individuation process.

Structurally, self- and object images become differentiated, but they have a varying relationship to each other according to the substage of the separation-individuation process in question. In the differentiation subphase, for example, self- and object images may still have a partial common core (fig. 1). In the next stage, the early practicing subphase, we have a self-image surrounded by the object image (fig. 2). The practicing phase proper can be represented as a self-image having introjected the object image (fig. 3). Due to the increased capacity to recognize the reality of separateness, there is a need for the external object to reinforce or refuel the introjected object image (fig. 4).

Lastly, the wish and fear of merging in the rapprochement subphase indicate the need to control or coerce the external object or to be controlled and coerced by it (fig. 5). There is an increased need for the external object's presence to reinforce and protect the frail stability achieved by self- and object representations, in the absence of object constancy. The borderline patient's sense of identity and of autonomous functioning is therefore impaired.

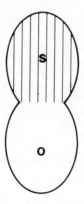

FIG. 1.—Early differentiation (S= self-image; O = object image)

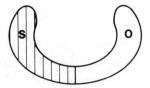

FIG. 2.—Early practicing (S= self-image; O = object image)

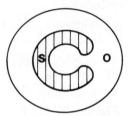

FIG. 3.—Practicing proper (S= self-image; O = object image)

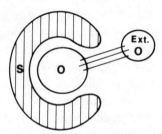

FIG. 4.—Symbiotic phase (S= self-image; O = object image; Ext. O = external object).

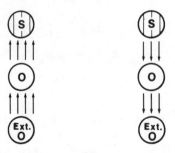

FIG. 5.—Rapprochement. Left, shadowing. Right, coercion (S= self-image; O = object image; Ext. O = external object).

SEXUAL IDENTITY

Logically, the deficient individuation process interferes with the learning and integration of sexual distinctions in the object representation and of gender identity as a component of the self-representation.

OBJECT RELATIONS

The borderline adolescent is unable to tolerate and perceive his parents realistically and maintain a sense of autonomy. In fact, he cannot tolerate his parents or his own anxiety. The patient's projections onto the parents or the parent's projections onto him distort his experience.

For example, a seventeen-year-old was hospitalized two weeks after his own mother had been hospitalized for a suicide attempt. In the preceding month he had wanted to work and was successful in getting employment on a newspaper. His mother, a chronically depressed woman, became so panicky about his moving out of the home and being more independent that she attempted to commit suicide and told him she would not be around anymore. After the mother's hospitalization, the son became upset and withdrawn, and for two weeks stayed at home, doing nothing. Finally, he had an abrupt outburst of temper, breaking chairs and furniture, and forcing his father, a passive and withdrawn man, to hospitalize him. Once in the hospital, he reorganized, feeling relieved to be away from the family. In those patients where endowment is adequate, the role of the family, specifically the relationship to the mother in the separation-individuation phase, seems to be crucial.

Object relations in the borderline adolescent are both arrested and pathological. The capacity to acquire socialization skills and signs of acculturation in handling aggression—a developmental task expected of the preschool child—is deficient in the borderline adolescent, as is the capacity to handle and establish peer relationships (a developmen-

243

tal task of the latency-age child). Social interaction is impaired because the borderline adolescent does not have a sense of autonomy and secure independent functioning due to his lack of object constancy. The awareness of the world at large and the sense of belonging cannot be well established because of the persistence of egocentric thinking. Furthermore, the struggle for emancipation and independence from the family expected of the normal adolescent, who is able to contain his anxiety and ambivalence toward his parents, is altogether absent in the borderline adolescent.

In what follows I shall first discuss the quality of relationship to external objects and then the structural qualities of object representations, using the terms defined by Sandler and Rosenblatt (1962).

RELATIONSHIP TO MOTHER

The borderline adolescent's relationship to the parents, and in particular the mother, is characterized by primitive forms of idealization or devaluation according to the need to split the good mother of separation from the bad mother of separation. In this manner the borderline adolescent attempts to satisfy his need for support, nurturance, and control in spite of his anger. Extreme forms of masochistic surrender, including what Anna Freud (1965) describes as altruistic surrender to the idealized mother or mother surrogates, may stem from this splitting mechanism in an effort to triumph and obtain love from the (perceived) cruel object.

RELATIONSHIP TO SIBLINGS AND PEERS

In borderline adolescents the quality of the relationship to siblings and peers is deficient. There is an unrelenting sibling rivalry and envy of siblings for sharing mother's attention. Peers are used as props for projection of internal objects; they do not have the growth-promoting role they have for the normal latency-age child. In addition, the borderline adolescent lacks the enjoyment and the gratification that the latency-age child finds in competitiveness with peers. Competitiveness, a sublimatory derivative of aggression, is in contrast permeated with primitive aggression causing intense anxiety that deprives the adolescent of gratification. Or, the aggression is felt as such a threatening emotion that inhibition of activity and withdrawal ensue.

TRANSITIONAL OBJECTS

Clinical observations indicate that borderline adolescents do not have a history of transitional objects in early childhood (Lobel 1978). The existence of a transitional object presupposes a positive object relation with the mother which can be internalized, so that the child's relation to his internalized object can be reproduced in an intermediate world of experience. It is not surprising to find that as children, for reasons of endowment and/or environment, borderline adolescents did not develop a positive sense of self in relation to a positive object (in the context of soothing and pleasurable experiences with the mother). Therefore, these patients did not have a transitional object at the appropriate age of eight to twenty-four months, or did not have one of the usual quality, such as a satin blanket edge, diaper, or furry soft toy. Instead, they continued to cling to the mother, searching for closeness experiences or positive refuelings, or they tended to represent their relationship to the bad mother of separation by attaching themselves to inanimate objects. The transitional object of the borderline child who eventually becomes a borderline adolescent often portrays a self-image or an ideal image similar in function to an imaginary companion; it serves to supplement a deficient self-image rather than reflecting a positive mother-child interaction.

INTERNALIZED SELF- AND OBJECT IMAGES

The borderline adolescent's unintegrated self- and object representations are in an unstable equilibrium and do not modulate one another. Neither the two self-images (self as happy and self as frightened) nor the two corresponding object representations (parents as loving and parents as deserting) are experienced as related to one object. Instead, contradictory self- and object images alternate so that one of the complementary parts is easily projected and displaced. (This

245

explanation will be referred to later in the clinical illustration of an adolescent and her family.)

At this point, I would like to describe the various behavioral forms that these projections may take in the patient-doctor relationship in psychoanalytic psychotherapy or in the relationship with the mother. There may, for example, be twinlike split self-images in which the therapist is perceived as having exactly the characteristics of the patient, but as a double, not as a fused self-image (which would be characteristic of psychosis). On the other hand, the therapist (the object) may be experienced as idealized and all-powerful, with the almost complete disappearance of the patient's self-representation, so that there is an obliteration of the sense of self and the patient becomes an echo of the mother. This could be understood as an extreme form of shadowing, with a renunciation of any existence beyond that of an echo.

A more primitive form of this splitting of self and object corresponds to the patient's experience that parts of the object acquire characteristics of himself, a projection of a part-object image. One analytic patient of mine, a borderline narcissistic personality, stated that it was her tough luck to have a therapist who had exactly the same face as her mother. In contrast, in other cases parts of the mother's physical characteristics may be introjected to form the patient's representation of himself. Another patient of mine, for example, felt that her neck became her mother's neck—short and ugly.

In the normal adolescent, with the widening variety of self-other relationships, the affective or motivational links between self and other are also modulated and increasingly intricately patterned. As discussed in the section on object constancy, in borderline patients this complex patterning has not been completed; the external object is needed. In borderline conditions, the use of the other as a mere prop through projection underlines that the internal images are not being modified to match external reality. Although the adolescent recognizes the existence of others in a separate world external to himself, he does not have the full commitment to test on his own the reality of his self- and object images. In fact, as observed in several adolescents, when the object becomes obtrusive or too discrepant, the patient reacts with massive ignoring, with fury, or by retreating to isolated activities, but without modifying his self- or object representations to a closer match with the external object (Fast and Chethik 1972).

The above description leads us to two consequences of the borderline patient's internal world of object relations. First, these patients cannot learn from experience and therefore are condemned to a chronic developmental interference unless appropriate therapeutic intervention is given. Second, supportive psychotherapy, which does not attempt to deal with the working through of primitive defense mechanisms, is not effective, as was indicated in the outcome of the Psychotherapy Research Project of the Menninger Foundation (Kernberg, Burstein, Coyne, Appelbaum, Horwitz, and Voth 1972). The borderline patients did poorly with supportive therapies and responded best to supportive-expressive modes of intervention.

THE OEDIPAL SITUATION

In contrast to the normal adolescent, who experiences a reactivation of the oedipal situation in derivative forms, the borderline adolescent's oedipal situation is distorted by the weight of the difficulties in the separation-individuation stages. The phallic stage is unstable, as the inability to separate from the mother enhances the incestuous ties; the boy has increased problems of disidentification with the mother which predispose him to homosexual behavior and other problems of core identity. The difficulty of separating to invest in another object is increased in the borderline adolescent because of the fear of annihilation by maternal abandonment (this reflects the lack of object constancy). In the borderline adolescent heterosexual relations are frequently characterized by extreme forms of sadistic control of the partner, multiple perversions, or altruistic surrender (Gunderson 1977).

FANTASIES

Masturbatory fantasies reflect the same point of fixation. In contrast to the normal adolescent, the borderline's masturbatory fantasies are characterized by bizarreness and regression. Sexual excitement may be derived from picturing partners defecating on each other or picturing sexual relations with both parents. There may be extreme forms of sadistic perverse fantasies with multiple objects.

247

COGNITIVE FUNCTIONING

In terms of cognitive functioning, the adolescent borderline fails to develop abstract thinking in terms of his social interactions, as well as to incorporate learning into a gestalt of living. Development of sublimatory channels is frequently deficient in relation to his potential capacity.

Although the descriptions of language in the borderline adolescent are rather inconsistent, the general agreement is that clinically there is no formal thought disorder, although primary-process thinking may be present in unstructured testing such as the Rorschach. This finding is not present in the normal adolescent.

PSYCHOTIC EPISODES

In contrast to the normal adolescent, the borderline adolescent is predisposed to brief periods of psychosis, which are characterized by paranoid symptoms, depersonalization, derealization, dissociation, and suicidal attempts.

Case Illustration

Fourteen-year-old Susan came to me for consultation at her parents' request. In my interview with them, the parents described how, while they were away for two weeks during the winter (the first time they had been away by themselves), Susan had attempted suicide by taking a bottle of barbiturates. Surprised by this behavior, they had returned early from their vacation.

During her parents' absence, Susan had complained of feeling depressed, lethargic, and bored. She stated to her sister that her parents should have taken her. Having ingested the pills, she told her older sister, who took her to the emergency room of a local hospital. After Susan's stomach was pumped she said she wanted to go to a warm place and not return to school. The patient was expressing her disturbed reaction to separation from her parents and indicated her potential for different levels of ego functioning, both characteristics of borderline personality organization outlined in the profile.

According to her parents, Susan had been a good student throughout her school years but was characteristically obsessed with a need to be the most outstanding student in her class lest "she feel like a nothing." She worked too hard and always complained that she had too much to do. At times she cried and stayed awake until 2 A.M. and then got up at 6 o'clock in the morning. Her mother would sit with her for one or two hours to help her with her homework. She complained that she did not do anything well enough; she had no hobbies, no interests, and a negative view of herself. For instance, she felt she was not good enough at tennis. These observations illustrate the patient's fixation to an omnipotent self-representation for the purposes of maintaining some sense of identity. Yet this self-representation was so unstable that it did not protect her from a feeling of emptiness, of being a nothing. Another coping mechanism she used to counteract the nothing feeling was coercive behavior, as in her forcing mother to stay with her while she did her homework. Because of her chronic unhappiness she had already been seen by a therapist on three occasions—at five, ten, and twelve years of age. After these consultations, however, the parents allowed her to refuse treatment.

FAMILY HISTORY

Possibly genetic predispositions are suggested by the patient's family background. The patient's father had had a depressive illness of long standing; the paternal grandmother had committed suicide. An older aunt had also suffered from severe depression, requiring professional treatment.

EARLY DEVELOPMENT

Susan was born with normal weight by breech delivery two weeks before her due date. The cord was around her neck, but there was no anoxia. She was bottle fed and walked at seven months of age.

Psychologically, the child who ambulates at an earlier chronological age may be more vulnerable to separation from mother, for his ego may experience as traumatic the awareness of mother's separateness. The baby confronts himself prematurely with the fact that mother is not constantly with him, and her lack of physical closeness may induce in him a sense of loss of self as she still is part of the self- and object system outlined earlier for the differentiation and early practicing phases.

Susan had no speech difficulties except a slight babyishness. Her vocabulary was advanced, and she was considered a highly intelligent child. She was seen at age five by a psychiatrist, and at that time she already stated that nobody loved her. She complained that her parents always left her alone, probably referring to her father's severe depressions and her mother's relative tension around her husband's illness. During her father's periods of deep depressions, Susan would try to console him. She wore a diaper at night until age five and had no friends her own age. For about six months, between the ages of four and four and a half, every ten days she awoke sobbing in the middle of the night. Although unable to say what was bothering her, Susan once asked her mother, "Where is mommy?" It was hard for the mother to convince her that she was right there. She had a distinct fear of darkness, needed a night light, and was very frightened of insects. All of these situations reflected her ongoing need for refueling so as to keep her sense of her self and the object, unstably held under the impact of her anger due to her frustration.

During her latency years, Susan was outgoing, manipulative, and phony in demonstrating affection. She would pick out a target to be artificially affectionate to, giving that "target person" her physical affection in order to gain a favor or attention. She acted like "Betty Boop," patted people on the cheek, talked somewhat babyishly, climbed all over the person, put her head on the person's thigh, and lapsed into generally infantile but cute behavior. This characterological development seemed to represent the acquisition of a pseudoself to maintain some object relatedness and satisfy some of her dependency needs. Ever since she had been sent to camp at age nine she had shown extreme separation problems. The first time she refused to go to camp. The second time she had to be brought back home after two weeks, and the third time she barely made it through the month. She was also reluctant to leave the house and preferred to maintain her few friendships by telephone contact.

Susan's relationship to her housekeeper, who had been in the home for many years, was very close. In fact, she had slept with the house-keeper until very recently and only recently had she become more distant from her. Again, patterns of separation are delayed and distorted, like her sleeping with her housekeeper until her early teens.

THE CONSULTATION INTERVIEW

Susan, a petite, dark-haired, bright girl, seemed extremely controlled in her behavior. She expressed her feeling of being tired of doing things: she wanted more free time—to go away, to swim, to play tennis. She found herself doing things she didn't enjoy and "there is always too much of it." Susan acknowledged that she had taken pills, but she talked as if this event had nothing to do with her and complained that her parents were bothering her and not letting her out of sight for a single minute. According to her, nothing else really bothered her, and she refused to acknowledge any other source of worry. She felt that currently she was happy and satisfied. These statements indicated her being at the mercy of sadistic, superego forerunners; the use of dissociation and denial with the preservation of reality testing was seen in her acknowledgment of her taking an overdose of pills.

In talking about her school, she said it was very competitive for grades. She always had the feeling that someone would do better. That annoyed her, as she knew that whenever she got a *B* she was capable of doing better. She denied any nervousness, anxiety, or obsessions. She described her mood as entirely dependent on whether Friday night comes or not. Friday night was her best night because she did not have to do homework immediately; Sunday was the worst night as it marked the beginning of the week. She felt it was a "dumb" thing to go to school five days and have only Saturday for herself. During this day she did not engage in any social interaction and just stayed at home by herself watching TV and doing homework.

She described herself as having the constant feeling of a "lot of things I have to do." Her parents and the housekeeper, she complained, were too much on her back—she seemed unaware that she might be contributing to their attitude.

Susan described her friends superficially. One friend was nice be-

251

cause they agreed in most things and the other one because they gossiped. (She had only telephone contact with these friends.)

When asked about her father, she responded, after a long pause, "I can't think of words to describe him." "He *let us* do things we want to do within reason. . . . As a little kid he gave *us* candy" (my emphasis). She could not differentiate between his relationship with her and with her sister or brother. Asked to describe her mother, she could not find any way to picture her. She just said, "She treats me different, but my parents basically treat us in a general way alike," an example of her inability to perceive external objects in their own terms.

She mentioned that she was the housekeeper's favorite. Nevertheless she stated that the housekeeper "purposely tried to get someone in trouble." She went on to complain: "Late at night she wants to know every detail in my life. She is evasive and likes to tell people about them. I used to go out of my way talking to her more than I did anyone else, but now she bothers me more." A paranoid quality seemed apparent in relation to the housekeeper, a toned-down expression of more flagrant paranoid ideation seen in more severe cases with less ego strength.

THE FAMILY INTERVIEW

During the family interview, Susan felt it was entirely her parents' problem to have her come to see a psychiatrist. As far as she was concerned, she had nothing to worry about. She said she was not going to talk to any psychiatrist, was quite adamant in feeling that she was not going to change, and claimed that her previous psychiatrists had all been stupid people. The last one, who had seen her when she had attempted suicide and had continued seeing her on a twice-a-week basis, was described as a "ridiculous figure. . . . He asked stupid things like what clothes I like, what food I ate, what courses I was taking at school, how long would it take me to catch up with school work." She attended the sessions just to see him run out of questions. She could not describe her previous experiences with psychiatrists.

At one point she indicated that her parents exaggerated. She appeared quite indifferent and in a kind of pseudoelated mood while her parents were crying, worrying about her, and feeling impotent in persuading her to see somebody in treatment. She just felt that her parents should "get off her back." She was completely unaware of how she actively encouraged the parents' involvement with her by her stating that her problems were her parents' fault, by involving her mother daily in her homework, and, last but not least, by her suicide attempt.

PSYCHOLOGICAL TEST RESULTS

The continuity of this patient's psychopathology will be illustrated. At age five, psychological testing indicated that on projective material, Susan became evasive when facing a difficult task. She would instruct the psychologist to ask her mother to answer the question. She used intellectualization to avoid fantasy stimulation. On the CAT, for instance, she requested a book about animals so that she could learn what they do.

The arbitrariness of her last Rorschach responses indicated that with fatigue and excessive stimulation her thinking gave way to mildly disorganized, idiosyncratic, and highly charged fantasies. Susan would regress under the impact of her self-disapproval and sense of impotence. As a consequence, a somewhat artificial compliance with the examiner replaced her more spontaneous behavior. She seemed depressed, feeling that all her own childish, preoedipal impulses were bad, which automatically reduced her sense of worth.

Susan's CAT responses contained several references to a mother who doesn't like to cook. In one response Susan actually said that the mother had died and that her role was taken by the more obliging housekeeper. When engaged in the task of identifying squirrels, Susan said. "I used to see squirrels on a tree, but I don't see them anymore." This confused picture of family relations suggested that Susan had little hope of being understood or helped by her parents. In her story, there is a little mouse who must dig underground to find her parents, suggesting both the need for her parents and the search she must make to locate them.

The repetition of the attachment percept suggested that sexualized closeness was also used to provide a substitute for the intimacy she wanted. She acted grown up in order to obtain attention from adults. Because of her marked tendency toward isolation and denial of her impulses, there was concern at the time of her acquiring a pseudoadult, compulsive structure, very much in the sense of a Winnicott's (1960)

253

"False Self." Almost ten years later, the characteristics of her personality had remained unchanged.

OVERVIEW

In summary, this is a young girl who had a genetic predisposition for severe emotional illness. She remained involved in the task of separation and individuation, with temporary loss of reality testing, impulsive behavior, and massive use of early defense mechanisms such as denial and projection. Projective identification was seen in the family diagnostic interview where the parents were depressed and helpless while she maintained her stance of pseudoindependence and pseudoeuphoria, and complained that her parents should "get off her back." Obsessive-compulsive defenses barely contained her sense of being a nothing. She showed a lack of direction and identity, a chronic sense of dissatisfaction, and an inability to establish more intimate relations both with friends of the same sex and with boyfriends. She maintained an infantile dependent attachment to the housekeeper, with whom she had lately become disappointed. Although she was fourteen years old, she was unable to separate psychologically from her parents. The similarities of her mental status examination at fourteen with the psychological examination at age five illustrated that the characteristics of her borderline personality organization had remained unchanged throughout a period of almost ten years.

Conclusions

A profile of the borderline adolescent has been presented by contrasting it with the developmental tasks normally achieved during the preschool, latency, and adolescent years. The chapter highlights specifically the deficits in the areas of object relations, reality testing, affects, impulse control, frustration, anxiety, and depression tolerance. The particular experience of self and object world is elaborated with the hypothesis of different structural implications to the vicissitudes of the separation-individuation phases. Relations to external objects, including transitional objects, parents, peers, and therapist, are discussed.

REFERENCES

Fast, I., and Chethik, M. 1972. Some aspects of object relationships in borderline children. *International Journal of Psycho-Analysis* 53:479–485.

Freud, A. 1965. *Normality and Pathology in Childhood*. New York: International Universities Press.

Frijling-Schreuder, E. C. M. 1969. Borderline states in children. *Psychoanalytic Study of the Child* 24:307–327.

Geleerd, E. R. 1958. Borderline states in childhood and adolescence. *Psychoanalytic Study of the Child* 13:279–295.

Grinker, R. R., Sr., Werble, B., and Drye, R. C. 1968. *The Borderline Syndrome*. New York: Basic.

Gunderson, J. G. 1977. Characteristics of borderline. In P. Hartocollis, ed. *Borderline Personality Disorders: The Concept, the Syndrome, the Patient*. New York: International Universities Press.

Kernberg, O. 1975. *Borderline Conditions and Pathological Narcissism*. New York: Jason Aronson.

Kernberg, O. 1977. The structural diagnosis of borderline personality organization. In P. Hartocollis, ed. *Borderline Personality Disorders: The Concept, the Syndrome, the Patient*. New York: International Universities Press.

Kernberg, O.; Burstein, E. D.; Coyne, L.; Appelbaum, A.; Horwitz, L.; and Voth, H. 1972. Psychotherapy and psychoanalysis: final report of the Menninger Foundations's psychotherapy research project. *Bulletin of the Menninger Clinic* 36:1–275.

Knight, R. P. 1953. Borderline states. In R. P. Knight and C. R. Friedman, eds. *Psychoanalytic Psychiatry and Psychology*. New York: International Universities Press.

Lobel, L. 1978. A retrospective study of transitional object use in borderline adolescents. Unpublished.

Mahler, M. S. 1971. A study of the separation-individuation process: and its possible application to borderline phenomena in the psychoanalytic situation. *Psychoanalytic Study of the Child* 26:403–424.

Masterson, J. F. 1967. *The Psychiatric Dilemma of Adolescence.* Boston: Little, Brown.

Masterson, J. F. 1972. *Treatment of the Borderline Adolescent: A Developmental Approach.* New York: Wiley.

Masterson, J. F. 1975. The splitting defense mechanism of the borderline adolescent: developmental and clinical aspects. In J. E. Mack, ed. *Borderline States in Psychiatry.* New York: Grune & Stratton.

Sandler, J., and Rosenblatt, B. 1962. The concept of the representational world. *Psychoanalytic Study of the Child* 17:128–145.

Senn, M. J. E., and Solnit, A. J. 1968. *Problems in Child Behavior and Development.* Philadelphia: Lea & Febiger.

Winnicott, D. W. 1960. Ego distortion in terms of true self and false self. In *The Maturational Processes and the Facilitating Environment.* New York: International Universities Press, 1965.

17 CONFLICT, CHARACTER, AND CONVERSION: STUDY OF A "NEW-RELIGION" MEMBER

ALEXANDER DEUTSCH AND MICHAEL J. MILLER

What kinds of people with what sorts of needs and vulnerabilities become members of cults or "new religions"? The following is a contribution to this broad question concerning unconventional religious adaptations raised in an earlier publication (Deutsch 1975). It is a study of a young woman, raised as a Catholic, who became a member of a new-religion group in her early twenties. In the course of our investigation, the influences of certain psychic conflicts and character trends on her attraction to group life and teachings became apparent, and these influences will be focused on in this chapter. The Case Report section contains relevant historical information, with an emphasis on her late adolescent turmoil which preceded her conversion. The interpretative comments that follow stress the conscious and unconscious needs and vulnerabilities that seemed to be at least partial determinants of her attraction to the church. Among the psychological features that will be highlighted are our subject's powerful sexual guilt and inhibition, seemingly related to a highly punitive maternal introject, her inordinate intolerance to aggression from within or without, leading to a reactive benevolence, and the apparent tendency to employ omnipotent thinking to neutralize threatening stimuli.

One of us met our subject (Jean) in the course of an earlier research project (Galanter, Rabkin, Rabkin, and Deutsch 1979). As she was cooperative, reasonably articulate, and had no obvious psychiatric history it was felt that she would be a good initial subject for investigation of religious-sect members through intensive individual case study.

She agreed to participate, and her decision was backed by church leaders. Both she and the leaders felt that objective scientific investigation would help demystify the church and counteract prejudicial accounts in the popular media.

The religious group joined by our subject has a large number of full-time adherents who live communally in houses, often near college campuses. Members spend their long workdays in activities which assure the financial and operational stability of the organization and help advance its growth. They spend a moderate amount of time in individual and communal prayer, but ecstatic or inspirational experiences that might create a gulf between a member and the community are not encouraged. The group considers itself an outgrowth of Christianity but teaches that Jesus was human and that his messianic mission has not been completed (Kim 1976). There will be a second Advent of the Messiah with the purpose of uniting all people and religions under God. Sexuality and marriage play central roles in church doctrine. The Fall of Man relates to the disobedience of God's will by Adam and Eve when, under the influence of Satan, they had sexual intercourse before God united them in marriage. Premarital chastity is an absolute in church life, and one's marital partner is frequently selected or at least approved by the group's leader who considers himself a prophet and an instrument of God's will who brings new vital teachings to mankind.

Method of Study

One of us (AD) interviewed Jean for five prolonged sessions (total of fourteen hours) over the course of two months. The interviews, basically clinically and psychodynamically oriented, were designed both to give the subject the opportunity to speak freely and develop themes that were important to her and to give the interviewer the chance to obtain data about specific topics and to refine progressively his understanding of the subject and her religious conversion. Following the fifth interview tentative formulations were made regarding Jean's character, conflicts, and development as well as the meaning of the cult in her life. Jean then took a battery of psychological tests (Wechsler Adult Intelligence Scale, Thematic Apperception Test [TAT], Rorschach, projective drawings, and Bender-Gestalt) with the psychologist (MJM), who

258

was blind to any of the data obtained from the interviews or any of the formulations made. The interpretations of the psychological materials were remarkably consonant with these earlier formulations but added new perspectives which were followed up in two subsequent lengthy interviews (total of six hours). In addition to these two separate methods of approach, Jean filled out various personality questionnaires (e.g., the Minnesota Multiphasic Personality Inventory) but these materials, while not contradictory to our formulations, did not contribute significantly.

Case Report

Jean was a moderately overweight, completely unadorned, but basically attractive twenty-seven-year-old woman who had been a member of a religious cult for four years. She was shy but friendly, and her words had a tendency to tumble over each other when she became anxious or excited. She was logical, coherent, and showed no formal signs of thought disorder. She was extremely responsible in filling out questionnaires and coming to her appointments on time in spite of her enormous work load in the church. However, she was by no means an automaton; she directed the interviews to issues she wished to discuss and protested strongly at one point when she felt that the line of questioning gave too much weight to psychological conflict as distinct from spiritual factors.

Born in a northeastern suburban community, Jean is the third oldest of five children. Her mother is a practicing Catholic who raised the children in her faith despite protest from Jean's father. Father, of Methodist background but irreligious, is a successful businessman. He did unremunerated work among the poor in the community and is highly respected. In spite of his many absences, which were symptomatic of the rift between her parents, and his distant and noncommunicative nature, Jean loved and idealized her father. Her family spurned her after her conversion, and he is the only family member with whom she had maintained contact.

It is very difficult for Jean to be critical of her mother, but the portrayal given is that of a cold woman, unempathic toward her children and especially toward our subject. There was a succession of older women, both relatives and mothers of friends, from whom Jean felt more warmth and acceptance than from her own mother. When she was a child, she and her mother would attend mass at different times, and she was envious of the warm Catholic families in her neighborhood who would worship together. She is not aware of any rivalry with her siblings (including a sister two years her junior who required much attention because of childhood illness) for her mother's affection. On the contrary, she was quite maternal toward her siblings and often felt herself to be more understanding than her mother. Indeed, she associated her long-term sense of mission to help people in need, spiritually and materially, to a special feeling of exaltation that she had had at age twelve while she was carrying her four-year-old brother who was unable to walk because a deep snow had fallen.

Jean's "goodness" was much in evidence in Catholic school during her childhood and preadolescence. She was a quiet, obedient student, well liked by her teachers. She believed in angels and miracles and all the doctrines of the Catholic church taught by the nuns at school. She felt privileged to be in this community of believers and superior to her friends who did not attend Catholic school.

In spite of this, Jean was not a diligent or ambitious student, neither in childhood nor in her later years. Part of the problem, she feels, was her "inability to compete" with her older brother and older sister who were excellent students. In association with this she remembers "sitting on the sidelines" while her older sister and father had intellectual discussions that went over her head. Through childhood and adolescence she did enjoy outdoor activities with her father, although there was no communication between them about personal matters.

Jean became conscience stricken at age twelve for reasons that are not clear to her. In obsessional style she drew up lists of "sins" she would have to correct. When her menarche arrived at fourteen she was quite upset: "My body was doing all these strange things . . . I was confused . . . I always hated my periods." During adolescence she was extremely shy with boys; she loved to dance, but after the dance would be embarrassed and have nothing to say.

Jean tends to implicate her mother in these problems. "If only I could have spoken to her about my periods or boys I would have been less confused." Her mother was experienced as proper, distant, nonindulgent, and mistrusting. She never spoke openly to Jean about sex but did warn her about drinking. Jean interpreted these warnings as cautions against lowering one's resistance to sexual advances while inebriated. Jean was particularly disturbed when her mother seemed to be mistrustful of her nonsexual friendships with boys. She could not, however, permit herself to feel angry with her mother or imagine that her mother was hostile toward her. If her mother disapproved it could only be for Jean's benefit and could only mean that Jean was wrong.

During her high school years, Jean's attitude and behavior in school altered in the direction of rebelliousness. She felt antagonistic toward her nun-teachers because they acted "superior" and "authoritarian." She began to develop negative feelings toward the Catholic church, believing that Protestant churches do more for "real problems" (i.e., helping people). She was frequently truant; she and her girl friends would wander through the city, go to movies, and talk about boys. It became increasingly evident in the interviews that a central factor in Jean's newly developed antagonism toward her teachers, school, and the Catholic church itself related to the nuns' exhortations regarding sexual behavior. She was quite upset when told not to wear patent leather shoes because they may reflect her body and undergarments and not to use white tablecloths because they would remind men of bedsheets. It seems that Jean must have experienced some overlap in the attitudes of her mother and her teachers, and it is likely that anger inadmissible toward the former was expressed toward the latter.

Jean attended college away from home during a period of student unrest, drug abuse, and permissive sexuality. She had a number of girl friends toward whom she tended to be protective and maternal, and she made passing grades. She began drinking moderately, but smoked marijuana only a few times since it made her feel "out of control." During her junior year she started seeing a young man regularly for the first time, and it was during this year, as their physical relationship intensified, that Jean's problems developed.

In the fall of that year, Jean became quite depressed. She experienced the world as bleak and degenerate; she felt hopeless, without guidance, and without knowing "who [she] was." She developed a fear of death, felt that "death was descending" upon her when she went to sleep, and had the persistent thought that she could kill herself. This thought was so pronounced that for a period she avoided going into kitchens by herself because she feared having access to knives. During Christmas vacation, at the height of her depression, she had a disturbing dream, which led to an (unsatisfactory) consultation with a psychologist upon her return to school. In the dream, her mother is chasing her through a destroyed area containing broken-down buildings, throwing bricks at her, and trying to kill her. The bricks cut her legs, which are bleeding. In her session with us, the brick throwing reminded Jean of the incident in the New Testament in which a prostitute is stoned and rescued by Jesus. The image of her mother trying to kill her remains, to this day, most disturbing.

The junior-year depression was followed and somewhat relieved by a revival of Jean's religious feelings. She liked her boyfriend but felt guilty and confused over their sexual relationship, preferring a platonic one. Attempting to prove to him that their sexual relationship was wrong, she searched the New Testament to find an unambiguous prohibition against premarital sex but somehow could not find the necessary statement (at least nothing that her boyfriend could not interpret in another way). Nonetheless, she decided after graduation to terminate their sexual relationship as well as her drinking and smoking, and she stuck to her resolve.

Jean began graduate work in one of the helping professions, planning to ultimately use her training in missionary work. A few weeks into the semester, she began looking for a church to affiliate with. She looked into a charismatic Christian group, but did not like its excessive emotionality. Jean then saw an advertisement for a lecture on "Christianity in Crisis." The title appealed to her, and her attendance at the lecture marked the beginning of her involvement with the group she eventually joined.

In discussing her attraction to life in the cult, Jean mentions several factors. She liked the people she met there, feeling they were warm, open, and dedicated. She was most impressed by the church teachings, particularly in regard to sexuality; she learned that the Fall of Man involved Adam and Eve indulging in intercourse before God united them in marriage, and she now had a clear reason why premarital sexual intimacy was forbidden. She was taken by the notion that the church would someday unite all people and all churches and bring everyone closer to God. She was gratified by the opportunity to spend long hours of hard work to help the mission. In this community of hard work, worship, and chastity, "God was more real" to her, and her depressions were less substantial and more easily transcended.

Since the point seemed crucial, the interviewer focused on Jean's preference for the group's teachings regarding sex compared with that of her Catholic upbringing. When the nuns made pronouncements about sexual matters, Jean experienced these teachers as arbitrary, petty, suspicious, and belittling. In addition, she later became confused when some priests expressed more liberal views in the area of sexuality, for example, in condoning divorce. The cult's approach was preferable in various ways. For one, the teachings were not arbitrary. Sexual prohibitions were based on a comprehensive view of human history which was fully explained. Also, the rules were not confusing but, rather, were clear and consistent. Further, in providing a historical, intellectually appealing background for sexual prohibitions, she felt she was being treated as an adult.

A few weeks after becoming acquainted with the communal group, Jean went home to tell her family of her decision to leave school and join it. She met with great opposition, particularly from her mother. She asked God for signs that she was making the right choice. The answer was provided for her by means of two "spiritual experiences," more powerful than any she had had previously, and these clinched her decision to join the cult. One of these was as follows: "When half-asleep she dimly heard a choir singing the words 'you are the only hope.' She then asked to hear only the women's voices and this wish was granted. She believed the voices came from the 'spirit world' or from angels."

Her mother has remained adamantly opposed to Jean's membership and thinks that her daughter was "brainwashed." She seems personally offended by Jean's conversion and has even expressed the feeling that Jean is killing her by remaining in the group. Jean scoffs at the notion that she was brainwashed, does not feel that her membership is an expression of antagonism toward her mother, and is upset that her mother feels that Jean does not love her. She would like to be friendly with her mother, but seems well able to do without her.

This last point may be related to a sense of acceptance that Jean has received from women in the group. Along these lines, after joining, she had a dream which she related in association to the dream of "mother trying to kill her," described above. In this second dream she has left an area of broken-down buildings and a woman hands her a copy of the New Testament. The broken-down buildings were similar to those in the first dream and the woman was the Chinese-American director of Jean's unit. In giving her thoughts about the dream, Jean again associates herself with the prostitute rescued by Jesus; she has now found acceptability because of her new purity.

Discussion

What was there about Jean that predisposed her to convert? In approaching this question through an examination of her conflicts, character trends, and development it is not our intent to reductionistically explain away the lifelong religiosity that was so fundamental to her. Loewald (1978), taking issue with Freud (1930), has put forth the thesis that a central core of this human trait might exist independent of conflict and defensive need. It seems clear, however, that psychic conflict did affect her religiosity and helped determine the particular form it took. In these comments, Jean's attraction to two aspects of the religious group will be emphasized: its teachings regarding sexuality and its universalistic messianic message. (It should be understood that these comments will focus on a few central psychological themes and that not all factors that may have had input into her conversion will be discussed.)

Jean, in her presentation as a chaste, moral, helpful, idealistic, shy, compliant woman struck us as a person who had an unusual degree of intolerance toward impulses relating to aggression and sexuality. Her evident inability to experience hostility toward her depriving mother or envy toward her younger siblings suggested that the early character trends of benevolence and altruism resulted, at least in part, from the warding off of these less acceptable feelings. This result may have occurred through a combination of defenses: repression of dependency and hostility; reaction formation; projection of her neediness onto her siblings; and identification with the helpless sibling (Brenman 1952; Freud 1946).

She had a reasonably serene adaptation as a good child until adolescence. The data suggest that at this point her sexual interests and the attendant competitive feelings drove a deep wedge between herself, on the one hand, and her mother and the nuns on the other. They were variously experienced as nonsupportive of her sexuality and critical, distrustful, and belittling. There is considerable evidence, however, that a good part of the struggle with the external authorities at this point reflected Jean's struggle with her own internalized authority (superego). Her private concerns about sin at age twelve, her guilt and inhibition in relation to sexuality, and the indication that once having distanced herself from the Catholic church she desperately needed backup for her feelings that premarital sex was wrong are reflections of this inner struggle.

These struggles were at their height during Jean's junior year at college. The concurrence of the symptoms of the fear of death and of knives and the dream of the murderous mother, coming at a time of heightened heterosexual exposure, suggests that the nuclear dynamic of Jean's adolescent turmoil and depression was guilt (Beres 1966) over heterosexuality with its oedipal implications. The image of the punitive mother appears to have been a repersonification (Blos 1967) of the harsh superego. Mother's actual nonsupportive behavior at the time might have fed into the imagery of the dream, in part by stimulating anger that would be repressed and projected. It also is reasonable to assume that Jean's superego had at its core a strong sadistic preoedipal component resulting from excessive frustration in relation to her mother with anger turned back on the self (Jacobson 1964). During this troubled period in her adolescence the lack of external support and guidance increased her sense of confusion, isolation, and helplessness.

The question arises, as it does in other cases of conversion to new faiths, as to why some individuals who experience their upbringing as too harsh manage to join a faith that might be quite totalistic and authoritarian. Salzman (1953) sees the conversion from one religion to another as being the product of an intense struggle with parental authority, resulting in the seeking of a new and higher authority which cannot be damaged by one's ambivalence. In another study, one of us found that converts to a cult with a charismatic leader felt comfortably free of parental authority and experienced the leader's authority as more reasonable and benign than their parents' (Deutsch 1975). Along these lines we would see Jean's conversion as representing a partial abandonment of a punitive internal authority with the substitution of a new internalizable authority experienced as less punitive. Jean required that this new authority provide strong external support for superego content (i.e., relating to sexual morality) which she had neither the desire nor the capacity to abandon. At the same time, she seemed to need a change in the authority figure and also in the form in which the authority's message was given to her; the new form allowed her to feel mature and not suspect or scolded. From the developmental point of view, the clinging to the old values and to the new authority suggests the inadequate accomplishment of the adolescent tasks of separation, individuation, and superego reorganization (Blos 1967).

That this new authority could be experienced as a powerful, loving, narcissistically gratifying female figure is suggested by Jean's hypnagogic experience of angel's voices just before she joined the church and the dream she had after joining. Gilberg (1974) has noted that for nuns the Catholic church often represents the yearned-for "good mother." It is being suggested here that the Catholic church was inextricably tied up with the image of the "bad mother," and for Jean the group represented the "good mother."

We have stressed how the teachings of this new authority in regard to sexuality fit Jean's needs. What about the other aspect that Jean was attracted to—the idea that someday all people and all churches would be brought close to God. To her the church represents benevolence, and working for it provides a powerful outlet for her altruistic, missionary impulses toward a messianic, universalistic creed. This may be clarified by examining certain aspects of her defensive style which were spotlighted by projective testing.

In general, psychological testing confirmed the impression that Jean was employing multiple hysterical and obsessional defenses to avert sexual and aggressive impulses. What was particularly characteristic of her TAT and Rorschach, however, was her tendency to transform potentially threatening percepts of all kinds, in a wishful and sometimes magical and arbitrary way, into pleasant ones. This defensive style was employed to neutralize percepts related to sexuality and, particularly, to aggression in a manner that we have labeled "benevolent transformation." Figure after figure on the TAT was seen as kind, wise, comforting, or helpful. As an example, card 18GF of the TAT shows two female figures seemingly engaged in struggle, with the hand of one grasping the throat of the other. Jean's response to this card was that a younger woman was helping her sister who was an invalid. Jean volunteered in a follow-up interview that at times she had changed her initial impression of a card. She felt that the cards, with all the gray unsmiling figures, were meant to be depressing and that she ought to put in something that would make them uplifting. Otherwise one negative feeling might lead to another, and in the end the feelings might be overwhelming.

The test material and her follow-up comments suggest that the defensive style of transforming threatening figures into benevolent, helpful ones could be used to neutralize threats of aggression from within or without and to deal with her own fear of helplessness. The style makes use of denial, reaction formation, and omnipotent thinking—wishing or saying something makes it so. The test material confirmed the impression that she has a low tolerance for aggression in herself or her environment and that she uses helpfulness as a defense against aggression. The omnipotent thinking seemed similar to that employed when she was able to produce a change in her hypnagogic experience as reported above. The defensive style appears to be analogous to the lifelong defensive posture adopted in relation to the potentially hostile maternal representation, a posture which had been rudely shaken by her junior-year dream.

Having pinpointed this defensive style of benevolent transformation, we can now make more specific suggestions about possible relationships between Jean's characterological needs and propensities and her affinity for a messianic universalistic creed. The indication that she must neutralize any trace of hostility within herself or her surroundings might relate to her attraction to a movement which aims to unite all people under God with the implication that differences and antagonisms will be erased. Also, the total immersion in such an idealistic movement and the affiliation with a leader experienced as totally beneficent and powerful might in itself be a comforting protection against hostility. It is also possible that her belief in the power of this movement might relate to her own omnipotent thinking. If she has the capacity to transform her world in a benevolent direction through wishful thinking, why cannot the idealistic movement she affiliates with, however small its size, make a more consequential transformation in the real world. Finally, the need and capacity for benevolent transformation could serve to erase any ambivalence or doubt in relation to her new creed or its leader.

Conclusion

Some of the psychological conflicts and character trends of a young woman that appeared to influence her conversion to a religious cult have been described. Guilt and confusion regarding sexuality and powerful superego conflicts seemed to be involved in her turning away from her religion of origin and her submitting to a new authoritarian religion which had suitable doctrines and restrictions in the area of sexuality. Her long-standing reactive character trends of helpfulness and idealism found expression in working for a movement with a messianic universalistic philosophy. She possessed an unusual defensive style which we labeled "benevolent transformation," combining denial, reaction formation, and omnipotence of thought, and used it to ward off poorly tolerated aggressive conflict. The implications of this style in relation to her affinity for a movement dedicated to rescuing mankind have been suggested.

REFERENCES

Beres, D. 1966. Superego and depression. In R. M. Loewenstein, L. M. Newman, M. Schur, and A. J. Solnit, eds. *Psychoanalysis—a General Psychology*. New York: International Universities Press.

Blos, P. 1967. The second individuation process of adolescence. *Psychoanalytic Study of the Child* 22:162–186.

Brenman, M. 1952. On teasing and being teased: and the problem of "moral masochism." *Psychoanalytic Study of the Child* 7:264–285.

Deutsch, A. 1975. Observations on a sidewalk ashram. *Archives of General Psychiatry* 32:166–175.

Freud, A. 1946. *The Ego and the Mechanisms of Defense*. New York: International Universities Press.

Freud, S. 1930. Civilization and its discontents. *Standard Edition*. 21:59–145. London: Hogarth, 1961.

Galanter, M.; Rabkin, R.; Rabkin, J.; and Deutsch, A. 1979. The "Moonies": a psychological study of conversion and membership in a contemporary religious sect. *American Journal of Psychiatry* 136(2): 165–170.

Gilberg, A. L. 1974. Asceticism and the analysis of a nun. *Journal of the American Psychoanalytic Association* 22:381–393.

Jacobson, E. 1964. *The Self and the Object World*. New York: International Universities Press.

Kim, Y. O. 1976. *Unification Theology and Christian Thought*. New York: Golden Gate.

Loewald, H. W. 1978. *Psychoanalysis and the History of the Individual*. New Haven, Conn., and London: Yale University Press.

Salzman, L. 1953. The psychology of religious and ideological conversion. *Psychiatry* 16:177–187.

18 PSYCHOPHYSIOLOGIC ASPECTS OF ADOLESCENCE: HEMIC DISORDERS

AKE MATTSSON AND DAVID P. AGLE

Adolescent behavior at times forces psychiatrists as well as parents to claim that the adolescent stage is a psychophysiologic disorder itself. Adolescents, pressured by rapid changes in biological, cognitive, and psychosocial development, are prone to focus attention on their bodily processes and communicate about them in a new, more sophisticated fashion. Following health classes or after browsing through medical shelves in the public library, many adolescents will suggest to their parents or physicians that they suffer from practically every illness in the book. Acne becomes the first sign of venereal disease, heart palpitation and occasional extrasystoles spell organic heart disease, pain in the extremities and joints is interpreted as early arthritis, and an increased need to urinate signifies diabetes or kidney trouble. The adolescents' achievement in formal, hypotheticodeductive thinking allows them to reason and speculate about their mental and physical inner worlds in a new, egocentric way. This cognitive gain partly explains their preoccupation with bodily functions and their common hypochondriacal concerns.

Criteria for the diagnosis of a psychophysiologic disorder in the current *DSM-II* classification (1968) and the 1966 Group for the Advancement of Psychiatry (GAP) classification of psychopathological disorders in childhood both follow Alexander's (1954) classical description of psychosomatic disorders, contrasting them with conversion hysteria. Psychophysiologic (or vegetative) disorders include those physical illnesses where emotional factors significantly contribute to the onset or course of the illness. Such disorders usually engage organ systems that are innervated by the autonomic or voluntary portions of the central nervous system. The physiological changes involved are those that normally accompany certain emotional states, but in these disorders the changes are more intense and sustained. Patients are usually not consciously aware of their emotional state, and organ dysfunction is without symbolic meaning, in contrast to the physical symptoms seen in conversion reaction. The psychophysiologic dysfunction commonly leads to permanent tissue-structure change, which may even become fatal. In contrast, conversion disorders involve voluntary innervated body structures and seldom progress to structural damage of the dysfunctional body part. Engel (1962) has stressed that psychophysiologic symptoms may occur when conversion symptoms have failed to dissipate anxiety. Thus, continuing anxiety states may activate biologic systems and result in physiologic changes such as tachycardia, hypermotility of the intestinal tract, or vasoconstriction and vasodilation.

An open-systems model of psychosomatic relationships (fig. 1) shows how extrafamilial (social) and intrafamilial stimuli or stress factors of a physical, social, or psychic nature impact upon a child or adolescent who is vulnerable to react with psychophysiologic symptoms. The vulnerability might be of an inborn constitutional or early acquired nature. A developmental phase, such as adolescence, often serves as a vulnerability factor. The psychophysiological arousal, related to the stress stimuli, engages various mediating mechanisms of the patient. These include psychologic (defensive) events, the limbic-

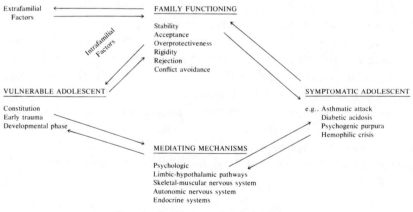

Fig. 1.—Psychosomatic relationships

hypothalamic pathways, and the activation of any of the three effector systems of the brain: the skeletal-muscular nervous system, the autonomic nervous system, and the endocrine systems. Through the action of the effector systems, responsive target organs become affected, and changes in cellular functions result. These, in turn, may lead to pathophysiologic conditions such as an asthmatic attack, a diabetic crisis, a hypertensive state, vascular extravasation with purpura, or spontaneous hemorrhages in a hemophiliac. Any psychophysiologic symptom brings about changes in the psychosocial relationships of the young person. Examples of positive and negative family interaction with an ill child include stability, acceptance, overprotectiveness, enmeshment, rigidity, rejection, and conflict avoidance. These family transactional characteristics have been succinctly described by Minuchin, Baker, Rosman, and Liebman (1975), with special reference to psychophysiologic conditions.

Psychophysiologic Aspects of Bleeding Disorders

Some hemic disorders will be used to illustrate how the bio-psychological stage of adolescence may influence the expression of physical disorders. The GAP report (1966) on a proposed classification of psychopathologic disorders in childhood notes under its heading "Psychophysiologic Hemic and Lymphatic Disorder" that "numerous physiologic concomitants of anxiety are seen in relation to this system, including variations in the blood level of leukocytes, lymphocytes, eosinophiles, glutathione values, relative blood viscosity, clotting time, hematocrit, and sedimentation rate. These ordinarily are reversible; chronic or recurrent states of leukocytosis or lymphocytosis may occur, however, as may alterations in other physiologic values which may be classified under this heading. Leukemia and lymphoma, as well as some cases of pernicious anemia, apparently may be precipitated by physiologic and interpersonal stimuli."

The influence of psychological stress and autonomic arousal on human clotting mechanisms remains incompletely explored (Ruxin, Bidder, and Agle 1972). Many attempts have been made to draw comparisons between humans and animals. Dog research, for instance, has shown that stress in the form of trauma, hemorrhage, cortisone

271

administration, and induced anesthesia cause elevation of blood fibrinogen levels. This results in hypercoagulability of the blood. Such a state can result in disseminated intravascular coagulation leading to renal damage, venus thrombosis, and other lesions. It has also been suggested that psychologic and physiologic stress can bring about an elevation of other clotting factors of the blood. It seems likely that short-term stress factors may increase the levels of fibrinogen and other clotting factors through stimulation of the pituitary–adrenal cortical and sympathetic-medullary axes.

Palmblad, Blomback, and Egberg (1975) found that prolonged human vigilance stress depressed blood levels of fibrinogen and of coagulation factors 5, 8, and 9. The urinary excretion of adrenalin and noradrenalin increased during the same period. Rapid increases in the blood levels of factor 8 (the antihemophilic factor) have been observed after adrenalin injections, which might be explained by a release of factor 8 from storage pools (Ingram 1961). It should be noted, however, that among severe hemophiliacs of the A or classical type, the antihemophilic titer (factor 8) is close to zero. Accordingly, there is little room for an increase or a decrease in factor 8 levels as a response to adrenalin secretion or to prolonged psychosocial stress. It is unknown whether increased cortisol production has an effect on factor 8 levels.

Anecdotal reports and nonsystematic studies have sought to link psychologic stress factors with the onset of some hemic and lymphatic disorders in childhood and young adulthood. Two bleeding disorders, often affecting children and adolescents, have been extensively investigated in regard to psychosocial influences on hemorrhagic symptoms. They include the syndrome of psychogenic purpura, or autoerythrocyte sensitization, and hemophilia due to factor 8 or 9 deficiency. Several studies of young patients with these disorders fulfill scientific criteria. They provide the child and adolescent psychiatrist with practical models of how psychosocial influences may precipitate or exacerbate hemorrhaging in vulnerable patients. This knowledge can be of assistance in providing psychiatric consultation to hematologists and primary-care physicians as well as direct help to the patients and their families.

Autoerythrocyte sensitization, or psychogenic purpura, is an intermittent purpuric state. For the most part, it afflicts adolescent and adult females and is manifested by episodes of painful, spontaneous bruising. The bruises, or ecchymoses, usually appear rapidly, following the onset of pain and inflammation. Usually no physical trauma precedes the lesions. An earlier suggestion that these patients were sensitive to their own red blood cells has been questioned by some investigators (Ratnoff and Agle 1968). In a series of carefully documented studies of close to forty women, they concluded that none of these patients had clotting defects and that psychological factors appeared important in the production of the ecchymotic lesions. Most of the patients related flare-ups of cutaneous purpura to emotional tension and stressful events. Hysterical and masochistic character traits were commonly seen, in addition to problems in dealing with hostility. In some patients, the skin test of autoerythrocyte sensitization could be influenced by hypnotic suggestion.

Psychogenic purpura often has its debut during adolescence. Frequently these young women report a history of physical or sexual abuse associated with a sadomasochistic relationship with a parent. The youngest patient with psychogenic purpura known to us was a fourteen-year-old girl who developed unexplained crops of purpuric and ecchymotic lesions of a month's duration on her trunk and extremities. She revealed to the psychiatrist that her father had forced her to have sexual intercourse with him from about ages eight through twelve. At that time the incestuous relationship ceased, apparently due to the patient's menarche and forceful rejection of her father's advances. At age fourteen, coinciding with her purpura, she was ready to talk about years of pent-up anger and shame related to the illicit past relationship. Her father only admitted to sexually fondling the patient. Several years of psychotherapy, while the patient resided in a group home, brought her relief from the purpura and better control of the dysphoric emotional state related to her traumatic past.

A seventeen-year-old high school senior student was evaluated after five months of spontaneously occurring crops of large ecchymoses, first on one arm, later all over her body. The bruises seemed to be associated with a culmination of emotional conflicts: for several years, the patient had felt unhappy and lonely, with suicidal ideation. The relationship with her mother was characterized by mutual distrust and hostility. Around the time of her first bleeding episodes her grandfather, to whom she was quite close, had died. In addition, her mother had been severely bitten in her arm by their dog, reportedly in the same body location as our patient's first ecchymotic occurrence. The patient recognized her long-standing difficulties in handling anger and self-assertive attitudes, as well as her depressive ideation. During a course of psychotherapy, the bruises ceased to appear and her emotional disorder greatly improved.

Another adolescent girl developed bruises within a week after the double trauma of visits to a brother dying of leukemia and to a sister-in-law whose leg had been amputated. In an additional female patient, the purpura appeared soon after she was shown her brother's amputated limb. Yet another teenager began to bleed after a humiliating experience with her peers in which she was accused of being in love with her priest.

Agle, Ratnoff, and Wasman (1967) have been able to induce purpuric lesions by hypnotic suggestion in several of the women with spontaneous purpura. This supports the notion that central nervous system influences, emotional or hypnotic, may release neurohormones which intensify or bring about inflammatory vascular reactions. These reactions may be of such a nature that vascular permeability is sufficiently increased to allow the leakage of blood. Many years ago, Wolff, Tunis, and Goodell (1953) described the production of swelling and ecchymoses near the temporal artery in patients suffering from severe migraine headaches. He also showed the accumulation of vasodilator polypeptides in the vessel walls and the perivascular tissues in the area of migraine pain. The properties of the polypeptides, named neurokinins, included the production of vasodilation, pain, lowering of the pain threshold, and increased vascular permeability. The implication of these findings for psychogenic purpura warrants further investigations.

The specific personality characteristics and psychological factors that often seem to trigger the appearance of ecchymoses in patients with psychogenic purpura are suggestive of the mechanisms of a conversion reaction (Agle, Ratnoff, and Wasman 1969). Many of the women have fulfilled the criteria for the diagnosis of conversion reaction as stated by Engel (1962). For example, emotionally stressful situations commonly preceded the onset or exacerbation of the disease state, and the patients often had a predisposition to express emotional problems in physical form. Symbolic (conversion) translation of mental conflicts into body language (a wish and the defense against its expression) often seemed present, as well as evidence of identification with past or present key persons who had suffered physical symptoms. In addition, sexual maladaptation, secondary gain, and marked suggestibility was seen among many of the adult women with purpura.

Following Alexander's (1954) lead, many writers have attempted to limit the concept of conversion symptoms to events mediated through the voluntary nervous system. They maintain that structural changes resulting from involvement of the autonomic nervous system should be classified as psychophysiologic reactions. More recently, Nemiah (1975) and Engel (1968) have reported that structural lesions may occur as a complication of conversion reactions. Engel stated: "There is now evidence that the conversion process may sometimes be one component in the development of a localized organic lesion which may then be considered a complication of a conversion. In such instances, a resulting lesion itself and the symptoms arising from it, neither have primary psychologic meaning as a wish or fantasy, nor serve a defensive function. Rather, it seems that the drive and defensive aspects of the conversion contribute to the timing and the choice of location of the manifestation but are not responsible for the nature of the ultimate organic lesion itself." Consequently, we have suggested that, in patients with psychogenic purpura, in some instances the lesion production is a complication of a conversion (Agle, Ratnoff, and Wasman 1969). In these patients, the true conversion symptoms would be the experience of a painful sensation, with the physical location determined by such psychological factors as identification, sadomasochistic gratification, and unconscious punishment to deal with guilt. As a result of these processes, the effector system of the autonomic nervous system becomes engaged, releasing the proposed bradykinin-like substances in the subcutaneous tissues. These induce vasodilation, increased vascular permeability, and extravasation of blood resulting in ecchymoses.

The psychiatric patterns observed in autoerythrocyte sensitization bring to mind the issue of religious stigmata. Of interest to adolescent psychiatrists is the report of Early and Lifschutz (1974) describing a ten-year-old Baptist girl who manifested religious stigmata periodically over a three-week period. These observations on stigmatization suggest a psychophysiologic route of bleeding similar in nature to the mechanisms described in psychogenic purpura.

There are similarities between the syndrome of psychogenic purpura and the so-called spontaneous bleeding episodes of patients with hemophilia (factor 8 or 9 deficiency). In our studies of hemophiliacs, we repeatedly found examples of situations in which psychological factors seemed to have an influence upon the course of the illness (Agle and Mattsson 1976; Mattsson 1975). Adolescent and adult hemophiliacs reported multiple episodes of apparently spontaneous bleeding which followed a situation that had been emotionally stressful to them. One example was a sixteen-year-old boy who stated that the night before he was to leave his home for a prolonged period he bled, apparently spontaneously, into the subcutaneous tissues of both feet. This bleeding caused an indefinite postponement of his trip. He further reported that he had many misgivings about leaving his parents at that time.

Many hematologists and pediatricians, as well as families of hemophilic boys, have attested to similar events of psychic stress preceding hemorrhages in the patients. Curiously, the emotional triggers often have been of a positive nature, such as anticipation of a pleasant event: a holiday, a birthday, or a camp meeting. Frequently parents describe their boys as "overenthusiastic" and "excited" in anticipating these events.

There is no evidence of significant changes in the levels of antihemophilic factors at times of stress. Some authors have therefore suggested that variations in the integrity of the capillary wall, occurring as an autonomic response to stress, may be responsible for certain periods of increased bleeding (Agle 1964). Similarly, Wolff and his associates demonstrated that the mucous membranes of the nose (Holmes, Goodell, Wolf, and Wolff 1950), colon (Grace, Wolf, and Wolff 1951), and stomach (Wolf and Wolff 1943) became congested and friable with anxiety, anger, and resentment. Such changes in the integrity of the capillary wall could have pathological consequences in the hemophiliac. Current investigations are examining the relationship of spontaneous bleeding in hemophiliacs to changes in platelet clumping capacities as influenced by emotional states.

Many hemophiliacs report an improved clinical state following a change from passive dependent behavior to more aggressive independence associated with adolescence (Mattsson 1975). At times these boys have become rebellious, physically hyperenergetic, and even "daredevils." Objective evidence—that is, noticeable decrease in the number of admissions to hospital, replacement therapy, and amount of time missed from normal activity because of bleeding—often support this claim. A dramatic example of this adolescent change is the following: A thirty-two-year-old hemophiliac with virtually no antihemophilic factor in his plasma had experienced about 300 hospital admissions before age fifteen and received over 500 units of plasma or blood. Since the age of fifteen, he had only four brief admissions. What had happened? This patient was the older of two children, having a sister eight years younger. He was told that it took his parents eight years to get up enough courage to have another child. His early years were described "as one bleeding episode and hospital stay after another." He enjoyed the attention of nurses and doctors while in the hospital and showed little interest in school and other activities outside his home. Occasionally he injured himself purposely to avoid unpleasant tasks, for example, cutting his finger so as not to have to dry dishes. However, he also remembered frequent episodes of apparently spontaneous bleeding before events that he later realized he had wished to avoid. Such situations included the first day of school, examinations, and some social events. Early in his fifteenth year, the patient spent the summer at his grandmother's home in a small town. After the summer, he refused to accompany his family to its new home in a large city, instead preferring to stay with his grandmother where he had begun to enjoy some independence. He befriended the high school coach, became a manager of athletic teams, began to date, and later obtained a motor scooter without his parents' knowledge. He turned it over several times because of his reckless driving. Yet, he missed school only once during these adolescent years—after having fallen down two flights of steps. He graduated with all A's, having completed three years of high school work in two. The patient was advised not to go to college because of his health problem. However, he did attend college, graduated, and moved into a junior executive position at around age thirty. He married and fathered three children. He was a hard-driving individual, with much self-control, and told us that he feared only one thing, namely, returning to the dependent state of his childhood.

Conclusions

Studies in psychogenic purpura and hemophilia illustrate how psychophysiologic mechanisms may influence bleeding disorders during adolescence. Both disorders have at least two characteristic features in common: (1) the clinical manifestations often seem related to emotional arousal of a general nature, presumably involving the cortical-hypothalamic-autonomic nervous system axis and the peripheral vascular bed; and (2) the biologically increased drives and independence strivings associated with adolescence seem to exert a more specific psychophysiologic influence among some adolescent girls with psychogenic purpura and some boys with hemophilia types A and B. These influences suggest symbolic, ideational conflicts. Among the girls with psychogenic purpura, there often is evidence of sexual trauma and intrapsychic conflicts, while some boys with hemophilia show conflicts relating to self-assertiveness and attaining independence.

The major psychologic difference between the two hemic disorders may be described as one of a cognitive or ego-impairment nature: the hemophilic adolescent boy knows he has a genetic, bona fide organic disorder whose symptomatic expression and management can be logically explained to him with the expectation of engaging his capacity for formal, operational thinking in a constructive, self-caring manner (Agle and Mattsson 1976; Mattsson, Gross, and Hall 1971). The adolescent girl with psychogenic purpura experiences mysterious, painful bouts of bleeding into her skin, which at best makes her unusual, arousing the pity and interest of the medical community. Usually she suffers from some ego or cognitive impairment as a result of classical neurotic processes: marked psychosocial traumas have caused an unawareness in her of conflicting ideation whose affective charge apparently is translated into psychophysiological symptoms and signs, often of a conversion nature.

These differences in the nature of the conflict and ego impairment help define treatment recommendations. Intrapsychic, conflict-solving psychotherapy is necessary for some young women with psychogenic purpura (Ratnoff and Agle 1968). On the other hand, the hemophilic adolescent boy with hemorrhagic episodes related to inevitable emotional stress or unnecessary dangerous physical activities often can be helped by more cognitively oriented sessions, not aimed at intrapsychic restructuring. In both instances, the psychiatrist will often recommend additional family counseling in order to promote a healthy family interaction necessary for the normal psychosocial maturation of the adolescent with a bleeding disorder.

REFERENCES

Agle, D. P. 1964. Psychiatric studies of patients with hemophilia and related states. *Archives of Internal Medicine* 114:76–82.

Agle, D. P., and Mattsson, A. 1976. Psychological complications of hemophilia. In M. Hilgartner, ed. *Hemophilia in Children*. Littleton, Mass.: Publishing Sciences Group.

Agle, D. P.; Ratnoff, O. D.; and Wasman, M. 1967. Studies in autoerythrocyte sensitization. The induction of purpuric lesions by hypnotic suggestion. *Psychosomatic Medicine* 29:491–503.

Agle, D. P.; Ratnoff, O. D.; and Wasman, M. 1969. Conversion reactions in autoerythrocyte sensitization. *Archives of General Psychiatry* 20:438–447.

Alexander, F. 1954. The psychosomatic approach in medical therapy. In *The Scope of Psychoanalysis*. New York: Basic, 1961.

DSM-II. Diagnostic and Statistical Manual of Mental Disorders. 1968. Washington, D.C.: American Psychiatric Association.

Early, L. F., and Lifschutz, J. E. 1974. A case of stigmata. *Archives of General Psychiatry* 30:197–200.

Engel, G. L. 1962. Somatic consequences of psychological stress. II. Decompensated states: somato-psychic-psychosomatic disorders. In *Psychological Development in Health and Disease*. Philadelphia: Saunders.

Engel, G. L. 1968. A reconsideration of the role of conversion in somatic disease. *Comprehensive Psychiatry* 9:316–326.

Grace, W. J.; Wolf, S.; and Wolff, H. G. 1951. *Human Colon*. New York: Hoeber.

Group for the Advancement of Psychiatry. 1966. *Psychopathological Disorders in Childhood: Theoretical Considerations and a Proposed Classification*. New York: Group for the Advancement of Psychiatry.

Holmes, T. H.; Goodell, H.; Wolf, S.; and Wolff, H. D. 1950. *The Nose*. Springfield, Ill.: Thomas.

Ingram, G. C. I. 1961. Increase in antihemophilic globulin activity following infusion of adrenaline. *Journal of Physiology* 156:217–224.

Mattsson, A. 1975. Psychophysiologic study of bleeding and adaptation in young hemophiliacs. In E. J. Anthony, ed. *Explorations in Child Psychiatry*. New York: Plenum.

Mattsson, A.; Gross, S.; and Hall, T. 1971. Psychoendocrine study of adaptation in young hemophiliacs. *Psychosomatic Medicine* 33: 215–225.

Minuchin, S.; Baker, L.; Rosman, B. L.; and Liebman, R. 1975. A conceptual model of psychosomatic illness in children. *Archives of General Psychiatry* 32:1031–1038.

Nemiah, J. C. 1975. Hysterical neurosis, conversion type. In A. M.

Freedman, H. I. Kaplan, and B. J. Sadock, eds. *Comprehensive Textbook of Psychiatry*. 2d ed. Baltimore: Williams & Wilkins.

Palmblad, J.; Blomback, M.; and Egberg, N. 1975. Experimentally induced stress in man: effects on blood coagulation and fibrinolysis. *Reports from the Laboratory for Clinical Stress Research*. Stockholm: Karolinska Hospital.

Ratnoff, O. D., and Agle, D. P. 1968. Psychogenic purpura: a reevaluation of the syndrome of autoerythrocyte sensitization. *Medicine* 47:475–500.

Ruxin, R. L.; Bidder, T. G.; and Agle, D. P. 1972. The influence of autonomic arousal on blood clotting time in patients receiving electro-convulsive treatments. *Journal of Psychosomatic Research* 16:185–192.

Wolf, S., and Wolff, H. G. 1943. *Human Gastric Function*. New York: Oxford University Press.

Wolff, H. G.; Tunis, M. D.; and Goodell, H. 1953. Studies on headache. Evidence of tissue damage and changes in pain sensitivity in subjects with vascular headaches of the migraine type. *Transactions of the Association of American Physicians* 66:332.

19 PSYCHIATRIC ASPECTS OF PHYSICAL DISABILITY: IMPACT ON THE FAMILY

RAPHAEL GREENBERG

Despite great accomplishments in the conquest of infectious diseases, chronic illness and disability confront medicine with new problems. A patient who is suddenly disabled may often be expected to improve, but transverse myelopathy creates a static disability. Patients with arthritis, particularly rheumatoid arthritis, are afflicted with a disease process that not only cannot be arrested but also is likely to worsen as time passes. Each case must be evaluated socially, psychologically, and vocationally—in addition to medical and functional appraisal—before a realistic rehabilitation plan may be established for that individual.

Every minute of every day on this North American continent a child is born who is not quite perfect and will be chronically ill or mentally or physically handicapped. Of these half-million children born every year, some get the help they need; others do not, and they exist outside the mainstream of our health-worshipping society.

Within the family, the tenderness of parents protects these children, but as they grow up and prepare to face the world their battle for physical and psychological survival begins. Experience at a hospital devoted to children with long-term illnesses[1] makes one aware of the monumental impact of physical disability on the patient's family. Each family shares similar problems, among them lack of funds, isolation from the community of the healthy, prejudice, loneliness, boredom, and depression.

The presence of severe and chronic physical handicap in a family

Paper read before the 9th International Congress of the International Association for Child Psychiatry and Allied Professions, Melbourne, Australia, August 21, 1978.

member almost inevitably creates disturbance or disequilibrium in family life. As Szalita (1968) has described, handicap injures family cohesiveness, lowers self-esteem, and undermines prestige. Thus the family, as well as the afflicted individual, is exposed to innumerable forms of damage.

In preparing the child to cope with the world, some parents concentrate unduly on limitations in activity. Pity may then become the dominant factor and lead to overprotectiveness. Moreover, pity for the child often gives rise to self-pity in the parents—a painful backlash that compounds their difficulties in rearing the child. At the other extreme are parents who overlook the full implications of the child's condition and are too demanding, both on themselves and on the child. These attitudes interfere with the setting of realistic goals for the child's future. Parental bereavement with interminable mourning for the "child who might have been" is another common phenomenon encountered (Group for the Advancement of Psychiatry 1973).

Szalita (1968), commenting on the diverse reactions of families to the presence of a handicapped member, states, "Some families will consolidate their strength, meet the challenge, and create favorable conditions which might prevent the development of disease. In other families, this leads to fragmentation of the family and isolation of the individual patient."

In dealing with the physically disabled, particularly those with a lifelong handicap, cooperation between the patient's family and the team of workers who are trying to help him rehabilitate himself is more important than in any other medical situation. No matter how much we try to empathize with the position of the physically handicapped, we never succeed fully in putting ourselves into his place. One reason for this is that the physically handicapped individual tends to deny his disability, both consciously and unconsciously. This characteristic defense of the severely handicapped also operates in the patient's family.

I talked recently with a twenty-nine-year-old woman who has been paralyzed from the neck down since her spinal cord was injured in an automobile accident when she was seventeen years old. Thanks to remarkable results achieved in her rehabilitation, she is now able to use an electric wheelchair and to feed herself with the use of numerous appliances. However, her daily functioning still requires the services of two attendants. The fortunate economic circumstances of her family make such care possible, just as it made it possible for her to continue her schooling despite her severe disablement.

When I discussed the impact of this severe handicap on her family, she recalled some of her experiences with patients from Puerto Rico and Mexico whom she met in the Arizona hospital to which she was taken after her accident. These patients had also incurred severe injuries in accidents. When members of their families visited them, the patients and their relatives would talk about what they were feeling and often would cry together. After these visits, she observed that the family members would leave the hospital in a much better mood. But not so with the members of her own family; they did not show their feelings at all in their visits to her. Despite their unstinting devotion to her physical dependency needs during the twelve years that have elapsed since her accident, she could not recall an occasion when her own or her family's feelings about the disability were discussed.

Her case illustrates a problem that is characteristically encountered in the rehabilitation of the physically handicapped—the problem of dealing with their inner lives. The woman said that she divides her life into two periods—before and after the accident. Before the accident, sports and social activities were her main interests. Since the accident, she has become a different person. Had it not occurred, she probably would not have developed into the mature and intellectual individual she has become, nor would she have acquired her present knowledge of world literature. But the changes to which she referred do not entail the acceptance of herself as a cripple confined to a wheelchair. In her dreams and thoughts about herself, she views herself as a physically intact person.

Over the years, I have repeatedly observed that the physically handicapped person leads a double existence. In waking life, he denies his disability, asking, in effect, to be treated as if the limitation did not exist. Rather than face the loss of function as the central issue in his life, he may complain about some relatively minor problem.

It is essential to make the distinction between the person and the disability. Assuming that this can be done, it is actually appropriate and healthy to hate the disability. This distinction applies to the family of the patient as well as to the patient himself. The fact is that a disability is never totally acceptable, particularly one that is crippling one's life. It is possible, however, for one to become dispassionate about it, to accept it, and to recognize the impairment as part of one's life.

Some physically disabled persons, particularly those who do not confront themselves with the depth of their deprivation, isolation, and disappointment, may claim the opposite. In some of these cases, it may be more helpful to insist on the challenge inherent in the disability, rather than insisting on facing their deprivation. Cayley (1954), who became a tetraplegic as a result of an accident, emphasized the notion of challenge in reporting on her own rehabilitation. Viewing the disability as a challenge stimulates the patient to mobilize available resources in order to manage the difficulties and, as a result, creates an immediate source of enthusiasm. But this is usually only a temporary measure. Instead of stopping there, one must help the physically disabled and their families to confront realistically the meaning of the handicap and its effects on their lives.

Of course, personality structure, ego strength, and immediate environmental factors have some bearing, but the meaning of the disability depends largely on whether it is congenital or acquired. This distinction influences the nature of the confrontation process (Greenberg 1974).

There are differences of opinion on whether a congenital or an acquired disability presents a greater obstacle to adjustment. For example, Cayley viewed adaptation to an acquired disability as more difficult because it necessitates a change in one's body image, whereas the person who is congenitally disabled gradually adjusts himself in childhood to the fact that he is different from the normal person. "His original concept of himself is that of a handicapped person, even though at first he may not appreciate all the consequences of living with a disability" (Cayley 1954). Those who maintain the opposite opinion point out that those who are disadvantaged from birth must make relatively more effort in compensatory adjustments to a severe disablement than those in whom it was preceded by a period of normal development. The congenitally disabled (and those constricted from early infancy) feel that their lot is more unfortunate, and I agree with them.

Time and time again, I have heard a crippled youngster voice the wish that he could walk down the street like other people—just once! Bitterness, ill will, and envy, however disguised, appear to be more intense in the congenitally disabled. Pluck and courage of an exceptionally high order are required for them to achieve an education and master an occupational skill.

Congenital disability has a more profound psychological impact on the patient's family than an acquired disability. Giving birth to a congenitally defective child is often regarded by the parents as a stigma. I have observed that many families in this situation experience intense feelings of being the unwitting victims of an unjust fate. Some experience the birth of such a child as punishment for a bad deed or as evidence of poor genetic endowment. In such cases, considerable effort is required to raise self-esteem and improve the relationship with the disabled child. The parents are helped to view the disability as a discrimination of nature, rather than a punishment. This helps discourage tendencies to convey to the child the feeling that he comes from tainted stock.

Many outstanding books have been written about the physically disabled (Keller 1902; Mann 1939; Zweig 1939). An excellent account of the impact of severe physical disability on the contemporary family is *Journey*, by Robert and Suzanne Massie (1975), the parents of a hemophiliac boy. They pose a question that deserves consideration by all people. In a world where moral disabilities are far greater than physical imperfections, the Massies ask, who is the more seriously handicapped—the child who is trying to lead a normal life and survive despite his defect or the physically healthy person who is unable to accept that child?

The Massies illustrate that some families do react to severe disability as a challenge, almost as a mark of distinction. Their hemophiliac son, now an adolescent, says: "I am not afraid of adversity. Having suffered setbacks and bounced back, I think that my character has been improved with my difficult childhood. I have gained resilience, willpower, determination and appreciation for what I have, not regret for what I lack. How can I, or anyone, wish that the most important thing that ever happened to me had not happened?"

Families like the Massies—admittedly, exceptional families—apply themselves wholeheartedly to meet the challenge. They focus as a unit on the disability to such a degree that it actually becomes an asset for the afflicted member. The life of the family centers upon and is basically organized around that disability. Often such concentration exacts a high toll from other siblings in the family and may have other kinds of warping effects. But it does mobilize the family to achieve the maximum results in the rehabilitation of the disabled member. Without the family's cooperation with the patient's physical therapist or rehabilitation team, it is difficult for the patient to commit himself consistently to making progress and to realize his potential usefulness within the limits of his disability.

Some families, like some rehabilitation centers, engage in a form of collective denial. They do not allow the patient to experience depression, to share feelings of isolation, disappointment, and unhappiness. Keeping the patient in a cheerful frame of mind is regarded as helpful, since the psychological state does influence the physical. For example, the Massies mention that their son's bleeding time was affected by his immediate mental state; when his mood was favorable, bleeding stopped quickly. However, efforts to prevent feelings of depression and despair in the disabled create a serious dilemma because they militate against the working through of depressive states and feelings about the disability, which is a vital aspect of the rehabilitation program.

Except, perhaps, for their extreme use of denial, there is no evidence that those with severe physical handicaps differ psychologically from other population groups (Barker, Wright, and Gonick 1946). And their use of denial often appears to be fostered by the environment; people are not disposed to "hear them out." The views of many psychiatrists, including Sullivan, have created an unfriendly climate for the application of psychoanalysis in these cases. We have been warned, in effect: Don't touch the physically disabled. These people are not going to go through psychoanalysis. They don't want to expose themselves.

It took a long time before I was able to listen to the feelings that the physically disabled patients reveal about themselves. Nevertheless, when I was able to listen, I discovered that they were able to talk about their disabilities.

One day, shortly after beginning my work at Blythedale, I suddenly found myself encircled by a phalanx of wheelchairs. At first I wanted to run away, but all of a sudden I said, "God, how I hate it." Becoming aware of my hatred for their plight made a crucial difference. It helped me to develop the ability to listen to the physically handicapped and to intervene appropriately in those cases. After that, I found it possible to tell these patients, "You must hate this disability."

I also recall an interview with the mother of a nine-year-old boy who had been crippled by poliomyelitis. She thought that her son was making a good adjustment to his disability until one day, through the open door of his room, she witnessed him holding up his maimed hands before a mirror and repeatedly exclaiming, "I hate them, I hate them."

The mother became disturbed as she watched this scene. She did not recognize that a child who is able to feel this way about a handicap is actually making a step in the right direction.

Probably the most difficult task confronting us in working for the psychological realization of a handicapped person is to allow him to mourn. This is often a painful and prolonged process in the case of a severe disability (Szalita 1964), and, in order to help the person undergo it and come to terms with his loss of function or deformity, one needs to have empathy. In the process of developing appropriate responsiveness to a person who is striving to become free of his struggle with a severe disability, one has to come to grips with one's own fears of physical mutilation.

As Zweig (1939) pointed out, insight once gained into human nature grows in mysterious ways. Experiencing vicariously any one form of ugly suffering is a tragic lession through which one acquires understanding of all forms of suffering, even the most abnormal and that which is most foreign to the beholder. Affliction per se does not generate wisdom, but suffering that is accompanied by insight and a gradual emancipation from narcissistic self-involvement leads to empathy. Empathy in turn contributes to the resolution of grief and a new commitment to life.

Conclusions

Without some compassion, one cannot really be of significant help to the physically handicapped and their families. But one has to distinguish between two kinds of compassion. One kind, which is accompanied by anger and pain, is a form of self-protection and vulnerability that evokes angry feelings toward the person who provoked those emotions and wants him out of the way. One observes this attitude, for example, among hypersensitive hospital attendants who do not want to enter a room where a child is dying of leukemia; they feel so sorry for that child that they leave him alone. Other workers, on the contrary, come into the room; they want to be with the child. This kind of compassion, which is free of self-centeredness, plays an important role in clinical work with the physically disabled and their families. The practitioner who possesses it can respond readily to their patients' needs without having to shield his own sensibilities and without making their suffering his own burden. When we respond to their needs, we discover that they make constructive use of the help we give them.

NOTE

1. Blythedale Children's Hospital at Valhalla, New York, is a ninety-two-bed research center for the care of children with long-term illnesses. The hospital has teaching associations with several medical schools and other teaching centers.

REFERENCES

Barker, R. H.; Wright, B. A.; and Gonick, H. R. 1946. *Adjustment to Physical Handicap and Illness: A Survey of the Social Psychology of Physique and Disability*. Bulletin 55. New York: Social Research Council.

Cayley, C. K. 1954. Psychiatric aspects of rehabilitation of the physically handicapped. *American Journal of Psychotherapy* 8:518–539.

Greenberg, R. 1974. Psychiatric aspects of physical disability in children and adolescents. *Adolescent Psychiatry* 3:298–307.

Group for the Advancement of Psychiatry. 1973. *The Joys and Sorrows of Parenthood*. New York: Scribner's.

Keller, H. 1902. *The Story of My Life*. New York: Dell, 1965.

Mann, T. 1939. *Royal Highness*. New York: Knopf.

Massie, R., and Massie, S. 1975. *Journey*. New York: Knopf.

Szalita, A. B. 1964. De fysisk handicappede. *Nordisk Psykiatrisk Tidsskrift* 18:479–484.

Szalita, A. B. 1968. The combined use of family interviews and individual therapy in schizophrenia. *American Journal of Psychotherapy* 22:419–430.

Zweig, S. 1939. *Beware of Pity*. New York: Viking.

PART IV

THERAPEUTIC APPROACHES IN ADOLESCENT PSYCHIATRY

EDITORS' INTRODUCTION

All of the approaches to the study of the adolescent phenomena finally converge upon technical aspects of the therapeutic process. This is to be expected in a volume that is directed to clinically oriented readers who are constantly faced with the necessity of understanding and dealing with confusing and needy patients.

Perhaps some of our confusion is the outcome of the problems that confront us. The adolescent patient—with his poorly defined identity, his lack of coping techniques, and his vacillating self-esteem—does not give us much to grasp, that is, to fit into a conceptual scheme that permits us to plan therapeutic strategy. He presents us with a challenge that perplexes and yet promises to widen our clinical perspective.

The therapeutic frame of reference represents an area in which many different currents meet. The chapters in this section highlight this confluence. For example, developmental theory and family dynamics gain equal prominence. Such orientations naturally lead to the construction of specific technical maneuvers as well as the formulation of therapeutic goals. Another therapeutic area, usually neglected, is the psychopharmacological parameter. Here we attempt to right that wrong.

Otto F. Kernberg discusses several important problems in the psychoanalytic psychotherapy of borderline late adolescents. He believes that the severely disturbed adolescent requires psychoanalytic psychotherapy, similar to the adult patient, while with well-functioning adolescents the early focus in psychotherapy may be on normal developmental tasks. In the intensive treatment of severely disturbed adolescents, analysis of cultural stereotypes as secondary defenses against full emergence of identity diffusion in the transference is necessary. Structuralized borderline pathology requires individual treatment; severe family psychopathology, requiring therapy, should be treated by another therapist. Borderline adolescents suffer from lack of differentiation of internalized object representations and excessive involvement, failure to complete developmental tasks, and lack of integration of superego structures. Normal developmental tasks of adolescence do not require special modifications of therapeutic technique, but will as a consequence of the resolution of primitive transferences resume and be completed naturally during advanced stages of treatment. Finally, he points out that intolerance of painful subjective experience brings about action in the transference as a defense against experiencing and introspection. Regression in the formal structure of communication—to action—is the most important aspect of aggression in the transference of borderline patients and appears in therapy as projective identifications.

Edward R. Shapiro and Jonathan E. Kolb discuss the tactics of engagement of the family during the hospitalization of a disturbed adolescent. They believe that a successful outcome requires the cooperation and participation of the family, but outline the regression stimulated by the separation. The Multiple Family Meeting, designed to create an opportunity for the examination of shared experience and for the broadening of opportunities for collaboration, is described. Three dynamic themes emerge in this setting: the fight/flight mode, the dependency mode, and the hope mode. Recognition and understanding of these tensions allow for perspective and resolution.

Max Sugar focuses on therapeutic approaches to the borderline patient and describes a variety of parameters that may be used in addition to individual therapy when dyadic treatment is inadequate at a particular point in the therapeutic relationship. Sugar describes the use of group therapy, home as a mental hospital, family therapy, network therapy, and chemotherapy as addenda to intensive psychoanalytic psychotherapy in borderline personalities.

John L. Schimel presents an overview of therapeutic fads in child and adolescent psychiatry. He views the current preoccupation with the family as a rather overdetermined approach and presents balanced clinical ideas for therapeutic planning. He believes in flexibility toward parents and the family and recommends careful attention to the development of the therapeutic alliance.

Arthur D. Sorosky, as Special Editor, points out that adolescents are often the forgotten patient as recipients of psychopharmacological agents. Drugs are widely used in adolescents but an organized scientific base of information has not developed. Toward that end Dennis P. Cantwell discusses the use of stimulant medication, Theodore Van Putten describes prescribing antipsychotic drugs, Samuel Black deals with the minor tranquilizers, and Gabrielle A. Carlson describes the use of lithium carbonate.

OTTO F. KERNBERG

Paradoxically enough, the more severely disturbed the late-adolescent patient, the more the treatment should resemble that given to an adult patient. For adolescent patients who are functioning fairly well, the early focus in psychotherapy is on the normal developmental tasks of adolescence. With adolescents who are not functioning well, on the other hand, it is necessary to work on the severely distorted, primitive transference dispositions, and these are similar to those found in adult borderline patients. The implication is that, when—as with borderline patients—the normal developmental tasks of adolescence have not been accomplished, psychoanalytic psychotherapy as conceptualized for the treatment of adult patients best serves the purpose of resolving primitive transferences, primitive defensive operations, and the ego and superego distortions that militate against carrying out these developmental tasks. The resolution of borderline psychopathology by analytic means will permit the spontaneous resumption of normal developmental processes later on. It thus seems reasonable for me to begin by briefly outlining my approach to the treatment of adult borderline patients.

Treatment Techniques

GENERAL TREATMENT APPROACH

For patients with good ego strength, a satisfactory sense of identity, and a predominance of advanced or neurotic defense mechanisms centering upon repression—in short, for neurotic patients with relatively nonsevere character pathology—where for individual reasons a psychoanalytically oriented psychotherapy rather than psychoanalysis proper may be indicated, it is possible to obtain good treatment results with psychotherapy that combines various exploratory (or expressive) and supportive features. Under these circumstances, there are combinations of expressive and supportive technical tools that can be harmoniously integrated into the individual treatment. In contrast, for most borderline cases, I have stressed the indication for a treatment approach that is a purely expressive or interpretive psychotherapy, a psychoanalytic psychotherapy in a strict sense (Kernberg 1978a). Here, I strongly believe, the combination of expressive and supportive features is counterindicated and may seriously threaten the effectiveness of a psychoanalytic approach.

In borderline cases, because primitive transferences (Kernberg 1976) are immediately available, predominate as resistances, and, in fact, reflect the severity of intrapsychic and interpersonal disturbances, they can and need to be focused upon immediately, interpreting them in terms of "here and now." This leads into genetic reconstructions only at late stages of the treatment, when primitive transferences determined by part-object relations have been transformed into advanced transferences or total-object relations, thus approaching the more realistic experiences of childhood that lend themselves to genetic reconstructions (Kernberg 1975b, 1976). Interpretation of the transference requires that the therapist maintain a position of technical neutrality. There should be no interpretation of primitive transferences without a firm, consistent, stable maintenance of reality boundaries in the therapeutic situation; the therapist must be cautious not to be "sucked into" the reactivation of pathological, primitive object relations by the patient. Insofar as both transference interpretation and a position of technical neutrality require the use of clarification and interpretation and contraindicate the use of suggestive and manipulative techniques, clarification and interpretation are maintained as principal techniques.

Therefore, the similarity between psychoanalytic psychotherapy—which must remain purely expressive or exploratory—and psychoanalysis is much greater in the case of the borderline conditions than in the case of patients with milder psychological illness. One might say that, in psychoanalytic psychotherapy of borderline conditions, the tactical approach to each session may be almost indistinguishable from psychoanalysis proper, and that only from a long-term, strategic view-point do the differences between the two forms of treatment emerge. By the same token, the cleavage between psychoanalytic psychotherapy and supportive psychotherapy is sharp and definite in the case of borderline patients, while it is more gradual and blurred in cases with less severe illness. However, although the technical approach to borderline patients is similar to psychoanalysis, the therapeutic atmosphere is quite different: the significant replacement of verbal communication of the patient's intrapsychic experience by non-verbal communication that colors the therapeutic interaction creates a distinctive therapeutic situation. Technically, however, the therapist's approach remains psychoanalytic. In short, it is not possible to bring about significant personality modifications by means of psychotherapy in patients with borderline personality organization without exploring and resolving primitive transferences, and this requires a close adherence to the analytic approach, although not psychoanalysis proper. I think it important always to maintain a careful distinction between psychoanalytic psychotherapy and psychoanalysis.

What, then, are the differences between the psychoanalytic psychotherapy of borderline conditions and psychoanalysis proper? First, in contrast to psychoanalysis proper, transference interpretation cannot be systematic. Because of the need to focus on the severity of acting out and on the disturbances in the patient's external reality (which may threaten the continuity of the treatment as well as the patient's psychosocial survival) and also because, as part of acting out of primitive transferences, the treatment easily comes to replace life, transference interpretation in each session has to be codetermined by (1) the predominant conflicts in immediate reality; (2) the overall, specific goals of treatment; and (3) the immediately predominant transference paradigm.

Second, there is also a limitation on technical neutrality derived from the need to establish parameters of technique which include, in certain cases, a structuring of the patient's external life and the establishment of a teamwork approach with patients who cannot function autonomously during long stretches of their psychotherapy. Technical neutrality is therefore a theoretical baseline from which deviations must occur again and again—to be reduced, again and again, by interpretation.

Third, over long stretches of time, transference interpretation with borderline patients has to be carried out on the level of an "as if" analysis, that is, centering on the construction of hypothetical meanings of what is activated in the present interaction and reflecting the patient's present intrapsychic structures but not tracing them back to any particular time of his past. These structures are only indirectly linked to the past genetic determinants, hence, a limitation is introduced to the extent to which present, unconscious reality in the transference corresponds to the patient's past significant interactions. While transference always refers to unconscious fantasies from the past, the relationship between such fantasies and actual experiences in the past is closer in neurotic and normal than in borderline patients. By the same token, the meaning of the transference paradigms, particularly of primitive transference paradigms repeatedly activated in borderline patients, gradually shifts in the context of new, integrative meanings that emerge as the treatment goes on. The relationship between present structure, genetic development, and past developmental history is more indirect than in neurotic cases, and this brings about a qualitative difference from the conditions of standard psychoanalysis that is important to keep in mind.

The psychoanalytic psychotherapy of borderline personality organization thus centers on the analysis of the patient/therapist interaction, with transference interpretations that gradually transform primitive transferences into advanced ones and gradually permit a shift from constructions into genetic reconstructions. The position of technical neutrality, constantly challenged and undermined, is interpretively reinstated again and again, and while the analysis of the transference is strongly influenced by the patient's immediate reality situation and overall treatment goals, the therapist must consistently refrain from dealing with such immediate reality and moving toward such long-range goals in other than interpretive ways.

With the typical borderline patient, the therapist's reliance on verbal communication as a reflection of the patient's intrapsychic state is often overshadowed by the need to rely on the examination of the total therapeutic interaction. In earlier work (Kernberg 1975b) I have described three successive steps by which primitive transferences, reflecting part-object relations, may be interpreted in the transference and integrated into total-object relations, which then permit the gradual reconstruction of the patient's past in advanced stages of the treatment. Step 1 consists in the clarification of the primitive emotional relationship now enacted in the patient/therapist interaction; step 2, in the definition of the self- and object polarity of that interaction and their alternating attributions by the patient (so that he and the therapist seem to interchange roles); and step 3 in the integration of such part-object relations with their complementary, dissociated, and opposite part-object relations, so that, eventually, advanced or neurotic—in contrast to primitive—transferences develop which then permit analytic work along the standard methods corresponding to psychoanalysis proper.

SUPPORTIVE EFFECTS OF NONSUPPORTIVE TECHNIQUE

I have stressed the importance of maintaining an attitude of technical neutrality in order to be able to interpret the primitive transferences occurring in the patient/therapist interaction. If we define supportive techniques as Bibring (1954) had suggested, including emotional and rational support, suggestion, giving advice, manipulation of environmental variables or external situations in the patient's life, and the therapist's actively presenting himself as a model to be imitated (or simply his clearly taking a stand on one or the other side of the patient's intrapsychic conflicts), then the therapist's technical position cannot be neutral and his interpreting the transference must suffer. I cannot emphasize strongly enough that a heavy price is paid whenever the therapist yields to these temptations. Immediate improvement is heavily paid for with the patient's later rationalizations of transference developments that cannot be resolved fully and thus limit the fundamental personality changes attempted in this treatment.

However, as Loewald (1960) has pointed out with reference to the standard psychoanalytic situation, the therapist's function in interpreting the patient's emotional reality itself reflects that his ego is functioning at a more integrative level than the patient's ego is capable of at the time of transference regression. The patient's identifying himself with the interpreting function of the therapist is therefore a growth experience. The patient identifying himself with the therapist under such conditions implies, Loewald observed, an identification with an object image of the therapist and with a self-image as well, that is, the image of the patient himself as perceived by the therapist.

To put it differently, the patient's identification with the therapist's interpreting function reflects an identification with a dyadic object relation of a good or helpful kind. This process, which normally occurs in subtle and unobtrusive ways in the treatment of neurotic patients, is strongly accentuated in the psychoanalytic psychotherapy of border-line conditions, where identity diffusion interferes with precisely the integrative function that the therapist can provide. Insofar as the actual age difference between an adult psychotherapist and an adolescent borderline patient magnifies this discrepancy, certain supportive effects of a purely analytic technique are significant in the treatment situation. Naturally, various transference distortions interfere with this identification process, and the more consistently the primitive transferences are interpreted the more this supportive effect of the psychotherapy can become operative.

It is very important for the therapist working with borderline patients to be able to integrate both cognitive and emotional aspects of chaotic, dissociated, primitive transferences in his understanding of the therapeutic situation. He brings together, by means of his interpretive comments, what is actively split off, dispersed, or dissociated in the patient. Winnicott, with his concept of the "holding environment" (1965), stressed the emotional implications of a nonintrusive empathy with the patient. Bion, with his concept of the analyst as a "container" (1970), stressed the therapist's cognitive function in providing the patient with a model of an "apparatus for thinking thoughts" that the patient cannot, initially, tolerate within himself.

Whereas the basis for potential growth provided by this integrative, cognitive-emotional function in the therapeutic situation is more important with borderline patients than with the standard psychoanalytic cases, this function may, at the same time, stir up the most intense experiences of hatred and envy in borderline patients: hatred because significant learning about oneself—as opposed to defensive dissociation—is always painful, and thus the therapist's helping attitude, paradoxically, is painful as well; and envy because primitive aggression frequently takes the form of envious strivings to destroy the therapist as a giving maternal image. Therefore, the interpretation of the patient's unconscious need to reject or destroy the therapist's integrative function may be an important aspect of interpretive work within an essentially technical neutral position.

Technical neutrality means equidistance from the forces codetermining the patient's intrapsychic conflicts and not lack of warmth or empathy with him. One still hears comments implying that borderline patients need, first of all, empathic understanding rather than a focused theory and cognitively sharpened interpretations based on such a theory. All psychotherapy requires as a baseline the therapist's capacity for authentic human warmth and empathy, and these qualities are preconditions for any appropriate psychotherapeutic work. Empathy, however, is not only the therapist's intuitive emotional awareness of the patient's central emotional experience at a certain point; it must also include the therapist's capacity to empathize with what the patient cannot tolerate within himself. Therapeutic empathy, therefore, transcends that involved in ordinary human interactions and also includes the therapist's integration, on a cognitive and emotional level, of what is actively dissociated or split off in borderline patients.

Special Problems in the Psychotherapy of Adolescents

The clinical experiences underlying this and the following sections of this chapter were carried out with fifteen-year and older patients, that is, they focus on issues in the psychoanalytic psychotherapy of borderline late adolescents. Paulina Kernberg's recent review of the pathology of early adolescent borderline patients (1978) offers complementary views and findings.

DIAGNOSTIC CONFUSION AND CULTURAL STEREOTYPES

There is still a tendency in the literature to confuse normal and neurotic identity crises in adolescents with the severe syndrome of identity diffusion that, together with a predominance of primitive defensive operations, characterize borderline personality organization. This confusion is particularly damaging in the psychotherapy of borderline adolescent patients. The syndrome of identity diffusion, the severe pathology of object relations with predominance of part-object transferences, and the lack of superego integration (with failure in the capacity to assume responsibility, concern, investment in values, and basic honesty) all reflect typical borderline personality organization and are not normal characteristics of adolescence. Unless the therapist keeps this in mind, it will become much easier for the adolescent patient under the influence of his psychopathology to be tempted to exploit the therapist's unawareness and to take refuge in stereotyped assumptions of adolescence as a natural time of chaos, confusion, irresponsibility, and lack of capacity for investment in object relations in depth.

I have earlier (1978b) explored the differential diagnosis of normal adolescent turmoil and borderline personality organization. I have proposed the following criteria for the differential diagnosis of borderline personality organization. First, the presence of identity diffusion, that is, of a lack of integration of the concepts of the self and of significant others (in other words, of self- and object representations); second, the predominance of a constellation of primitive defensive operations centering around splitting; and third, the maintenance of reality testing. The first two criteria differentiate borderline conditions from the symptomatic neuroses and nonborderline character pathology, which present a solid ego identity and a predominance of defense mechanisms centering around repression; the third criterion differentiates borderline conditions from the psychoses. Reality testing refers to the capacity to differentiate self from nonself and intrapsychic from external origin of stimuli, and to the presence of empathy with ordinary social criteria of reality in interpersonal situations.

In applying these criteria to the initial evaluation of adolescent patients, the clinician is faced with various complicating features. First, the relative severity of the disorganizing effects of symptomatic neuroses in adolescence, typically of severe anxiety and depression, may affect the adolescent's overall functioning at home, in school, and with peers to an extent that may resemble the more severe social breakdown typical of borderline conditions.

Second, the presence of identity crises, characterized by rapidly shifting identifications with this or that social ideology or group (so that what appears on the surface as "radical changes" in personality may appear in the course of a few months), raise the question of whether the much more severe syndrome of identity diffusion is present.

Third, severe pathology of object relations that reflects an underlying syndrome of identity diffusion may be misinterpreted as a reflection of neurotic conflicts regarding dependent and rebellious needs, resulting in a failure to recognize the severely pathological nature of conflicts with parental authorities, with siblings, and at school. To the contrary, nonborderline neurotic conflicts with parents and authority may intensify and activate the potential for primitive defensive operations in an essentially nonborderline patient, so that what appears as omnipotent control, projective identification, and devaluation may become prevalent in certain object relations of some nonborderline patients.

Fourth, antisocial behavior in adolescence may be both an expression of a "normal" or neurotic adaptation to an antisocial cultural subgroup (and thus be relatively nonmalignant) or reflect severe character pathology and borderline personality organization appearing as an adaptation to an antisocial group. Accordingly, the frequently misused label "adjustment reaction in adolescence" is not so much a diagnosis as an alarm signal indicating the need to evaluate in depth the personality structure of an adolescent in social conflicts.

Fifth, normal neurotic and infantile narcissistic reactions that are so frequent in adolescence may mask a severe narcissistic personality structure, particularly when there are no antisocial features to immediately alert the diagnostician to the evaluation of narcissistic, in addition to antisocial, pathology. Narcissistic pathology may present not as typical conflicts around omnipotent control, grandiosity, and devaluation, but rather as a strange oscillation between excellent school functioning and puzzling failure in competitive tasks.

Sixth, the normal emergence of multiple perverse sexual trends in adolescence may imitate the condensation of genital and pregenital features (with the predominance of aggressive conflicts) that is typical for borderline personality organization: I have earlier (1975a) pointed out that the nature of the predominant unconscious conflicts is not a good diagnostic element.

Seventh, and finally, the more slowly developing psychotic conditions, such as chronic schizophrenia reactions, may mask as borderline conditions because of the predominance of severe pathology of object relations, social withdrawal, and severe character pathology in general. Also, while hallucinations are rather easily diagnosed, insidious delusion formation may at first be misinterpreted as, for example, hypochondriacal tendencies or excessive preoccupation with physical appearance.

I wish to underline the need for a careful initial evaluation of the adolescent who comes to treatment and, once the diagnosis of borderline personality organization has been made and psychoanalytic psychotherapy been indicated, the need to interpret consistently the manifestations of identity diffusion, primitive defensive operations in the transference, and superego pathology.

Because of the significant age difference and, therefore, the difference in role and status between the adolescent patient and the adult psychotherapist, the former usually was tempted to define himself as "an adolescent" relating to a stereotyped "adult." For example, the borderline patient's contention, with the slightest of justifications, that the therapist thinks, behaves, and treats him exactly as the patient's parents may be less a specific transference manifestation than an effort on the patient's part to avoid awareness of his confusion, suspicion, derogatory behavior, etc., regarding the significant grownups in his life by lumping them all together in simplistic stereotypes.

As part of the systematic examination of the therapeutic interaction, therefore, the therapist may have to examine the patient's denial of the therapist's individuality as well as his own by taking refuge in stereotyped behavior of a cultural subgroup. A position of technical neutrality does not mean that the therapist permits the patient to unload on him all the accumulated biases and stereotypes that both protect the patient against and yet reflect his identity diffusion. It is possible to clarify such distortions without telling the patient, "No, I'm not the way you see me." The general statement, "You have no reason to see me this way rather than in many other ways; therefore, there must be meaning to the fact that it is so important to you to see me in precisely this way," covers the issue.

Adolescent borderline patients often strenuously attempt to induce in the therapist the very attitudes they accuse adults, particularly their parents, of having toward them. This reflects particularly the mechanism of projective identification (Kernberg 1975a). Under these conditions, the therapist's alertness to such developments may permit him to interpret the patient's unconscious effort to make him into one more image of the parents. At the same time, the therapist may have to resist a tendency to behave in a way opposite to that the adolescent patient describes his family as behaving; the therapist must beware of trying to foster a good therapeutic relationship by seductive means. A seductive attitude toward adolescents is also fostered by the general idealization of adolescence, so prevalent in our culture, and by the therapist's unconscious efforts to defend himself against unconscious envy of adolescents by means of idealizing or imitating them.

Sometimes, simply the effort to resist the patient's attempts to stereotype the therapist as conventional may induce in the therapist a wish to show the patient that he is nonconventional. In a deeper sense, of course, the therapist has to be nonconventional in standing up to cultural stereotypes enacted in the transference; but his nonconventionality should emerge by means of his absolutely serious, fearless, consistent, and personal way of raising questions regarding what is going on in the treatment and his refusal to allow the patient to seduce him into certain role models. A serious, concerned, nonseductive, nonidealizing, moral yet nonmoralistic, nondemonstratively unconventional attitude provides the ingredients of technical neutrality.

In summary of this point, the analysis of cultural stereotypes as secondary defenses against full emergence of identity diffusion in the transference is an important aspect, particularly in early stages of psychotherapy with borderline adolescents.

PSYCHOANALYTIC PSYCHOTHERAPY AND FAMILY STRUCTURES

There seems to be mounting evidence, derived from the clinical situation and research, that borderline adolescents come from severely pathological families (Goldstein and Jones 1977; Shapiro, Zinner, Shapiro, and Berkovitz 1975). For practical purposes, the question is often raised to what extent the borderline adolescent patient simply reflects severe family psychopathology or internalized, structured illness. I think that whenever a careful study of the adolescent patient demonstrates the existence of the syndrome of identity diffusion and of predominance of primitive defensive operations, we must assume, regardless of what the family contributions to his illness has been in the past, that the patient has a bona fide structuralized borderline pathology that will require intense individual treatment.

For the purpose of carrying out psychoanalytic psychotherapy as defined, however, I think it is crucial that the psychotherapist have an exclusive psychotherapeutic relationship with the adolescent, and that family therapy, if indicated, be carried out by another therapist. If the patient is to be involved in that family therapy, the family therapist should have the family's and the adolescent patient's authorization to communicate his observations to the patient's psychotherapist, thus establishing a teamwork approach similar to what I have recommended for those borderline patients whose severe acting-out potential cannot otherwise be controlled (Kernberg 1975a).

The general implication of what I have said is that, while the family, particularly the parents, may have had fundamental contributions in inducing borderline psychopathology in their child and in maintaining it presently, the diagnosis of borderline personality organization implies severe, long-standing pathological intrapsychic structures that now have an autonomous existence of their own.

The predominance of primitive defensive operations, particularly projective identification, omnipotence, devaluation, splitting, and denial, may permit the adolescent borderline patient to induce complementary pathology in the key family members with whom he lives and bring about self-fulfilling prophesies in all his interactions that can become a most powerful resistance in the treatment. It is important for the therapist to evaluate the extent to which the patient is responding to pathological pressures from his parents and to what extent he is inducing such pressures in them.

The answer to these questions is usually found in the transference developments, particularly in the patient's unconscious efforts to reproduce his parents' behavior in the therapist. Systematic analyses of such attempts in the transference may be the first step in helping the patient become aware of how he perpetuates pathological conditions at home. For example, the patient's pathological submission to sadistic behavior of his parents as perceived by him is usually reflected in the recreation of the situation with inverted roles in the psychotherapy. Unconsciously, adolescent patients may treat the therapist in omnipotent and sadistic ways, projecting onto him their masochistically suffering, mistreated, devalued self-representation, while identifying themselves with a triumphant, sadistic, grandiose parental image.

The therapist's conception of primitive transferences as reflecting the activation of such part-object relations with roles reversal will permit him to interpret this transference relationship and then apply his interpretation to the patient's relations with his family. In more general terms, the systematic analysis of the therapeutic interaction, with a sharp focus on the activation of primitive part-object relations in it, is the first step leading to the interpretation of the patient's pathological interactions in his home. However, it is important to keep in mind that such interpretation is not a genetic reconstruction and that, in turn, the present pathological interactions with the parents may also reflect a part-object relation. This part-object relation may be defensively split off from opposite, contradictory part-object relations that need to be examined first, before an understanding can be gained of the total underlying pathogenic object-relation against which both the present relation with the parents and the respective transference developments are defenses.

BORDERLINE PATHOLOGY AND DEVELOPMENTAL TASKS OF ADOLESCENCE

By definition, late-adolescent borderline patients have not accomplished the normal developmental tasks of adolescence, particularly (1) the achievement of an integrated self-concept or a sense of ego identity; (2) the consolidation of a normal sexual identity, with the predominance of a heterosexual identification, subordination of partial polymorphous to genital strivings, and the beginning integration of tender and erotic trends into a relatively stable object relation, reflected in the capacity to fall in love; (3) the loosening of the ties to the parents, in reality linked with the appropriate differentiation of sexual and generational roles in the expanding social interactions with other adults and peers (and the corresponding, intrapsychic individualization and stability of object relations); and (4) the replacement of infantile superego regulations by a relatively abstracted and depersonified, firmly internalized, yet flexible system of unconscious and conscious morality that integrates adult sexual tolerance with firm repression of direct oedipal strivings.

In contrast to a real loosening of ties to the infantile objects, reflected normally in increasing distance and yet deepening object relations with the parents, borderline adolescents, suffering as they do from lack of differentiation of internalized object representations, evidence an excessive involvement, violent rebelliousness, overdependency, and general chaos in the—relatively unstructured—interpersonal relations at home.

Similarly, in psychotherapy, not only does the patient overidentify the therapist with his parental images or defensively experience him as different in a fantastic way, but a chaotic alternation of mutually split-off, partial parental, and combined father/mother images and a defensive refusal to really experience the therapist as different from the parents and as a differentiated person in his own right develop. Differences, for the adolescent borderline patient, can often only signify more threatening chaos, while the individuality of the therapist cannot be grasped.

This situation can easily mislead the therapist to assume that the adolescent patient needs new identification models and that direct educational efforts may be warranted by means of which the therapist establishes himself as new and different. The developmental task of the borderline adolescent who needs to complete his processes of individuation and differentiation are better served by the interpretation and working through of primitive transferences. Otherwise, new surface adaptations of the borderline adolescent to the therapist may evolve, activating an "as if" quality in the therapeutic interaction and the presence of what Winnicott (1965) called the "false self."

In contrast, resolution of primitive transference by analytic means and resumption of normal growth processes in borderline adolescents go hand in hand. The implication is that, when in advanced stages of the treatment the adolescent patient gradually recognizes the therapist as a differentiated individual, the integration of and differentiation from the parental images will occur in parallel fashion.

To illustrate this process with the vicissitudes of two defensive operations that span the developmental field of primitive and early, as well as sophisticated and advanced, defense mechanisms, the changes in idealization and devaluative processes will follow naturally the resolution of primitive transferences in the therapeutic situation. Thus, the primitive idealization of poorly differentiated adult or peer models that represent split-off part-object relations will gradually shift into the integrative idealization processes that reflect reaction formations against guilt and, later on, into the normal projection of sophisticated idealized values and aspirations that emerge in normal falling in love and the idealization of admired teachers. And the primitive devaluation of the parents (the counterpart of split-off primitive idealizations) will gradually become integrated into an age-appropriate, hypercritical but ambivalent recognition of their realistic features, a disappointment reaction that now contains elements of guilt and mourning and acceptance of the loss of primitive idealized parental images.

If and when an analytic stance is maintained consistently, the real relation with the therapist will eventually become the testing ground of a resumption of normal developmental processes.

Another area of severe borderline pathology, namely, the lack of integration of superego structures, may superficially resemble the normal adolescent features of partial redissolution and reprojection of the superego (Jacobson 1964). The emergence of primitive, dissociated sexual and aggressive drive derivatives in borderline conditions may mask as the instinctual irruptions of normal adolescence. It is, at first, difficult to differentiate drive derivatives that emerge in consciousness in the context of an integrated self-concept and object constancy from drive derivatives that express dissociated part-object relations. However, a consistently analytic approach to this material, the therapist's exploring the homosexual and polymorphous perverse impulses in the light of their functions within part- or total-object relations activated in the transference, will differentiate normal developmental drive irruptions from structured part-object relationships and permit the integration of object relations rather than the premature suppression of certain drive derivatives.

The neurotic or normal adolescent will, rather soon, repress certain polymorphous perverse drive derivatives and integrate others into his conscious ego. The borderline adolescent patient, in contrast, may have to experience consciously and express in the transference (or in transference acting out) sexual and aggressive drives that are dissociated and/or condensed in various ways, over many months or years of treatment. Here, the normal integrative and repressive tasks of adolescence will eventually follow the integration of the self, of the superego, and of repression barriers of the ego. In other words, integration of part- into total-object relations will eventually bring about the replacement of dissociative by repressive defenses.

In short, I believe that in these cases the normal developmental tasks of adolescence do not require special modifications of the psychotherapeutic technique proposed for borderline personality organization in general but will, as a consequence of the resolution of primitive transferences, be resumed and completed naturally in the advanced stages of the treatment.

Types and Management of Acting Out

I shall now examine further the nature of the basic interaction of patient and therapist, which by definition constitutes the primary focus of systematic exploration in psychoanalytic psychotherapy. It needs to be stressed that my focus upon this interaction is very far from a simplistic, psychosocial model of interaction that relates present interpersonal interactions to past interpersonal interactions of the patient on a one to one basis. In the case of borderline personality organization, the present interaction expresses pathological intrapsychic structures that reflect primitive types of interaction of a fantastic nature— fantastic both in the sense of the unreal, emotionally threatening, and uncanny, and in the sense of a fragmented, distorted, part-object relation—that only indirectly reflects the actual pathogenic relations of the past. The focus on present interactions in the case of the treatment of borderline conditions really starts out as the focus on the intrapsychic life of the patient as it is expressed in the therapeutic interaction. Rapidly, particularly with adolescent borderline patients, their intolerance of painful subjective experience brings about action in the transference as a defense against experiencing and introspection. The importance of the psychotherapist's technical neutrality lies precisely in the need to maintain an objective frame in the present interpersonal situation, so that its distortion by action reflecting a primitive transference relationship can be highlighted.

Borderline personality organization always reflects severe character pathology and, therefore, a predominance of expression of unconscious intrapsychic conflicts in the form of chronic, repetitive behavior patterns and expression by nonverbal means in general. Therefore, the nonverbal aspects of the interaction with the therapist supply fundamental information, replacing to quite an extent what the content of verbal communication conveys in the standard psychoanalytic situation. In other words, the expression of dissociated or split-off units of self- and object representations interacting under the organizing influence of a certain affect state attaches itself, so to speak, to the actual interaction of self and object in the therapeutic encounter.

By means of his nonverbal behavior, especially by a particular use of language as action and as a means of controlling the interpersonal situation, the patient attempts to activate his intrapsychic part-object relations in the present interpersonal one. In fact, primitive transferences may be conceived as mutually dissociated units of strange, bizarre, primitive units of interaction that the integrative understanding of the therapist transforms by his interpretations into the patient's subjective experience. One might say that in this transformation of intrapsychic conflict into interpersonal action the patient is resorting to a means of communication and relationship that, genetically speaking, predates the predominance of communication by verbal means: regression in the formal structure of communication is perhaps the most important aspect of regression in the transference of borderline patients.

To reformulate all this in a still different way, the patient's expression of his intrapsychic past in terms of interpersonal action, rather than in remembering (in thoughts or feelings), illustrates the prevalence of acting out as a predominant characteristic of transference developments in borderline patients.

Acting out is a concept that has been stretched to include a broad range of phenomena: from the appearance of concrete acts or behaviors in the course of psychoanalytic or psychotherapeutic sessions (acts or behaviors that express an emerging transference disposition that the patient cannot yet tolerate subjectively); to the development of complex behaviors toward the therapist or analyst that express, in a conscious emotional development toward him, the aspect of related past pathogenic conflicts that is still repressed as an awareness of a past (in contrast to present) experience; to the development of behaviors outside the analytic setting that correspond to split-off aspects of the transference; to the patient's disturbed interpersonal relations that drain off significant intrapsychic conflicts during the treatment in general (Atkins 1970; Fenichel 1945; Freud 1968; Greenacre 1950, 1963, 1968; Grinberg 1968; Kanzer 1957, 1968; Limentani 1966; Moore 1968; Rangell 1968; Rosenfeld 1966).

Psychoanalytic discussions of the origin, mechanism, and functions of acting out are constantly complicated by this broad range of phenomena. Efforts to restrict the meaning of the term or to redefine subsets of it (for example, "acting in" as a temporary behavior expressing transference in actions in the treatment hours) have not been, it seems to me, particularly helpful.

I have found it useful to consider acting out in the broadest sense as an essential aspect of transference developments in borderline patients, and, insofar as the rapidly changing social and interpersonal world of the adolescent temporarily decreases the stability of social structures around him and fosters the expression of old and new experimental behaviors in all areas, acting out in this broad sense is particularly prevalent in borderline adolescents. One crucial task is to diagnose when "living out," as a broad disposition, becomes acting out in a narrow sense, that is, the expression in action of transference material that cannot yet be tolerated in subjective awareness.

It is helpful, at the beginning of the treatment, for the therapist to evaluate to what extent severely pathological behavior patterns need to be controlled in order to permit psychotherapy to get under way and, if in his judgment the psychotherapeutic relationship will not be able to contain predating impulsive behavior patterns that threaten the adolescent's life or the treatment, to establish a team approach, with another team member carrying out the responsibility of providing sufficient social structuring to permit stability of the therapeutic situation. It needs to be stressed that there are cases not only where some external control needs to be established to restrict certain behaviors but where, to the contrary, the structuring of external reality reflects an effort to increase the adolescent's participation in ordinary life and to provide new challenges to him in order to avoid allowing the treatment situation to become the patient's only meaningful social experience.

When can severely pathological behavior that predated the beginning of psychotherapy and continues, apparently unchanged by the psychotherapeutic relationship itself, be considered acting out? First, if and when significant changes occur in such preexisting behavioral patterns they should be explored in terms of the developments in the transference. It is important that the therapist really explore their significance rather than implicitly reward or punish behaviors that are, respectively, favorable or unfavorable. The reasons for positive changes need to be explored with the same technically neutral attitude as the reasons for deteriorating patterns.

Second, the development of a striking contrast between a psychotherapeutic relationship in which "nothing seems to happen," on the one hand, and dramatic actions occurring in the patient's external life—regardless of whether such dramatic actions predated the treatment or not—on the other, usually is a clear expression of transference developments. Here, the typical situation of borderline pathology obtains in which the patient, incapable of tolerating the intrapsychic experience of his conflicts, has to express them in actions, particularly in splitting of the transference. The availability of the therapeutic relationship should, ideally speaking, provide a new channel for expression of dissociated or repressed urges. When this does not occur, when, to the contrary, an atmosphere of emptiness in the psychotherapeutic relationship prevails, this needs to be interpreted systematically. Emptiness does not only mean that the patient feels he has nothing to say or to tell the therapist and that a general paralysis seems to have developed in the sessions. Emptiness may also be expressed as the use of language to develop a smoke screen in the hours, the filling up of the void of the hours with statements that reflect the patient's learning to speak the psychotherapy language. The therapist's consistent exploration of the reality and meanings of his interaction with the patient will provide the frame against which emptiness or fake contents reflect, in contrast, the specific part-object relationship activated in the transference that needs to be interpreted as the split-off counterpart of where the action seems to be, namely, in the patient's outside life.

Third, acting out should be interpreted under the subtle yet frequent conditions in which action takes place in the hours and has the effect of distorting, fragmenting, or temporarily destroying the reality aspects of the patient/therapist relationship. This third category of conditions is really the most important aspect of work with primitive transferences. What follows are some special types of acting out in this third, restricted, sense, and they should also illustrate the general principles involved in transference interpretation with borderline patients.

TRANSFORMATION OF A PART-OBJECT RELATION IN THE TRANSFERENCE INTO ACTION

A patient, a seventeen-year-old girl, swallowed a Darvon® pill before entering her session. She was not addicted to any drug per se but would take multiple drugs occasionally as a way to make herself feel good. This pattern predated the beginning of treatment but had now changed into the patient's casual report to me that she had taken a pill before a session. It was our understanding on initiating the treatment that I expected her to be off all drugs and that I would not prescribe any medication for her as part of our treatment arrangement. In fact, by this time, there had been several episodes of relatively severe anxiety and/or depression that could be resolved by interpretive means alone, illustrating in the process the defensive nature of the patient's request for medication.

Efforts to stimulate the patient to explore her understanding of taking a Darvon® pill this time led nowhere, except to the patient's saying, "You know, I do this quite frequently." She denied any particular feelings regarding coming to the session or surrounding the impulsive decision to take a pill. She had looked rather relaxed and at ease on entering the session. However, as I sat back, implicitly inviting her to continue talking, she became increasingly more uneasy, finally expressing her fear that I would criticize her for having taken the pill.

At first, I did not know how important it was to focus on her taking the pill and was expecting new subject matters to emerge. Now, however, I felt that this was, indeed, the predominant subject matter at this point and speculated that the patient might have taken the pill as an expression of defiance or to provoke me into critical behavior toward her and thus to allay her feelings of guilt for experiencing herself in a good relation with me (we had clarified in the past that there were deep-seated internal prohibitions against a good relation with me as a fatherly image).

I also speculated that the patient's honestly telling me that she had taken the pill contrasted with her secretive behavior in the past, but then I felt that it was an honesty not leading anywhere else and perhaps an expression in action of her sense that honest relationships led nowhere. At that point, the patient started discussing entirely different matters. I could not connect these in my mind with her having taken the pill, and I felt distracted by my thoughts about her having taken the pill and then guilty for not paying full attention to the new issues she was commenting on.

A few minutes later the patient suddenly glanced at me inquisitively and said that she was boring me. In response to my asking what made her think so, she said that I looked puzzled and distracted. I acknowledged that she had made an accurate perception and expressed my puzzlement over her change of subject and the casual nature of her comment about having taken the pill—as if she were indifferent to its meaning—in contrast to her concern over my being indifferent to something she was saying after that. I added, however, that she was right in observing that, as a consequence of having taken her more seriously than she had, I had become distracted. The patient said that she felt that I was paying attention to her only when she had a problem. I commented that I now wondered whether she had taken the pill and told me about it as an expression of her sense that only if she misbehaved would I pay any attention to her. At this point, she evidenced surprise and became thoughtful; she remembered that indeed she was worried about whether she would have anything important to tell me before she decided to take the pill. I now experienced our interaction as reflecting, at the level of this transferential aspect, the relationship between an indifferent mother who only pays attention to her child when the child misbehaves, while the patient was reenacting the role of

313

the defiant yet guilt-ridden, submissive yet suspicious, child. Further material in the hour confirmed that impression. This case illustrates a relatively simple transformation of an emotional experience into an action, with concomitant initial denial of the emotional experience. The following is a more complex form of acting out.

ACTION AS AN ACCRETION OF MEANINGS

An eighteen-year-old borderline girl who repeatedly burned herself with cigarettes (and who had been treated on several occasions for third-degree burns on her arms and legs) casually mentioned in a session that she might feel like burning herself during the time of a forthcoming absence of her therapist for a two-week period. Her comment, made casually in the context of an ongoing discussion over many weeks of whether she would be able to control her tendency to burn herself if she were permitted to stay outside the hospital (where she was an inpatient), led into renewed discussion of whether outpatient treatment for her would be feasible at this point. The realistic concerns of the therapist contrasted with the patient's apparent total indifference to the situation and with her attitude of expectation that all those who were taking care of her naturally would be worried and do something to prevent her from burning herself. On repeated occasions the therapist had explored with her the implicit atmosphere of violence and blackmail that she created around herself, innocently forcing her parents, her therapist, and her social worker to go into elaborate analysis of how to deal with her while she smilingly announced the tempting thoughts about burning herself. At the beginning of one of the last sessions before the therapist's absence, the patient said that she had made plans for spending the time of his absence at the house of a religious group that had been very supportive to her in the past and that would provide her with spiritual stimulation over this time.

The therapist's reaction to this announcement was a momentary flash of anger and then a feeling of helplessness, followed by a temptation to resign himself to let her do as she pleased without further exploration of the issue. In the course of my discussing this particular session with the therapist, it emerged that to fully understand the patient's comment the following information needed to be kept in mind. The patient was changing her plans suddenly and, by the same token, discarding with one gesture all the serious and lengthy discussions that had taken place between her parents, herself, and her social worker regarding the period of the therapist's forthcoming absence. The therapist had provided her and the social worker with the name of another psychiatrist who would be available if needed during his absence, and these plans also seemed irrelevant now. In addition, the patient had, indeed, spent some weeks in the past at that religious house, particularly at a time when violent rebelliousness against her parents was expressed in a combination of frequent escapes from the home, self-mutilating behavior, and search for ideal substitute parents, all of which had been explored in great detail in earlier stages of the psychotherapy.

Thus, her casual comment about her plans reflected her eliminating, symbolically speaking, the substance of an important aspect of her psychotherapy. In addition, the comment also reflected a very concrete depreciation of the psychotherapist as the key element in the changed constellation of her life: it was as a consequence of psychotherapy that the diffuse, destructive, chaotic behavior in all aspects of her life (of which living at that religious house was part) had been changed.

More concretely, the patient's statement reflected an almost studied thoughtlessness, presented in a natural and yet pseudothoughtful way that belied the impulsive and unreflexive nature of it. And also, attempting to seriously convince the therapist of this new plan arrived at all of a sudden (in between two sessions) illustrated, by contrast, the spurious way in which the patient seemed to have been using verbal communication to convey apparent thoughtfulness in the sessions immediately preceding this one.

What needs to be stressed is the easy, relaxed, well-organized way in which the patient presented a plan that was completely dissonant and destructive in terms of everything that had been going on in the treatment. And she did it in a few seconds, while the analysis of the implications of that statement took literally an hour of my consultation.

In other words, that statement represented a microscopic but extremely violent and severe form of acting out that reflected, rather than a condensation of various meanings into one, an intense accretion or compression of multiple meanings in such a fast and immediate way that it temporarily exploded the therapist's capacity to hold, contain, or integrate the total object relationship enacted at that point.

Such episodes are quite frequent in the treatment of borderline adolescent patients, and the immediate impact of the patient's behavior on the therapist may be precisely that kind of rage, helplessness, and discontinuity of the emotional relationship that the patient unconsciously attempts to avoid experiencing subjectively. This is the emotional reality that has been translated into action and into violent projective identification affecting the therapist.

The optimal way of dealing with this kind of acting out is for the therapist to spell out gradually and very fully all the meanings of the behavior, including the reasons for expressing in action what the patient cannot tolerate in self-awareness. The net effect of an interpretive attempt at such points is that a brief comment by the patient may have to be followed by lengthy statements from the therapist. It is as if the therapist, in a gradual reconstruction, would have to spell out what, in action, was compressed into a minimum of time, and the patient may often accuse the therapist of making a mountain out of a molehill. What is required from the therapist here is the combination of a full emotional awareness of his own reactions to the patient's action, the capacity to contain this reaction within himself without, in turn, having to act on it, and then the gradual development or recreation of all the emotional aspects of the relationship that were compressed into such brief action.

THE ISOLATION OF MEANINGFUL COMMUNICATION WITHIN CHRONIC ACTION IN THE TRANSFERENCE

The situation to be described here represents the opposite polarity of the accretion of meaning in sudden actions just described. I am referring here to borderline patients who, in concrete developments within one hour or a brief sequence of sessions, provide the key to the understanding of complex transference paradigms that appear as a chaotic although strangely repetitive sequence over a period of weeks or months.

One borderline adolescent patient with severe schizoid and masochistic features come to understand, at one point, how she experienced her mother as getting depressed every time the patient was successful or felt happy. Her mother, the patient felt, could not stand the patient's growing up and becoming independent and would mercilessly bombard the patient with questions, criticism, and ironical comments until she made the patient feel completely helpless and defeated. But when the patient was feeling resigned and depressed mother became very warm and supportive; in fact, the patient felt that when things were going poorly there was really nobody who could be as warm and giving as her mother.

This understanding, gained in the context of an integrative analysis of various part-object relations that reflected mutually split-off aspects of this same general transference paradigm, was followed by a period of rapid improvement, gain of self-confidence, increasing autonomy, and the capacity to study and broaden her social life. However, a few months later the patient reverted to periods of chronic dissatisfaction with the therapist and repetitive complaints that the therapist was controlling, rigid, dominant; that he could not tolerate the idea of the patient's becoming more independent, etc. The interpretation of this experience as an attribution to the therapist of the characteristics of her own mother led nowhere; on the contrary, the patient seemed to enjoy herself in ironic paraphrasing of the therapist's interpretations—of outguessing him step by step—and a long period of time ensued in which no understanding gained in the hours seemed to have any meaning.

Retrospectively, it seemed rather easy to interpret the patient's attitude of refusal to listen, of almost joyful destruction of everything received from the therapist, as a repetition of the relationship with mother with inverted roles. The patient now had become a sadistic, intruding mother who could not tolerate the therapist's success. However, during the many weeks in which this pattern was successfully enacted by the patient, the therapist's only hold on his own conviction that this was the meaning of her behavior was given by his keeping in his mind the understanding of the total transference transitorily gained in an earlier episode. Here, the acting out consisted not only in creating a smoke screen that would destroy earlier understanding the patient had achieved but also in the very isolated nature of understanding that the patient could tolerate in herself. In short, isolation of brief moments of understanding in depth may be in itself a form of acting out, an expression of the intolerance of learning as a continuous process because of, for example, severe unconscious guilt.

The Central Function of the Therapist as a Dyadic Polarity and the Dangers of Countertransference Acting Out

The therapist's efforts to integrate effectively and cognitively what is going on by using his subjective experience as a starting point must expand with his understanding of whatever object evidence becomes available to him through the very process of chronicity, of repetition—the diachronic sequences within the repetitively predominant transference paradigms that are so typical of borderline conditions. To maintain a perspective of understanding throughout time permits the therapist to transform his subjective experience into an interpretive statement. The main risk is the therapist's overdependence on his emotional reactions, which may in turn reflect countertransference issues in a restricted sense, that is, the effects of the therapist's unconscious transferences to his patient.

There are narcissistic temptations involved for the therapist when he puts himself at the center of understanding the patient/therapist interaction. Many borderline patients, particularly those with severely narcissistic tendencies, will accuse the therapist of grandiosity, of injecting himself artificially into a situation that, as far as the patient can see, has no emotional relevance for him at all. The therapist's reevaluating the knowledge he has about the patient's present life outside the hours, his keeping in mind the overall problems that brought the patient to treatment and the respective therapeutic goals, and, above all, his unshakable common sense in terms of starting out, before any kind of theoretical speculation, with a solid evaluation of the immediate reality of the therapeutic situation will help him to stand up to the many threats to his objectivity.

Perhaps the most difficult understanding to be acquired in the therapeutic interaction is that of the therapist's subjective experience as a reflection of a projected aspect of his patient's self-experience. In other words, it may be more difficult for the therapist to tolerate what is in part induced in him—by the patient by means of projective identification—while the patient enacts the experience of his object representation than when he represents directly the object representation of the patient's self-representation. Insofar as the patient usually sees himself as the victim of a frustrating, overwhelming, unavailable, or sadistic object, the identification with the patient's self-image at such points may be quite threatening to the therapist's containing that reaction within himself and using it for interpretive functions. Again, the theoretical understanding of the nature of reciprocal activations of part-object relations, of primitive self- and object representations in an alternating way, should help the therapist organize his experience at such moments. The therapist's tolerating his emotional experience without having to transform it into action, deriving his interpretation from this situation rather than acting upon it directly, is a major factor in helping the patient transform action into subjective experience.

Conclusions

I have first tried to spell out a theory of psychoanalytic psychotherapy that stems from standard psychoanalytic technique as a basic model or paradigm. Within this theoretical frame of reference, I have differentiated psychoanalytic psychotherapy of borderline conditions from psychoanalytic technique per se and illustrated some key aspects of this psychotherapeutic technique with clinical considerations that apply particularly, if not exclusively, to the treatment of late-adolescent borderline patients. I have stressed that the resolution of borderline pathology takes precedence over the direct focus on adolescent developmental tasks and that the structural changes that derive from resolution of primitive transferences will permit normal development to resume naturally as part of the advanced stages of treatment. Finally, I have illustrated some frequent patterns of subtle but crucial forms of transference acting out.

REFERENCES

Atkins, N. 1970. Panel report: action, acting out and the symptomatic act. *Journal of the American Psychoanalytic Association* 18:631–643.

Bibring, E. 1954. Psychoanalysis and the dynamic psychotherapies. *Journal of the American Psychoanalytic Association* 2:745–770.

Bion, W. R. 1970. *Attention and Interpretation*. London: Heinemann.

Fenichel, O. 1945. Neurotic acting out. *Psychoanalytic Revue* 39:197–206.

Freud, A. 1968. Symposium. Acting out. *International Journal of Psycho-Analysis* 49:165–170.

Goldstein, M., and Jones, J. 1977. Adolescent and familial precursors of borderline and schizophrenic conditions. In P. Hartocollis, ed. *Borderline Personality Disorders*. New York: International Universities Press.

Greenacre, P. 1950. General problems of acting out. *Psychoanalytic Quarterly* 19:455–467.

Greenacre, P. 1963. Problems of acting out in the transference relationship. *Journal of the American Academy of Child Psychiatry* 2:144–175.

Greenacre, P. 1968. Symposium. The psychoanalytic process, transference, and acting out. *International Journal of Psycho-Analysis* 49:211–218.

Grinberg, L. 1968. Symposium. On acting out and its roles in the psychoanalytic process. *International Journal of Psycho-Analysis* 49:171–178.

Jacobson, E. 1964. *The Self and the Object World*. New York: International Universities Press.

Kanzer, M. 1957. Panel report: acting out and its relation to impulse disorders. *Journal of the American Psychoanalytic Association* 5:136–145.

Kanzer, M. 1968. Ego alteration and acting out. *International Journal of Psycho-Analysis* 49:431–435.

Kernberg, O. 1975a. *Borderline Conditions and Pathological Narcissism*. New York: Aronson.

Kernberg, O. 1975b. *Transference and Countertransference in the Treatment of Borderline Patients*. Strecher Monograph Series, no. 12. Philadelphia: Institute of the Pennsylvania Hospital.

Kernberg, O. 1976. Technical considerations in the treatment of borderline personality organization. *Journal of the American Psychoanalytic Association* 24:795–829.

Kernberg, O. 1978a. Contrasting approaches to the psychotherapy of borderline conditions. In J. Masterson, ed. *New Perspectives on Psychotherapy of the Borderline Adult*. New York: Brunner/Mazel.

Kernberg, O. 1978b. The diagnosis of borderline conditions in adolescence. *Adolescent Psychiatry* 6:320–338.

Kernberg, P. 1978. Borderline conditions: child and adolescent aspects. Paper presented at the 25th annual meeting of the Academy of Child Psychiatry, LaJolla, California, October, 27.

Limentani, A. 1966. A re-evaluation of acting out in relation to working through. *International Journal of Psycho-Analysis* 47:274–282.

Loewald, H. 1960. On the therapeutic action of psychoanalysis. *International Journal of Psycho-Analysis* 41:16–33.

Moore, B. 1968. Symposium. Contribution to symposium on acting out. *International Journal of Psycho-Analysis* 49:182–184.

Rangell, L. 1968. Symposium. A point of view on acting out. *International Journal of Psycho-Analysis* 49:195–201.

Rosenfeld, H. 1966. The need of patients to act out during analysis. *Psychoanalytic Forum* 1:19–29.

Shapiro, E. R.; Zinner, J.; Shapiro, R. L.; and Berkovitz, D. 1975. The influence of family experience on borderline personality development. *International Revue of Psychoanalysis* 2:399–412.

Winnicott, D. W. 1965. *The Maturational Processes and the Facilitating Environment*. New York: International Universities Press.

21 ENGAGING THE FAMILY OF THE HOSPITALIZED ADOLESCENT: THE MULTIPLE FAMILY MEETING

EDWARD R. SHAPIRO AND JONATHAN E. KOLB

The hospitalization of the acting-out adolescent is a traumatic and disruptive event in the life of a family. It usually represents the end-point of a lengthy, turbulent period of upset involving the family as well as various outsiders. Parents then bring their child to another outsider—the hospital—in the midst of complex negative feelings about themselves and their child. They feel angry, guilty, helpless, and con-fused. The adolescent is usually angry and bewildered. The entire family approaches the treatment staff in a regressed state, with a mixture of demands, fears, expectations, and hopes. The adolescent, accustomed to experiencing his conflicts as external, is prepared to find in the staff the same depriving, inconsistent, critical, unavailable adults he has found (or created) in his family and in the outside world. Parents are prepared, on one hand, to be criticized and blamed for their per-sonal failures as parents and, on the other, to relinquish their burdens to more sophisticated and, in fantasy, more omnipotent, nurturing professionals. The situation is ripe for unrealistic expectations and misunderstanding.

The engagement of the family in a cooperative attempt to facilitate the treatment of the child is an important ingredient in a successful outcome. The therapist and treatment staff who attempt to treat the adolescent without a solid alliance with the family may not only fail to mobilize the potential healing power within the family group (Shapiro 1978) but may also run the risk of mobilizing a loyalty conflict within the child (Boszormanyi-Nagy 1972).

Regressive responses of all family members toward the treatment staff are characteristic of the early stages of hospitalization, but these responses differ in the parents and child. While hospitalized adolescents recreate elements of family turmoil in their regressive interactions with staff, parents develop a regressive identification with their adolescent child as they disavow and externalize uncomfortable aspects of their own experience as parents onto the staff. Recognition and interpretation of these differing resistances can facilitate the establishment of an alliance with all family members which mobilizes powerful intrafamilial supports and allows parents to join the staff in the provision of an environment which is supportive to the treatment of the entire family.

The clinical material from which these observations are made is derived from families of acting-out adolescent patients (male and female) who are hospitalized on a ten-bed inpatient treatment unit at McLean Hospital. Therapeutic modalities include intensive individual psychotherapy for the adolescent, weekly marital therapy for the parents, weekly family therapy for all family members, and a weekly multiple family meeting for all families. In addition, there are group meetings for the adolescents in which peer and authority relationships are studied, and frequent staff meetings to examine both staff tensions and responses to tensions within the patient group. The milieu is actively structured to provide necessary ego support to the adolescents, with firm limit setting and a carefully monitored privilege system as an integral part of the program.

Alliance and Resistance

The psychoanalytic definition of a "working alliance" (Greenson 1965; Zetzel 1958) requires that the patient be able to maintain a continuous sense of a shared work task and a positive relationship with the therapist despite regressive evocation of disturbing wishes, fantasies, and affects in the transference relationship. This alliance requires the patient to sustain his capacity to observe as well as experience within the treatment setting (Sterba 1934). In the turmoil surrounding the hospitalization of acting-out adolescents, frustration and consequent regression occur in all family members. The intensity of these pressures may lead to an intense and complex transference to treatment staff in which family members may lose both their capacity to observe and their general perception of the treatment staff as helpful.

For example, under the pressures of hospitalization, adolescents in general and borderline adolescents in particular can impair a working alliance by "splitting" relationships to treatment staff (Adler 1973). Staff members who work with such patients are trained to be cautious of special relationships (both good and bad) and to guard against encouraging attempts to avoid frustrating encounters by dissociation and splitting. Therapists are taught to consider the possibility that descriptions of negative reactions to staff may represent a displacement from frustration in the therapy. In an inpatient setting, therapists often hear such displacements in regard to nursing staff ("they're inconsistent, untrained," etc.) or administrators ("he's unfair, rigid, doesn't listen," etc.). Therapists must decide whether to work with these issues in displacement by exploring these outside relationships or to attempt to bring these responses back into the therapeutic relationship itself. An important aspect of any psychiatric hospitalization is the provision of an environment in which the anxiety which leads to splitting can be contained and in which negative projections and externalizations can be examined and integrated without being acted out.

In a treatment program where the therapy of parents is separated from that of the adolescent, characteristic resistances to a working alliance are described as occurring in relation to different aspects of the treatment team. Rinsley and his coauthors (Rinsley and Hall 1962; Rinsley and Inge 1961) describe a major resistance of the adolescent as his "need to view the treatment structure as an adversary with whom he or she is locked in combat." They describe parental resistances as "attempts to defeat the casework process" by (1) deflecting the caseworker's attention toward the adolescent's relationships in the hospital and away from their own interactions with the child, and by (2) avoiding any significant degree of emotional involvement with the hospital. While these authors seem to recognize these resistance patterns as displaced aspects of conflict within family members, they do not utilize the fact that the caseworker on the parents' side and the therapists and nursing staff on the adolescent's side can be seen to represent a joint transference object for parents and child—namely, the treatment staff. Separation into what appear to be separate transference relationships removes from view the shifting struggles within the family group to externalize onto a common focus aspects of intrafamilial conflict.

Family Regression and the Sources of Anxiety

Clinical investigations of hospitalized, nonpsychotic adolescents and their families (Berkowitz, Shapiro, Zinner, and Shapiro 1974; Shapiro, Zinner, Shapiro, and Berkowitz 1975; Zinner and Shapiro 1972) reveal that externalization and projective identification are characteristic defenses in these families at times of turmoil, and that the adolescence of these children often revives conflicted aspects of the parents' own childhood and adolescence. Unconscious parental identification with aspects of the adolescent in turmoil may lead to misinterpretation of the adolescent's needs because of unconscious parental projections. In such an interaction, family members split off disavowed or cherished aspects of themselves and project them onto others within the family group. Family members relate to the projected aspects of themselves in the same manner as they would were these projections internalized. Hence, internalized conflict within individuals may be externalized, assuming the form of interpersonal conflict among family members. Frequently, the tension between parents and the aspects of themselves projected onto their children recaptures aspects of the lost nuclear family relations of the parent when he was a child.

The content of these projections can include (1) aspects of drive and superego in families with antisocial adolescents, where parental intolerance of their own impulses leads to projection (and covert sanctioning) of impulse expression in their children, and where children simultaneously disavow and project aspects of their own superego functions onto their parents (Johnson and Szurek 1952; Zinner and Shapiro 1974); (2) unintegrated and dystonic aspects of self-representations often related to issues of dependency and autonomy in families with borderline adolescents where, for example, parental dependency may be disavowed, perceived as bad, and projected onto the adolescent, leading to a misinterpretation of the adolescent's requests for support as hostile, draining demands (E. R. Shapiro et al. 1975; Zinner and Shapiro 1975); and (3) aspects of self-esteem in families with narcissistic adolescents, where certain family members become inordinately dependent on the behaviors of others within the family to support and stabilize their own sense of self-worth (Berkowitz et al. 1974).

In the presence of the adolescent's own ego deficits and sense of identify diffusion, these family pressures contribute to the adolescent's difficulty in sustaining a working alliance in individual therapy. Under the pressure of drive discharge and inadequate impulse control in many of these adolescents, reality testing may be lost and the therapeutic relationship endangered. In addition, unrestrained expression of the patient's transference rage may evoke confusing countertransference responses of anger, guilt, and anxiety in the therapist which can interfere with his capacity to observe. Adding conjoint family therapy to individual therapy is one way to provide a place where contributing family tensions can be observed and where the individual alliance can be strengthened and supported (Shapiro, Shapiro, Zinner, and Berkowitz 1977).

In the family therapy session, the focus of tension is shifted from therapist and adolescent to parent and adolescent. Regressed interactions between family members may reveal elements of conflict similar to those appearing in the individual negative transference, thus providing both therapist and adolescent with a new perspective. This perspective supports the capacity of both participants to observe, facilitates the therapist's ability to be helpful, and strengthens the working alliance.

Parents of the hospitalized adolescent are, in some ways, in a similar position to that of the individual therapist. The intensity of the regressive struggle between their children and themselves prior to hospitalization evokes in them powerful responses of guilt and anxiety which interfere with their capacity to be helpful as parents. The transference repetition of this family struggle in the relationship between hospitalized adolescent and treatment staff provides parents with an opportunity to utilize their own capacities to observe and offers a potentially useful perspective on their own responses.

The Multiple Family Meeting

The Multiple Family Meeting (MFM) was developed in an attempt to create a place for both the examination of shared experience and the broadening of opportunities for collaboration. On our unit, the MFM is a seventy-five-minute meeting attended by all members of all families as well as staff, consisting of the director (representing the hospital), the administrator (representing the unit administration), one resident (representing the therapists), and the nursing staff on duty (the last, a rotating group). The group often comprises as many as forty-five people and is approached by the staff in a nondirective, group-interpretive manner.

The meeting is seen as distinct from the more highly structured, active, milieu treatment characteristic of the day-to-day life on the unit. The group's task, as defined by the staff, is to explore and attempt to understand the experience of families and staff on the unit. Given the ambiguity of the task, group members lean on the structures and roles already present within the MFM. Themes often emerge which are organized around families, with subgroups of adolescents, parents, fathers, mothers, and siblings finding shared responses in relation to other subgroups and to the staff. Since the group consists of families with a hospitalized adolescent who are in a relationship with treatment staff, the meeting offers an opportunity to witness and understand tensions in these relationships which cross family boundaries. Because of its position as the meeting which brings together all elements of the treatment program, the MFM acts as a microcosm of the unit, wherein ongoing tensions get dispersed and dramatized. Major events in the life of the unit (escapes, returns, etc.) often cluster around the meeting time.

Examination of family members' use of treatment staff in the MFM suggests that the adolescents recreate aspects of their family experience in their struggles with staff, while parents intensify their identification with the adolescent, unconsciously projecting aspects of their own conflicted parental functioning onto the staff. From this perspective, parental focus on the adolescent's interaction with the staff may be seen not as an interference but as an opportunity to help family members understand, in displacement, previously overwhelming intrafamilial tension. It is our impression that the themes which emerge in this setting are representative of characteristic but often unobserved tensions which develop between families and staff when an adolescent is hospitalized.

Our study of the MFM reveals that these complex interactions may be loosely grouped within Bion's (1961) descriptions of "basic assumption group" modes of fight/flight, dependency, and hope ("pairing'') (Shapiro, Zinner, Berkowitz, and Shapiro 1975). These modes of unconscious resistance have been observed to occur in groups of relative strangers (McGlashan and Levy 1977). In the MFM, however, the presence of adolescents, parents, and staff adds an additional complexity to these three modes of functioning (see table 1).

FIGHT/FLIGHT MODE

The fight/flight mode appears to be related to dissociation of impulse and prohibition and appears in the MFM when issues of limit setting are being explored. Limit setting is a complex task. It is often experienced by the adolescent as punitive deprivation, evoking intense rage. In the presence of staff members' conflicts about their own aggression, limit setting and the adolescent's angry response to it may evoke guilt and anxiety in staff members which will be recognized by the adolescent, leading to a confirmation of his fantasies of being abused and deprived.

Limit setting is a parental task, the failure of which is seen in almost every family with a borderline or acting-out adolescent. The struggles of staff to master this function provide opportunities for empathic understanding of parental tension. The wish to remain in a positive relationship with the adolescent, combined with anxiety about one's own relative impotence and guilt about one's hostility, makes the setting of limits extraordinarily difficult. When the relationship between staff and adolescent is not strong enough to master these anxieties, the regressive interaction that ensues around this issue appears to create the stereotype of the impulsive adolescent and the controlling parent.

In this mode, adolescents find themselves united in a state of anger and impulsiveness with no self-control. They and their parents focus their attention on the perceived imperfections, incompetence, arbitrariness, and inadequacy of treatment staff and behave as if the task of the group were not to understand but to criticize and blame the staff. The group acts as though all the impulses were in the adolescents and all the capacity to worry and control in the staff. In response to the aggressive attack, staff members may experience a loss of confidence in their own intuition, guilt and anxiety about their inadequacies, and anger at the group for its attack. Anxiety and anger about a sense of relative impotence may result in punitive wishes or reaction formations against these wishes (e.g., excessive kindness).

In this interaction, adolescents disavow and project onto the staff aspects of their own superego and reexperience with the staff their disappointment and fury at parental imperfections. In addition, parents project and disavow their own punitive wishes and displace onto the staff their unrealistic expectations of themselves. The task of the staff in this situation is to recognize and interpret both the dissociation of drive and prohibition and the displacement of unrealistic expectations and excessive guilt.

DEPENDENCY MODE

Parental search for answers is characteristic of the initial engagement in treatment. It is in some sense equivalent to the adolescent's demands for gratification. There are, of course, no adequate answers, just as there is no gratification which will allay primitive fears of helplessness and deprivation. The temptation to offer a parent an answer is a seductive one. It places parents in a dependent position and staff in an expert one. It rests the solution of conflicts on the authority of the staff, provides the illusion of tension relief, and weakens the authority and potential strength of the parent-child relationship. To the extent that it is possible to avoid the dependency on staff and strengthen the parent-child relationship, it is the task of the staff to help contain the family's anxiety and join them in a search for less conflicted functioning. The regression that lies behind the understandable wish for magical answers is not helped by providing diagnoses or advice or even by exploring parental conflicts in isolation from the rest of the family. Regression is shared in these families and derives from conflicts which can be understood in the family context.

Parents who bring their children to the hospital do so out of a wish to be better parents. Often they have attempted every means at their disposal to help their child, and despite their overt request for staff to take over their role, their underlying wish is for assistance in learning to be more useful to each other. It is often, however, in response to a regressive wish for magical solutions that the dependency mode evolves in the MFM.

329

TABLE 1

REGRESSIVE INTERACTION IN THE MULTIPLE FAMILY MEETING

	Fight/Flight	Dependency	Hope
Adolescent experience ...	We're not crazy, your staff is driving us crazy by ineptness and inconsistency (impulsive actions, direct drive expression, no self control)	We're hopeless and confused nothing makes any sense; we're spaced out, without ideas	We're thinking about future plans, school, etc.; we're wasting our time here, should get on with our lives; the past is past
Staff experience	Loss of confidence in own intuition; anxious about impotence; excessive need to control, judge; angry at patients, need to demonstrate power and control, may be punitive or react defensively to punitive wishes (excessive kindness, forgiveness); pressure leaders to act	Anger at patients for not having ideas; out of touch; maybe drugs will help; leader do something (limits); somebody (therapist?) must know what's going on; demands are enormous and we are overwhelmed	Treat patients gently, don't rock the boat; social recovery overvalued: if he's better, I am a good caretaker; or, all hopeless and memory of the past resides in the staff
Parent experience at home before hospitalization ...	Similar to staff; guilt, feeling responsible and incompetent, angry at adolescent, may be punitive or defensive about punitive wishes; excessive need to control	Similar to staff; may be the courts, school, or hospital will help; somebody must understand, we want answers; demands are enormous; we are overwhelmed	Similar to staff; my self-esteem is tied up with his success; if he's troubled, I'm a bad parent

Parent experience in hospital	Identify with adolescent; staff should be more perfect; staff is responsible for patient behavior; staff is too arbitrary and inflexible	Identify with adolescent; we need answers and are confused and hopeless	Identify with adolescent; let's plan the future and leave the past behind
Interpretation for staff and family	(1) Examine unrealistic self-expectations; evaluate excessively guilty response to punitive wishes; (2) examine dissociated impulse and prohibition: (to staff/parents) "Only adolescents have impulses" (to adolescent) "Only parents/staff can worry and exert control"	Examine unconscious dependent wishes ("There must be someone who can fix this mess"); help accept powerlessness and helplessness within onself	Examine own needs for adolescent to succeed; examine own vulnerability to failure and intolerance of hopelessness and despair

NOTE.—Fight/flight, dependency, and hope are Bion's (1961) "basic assumption group" modes.

In the dependency mode, parents, adolescents, and staff alike share an experience of helplessness, confusion, longing for guidance, and an absence of ideas. Group members act as if the experience of helplessness were intolerable. Staff members experience the patients' demands as overwhelming and find themselves out of touch with the patients, angry at them for not producing ideas, and wishing either for magical solutions or omniscient understanding.

In this interaction, adolescents recreate their struggles over nurturance with the staff. Parents identify with their adolescents, projecting their guilt and anxiety over their inability to provide onto the staff. The task of the group under these circumstances is to examine the shared intolerance of the experience of helplessness, powerlessness, frustration, and ambiguity.

HOPE MODE

In the hope mode, group members experience themselves as thoughtful, reasonable, and hopeful about the future. The adolescent appears well organized and considerate. Group members forgive the staff its imperfections, find no questions unanswered, and suspect that they are wasting their time in the hospital when they should be getting on with the business of their lives. Adolescents and parents join in a shared denial of past turmoil and focus their attention on concrete plans about their lives and futures, with a fantasy that something creative will be generated from this collaboration. In this mode, staff members are tempted to treat the group gently, shying away from confrontation and questions. They have the tacit hope that things will stay quiet, that social recovery is enough, and that intrapsychic turmoil is resolved. Alternatively, staff members may find themselves alone with worries about impending disaster and memories of past turmoil.

On occasion, parents will repudiate the adolescents and attempt to join the staff in a pairing experience which also represents a search for hope. Such attempts constitute an avoidance of shared attitudes and affects between adolescents and parents in attempt to avoid painful experience.

These interactions represent a shared denial and an intolerance of hopelessness and despair. The task for parents and staff is to examine their own needs for the adolescent to improve. The task for all group members is to examine this shared intolerance of despair and to understand the need to exclude part of the group in a desperate search for hope.

Clinical Observations

In the following, we shall present two examples of staff-patient interaction which illustrate the themes we have described. In the first, an example of a ward riot, we shall illustrate the failure of a working alliance with family members and describe the three modes of regressive interaction between staff and patients as they emerged during the disturbance and the MFM. In this description, the focus will not be on the structure and limits of the unit (of obvious importance to the management of a riot) but on the dynamic themes underlying the complex relationships between families and staff. While limit setting and gradual restrictions are an integral fact of community life on an adolescent unit, the effectiveness of these limits depends on the strength of staff-patient relationships. Failure in these relationships and its contribution to the riot will be illustrated.

The second example is an extended excerpt from a single MFM which illustrates in detail the potential in such a meeting to utilize the understanding of the dynamics of this behavior to reverse the regressive pull and allow group members to join in a shared work task.

A WARD RIOT

Three weeks before a disturbance on the unit, several new families joined the MFM. Adolescents began to talk about a sense that their needs were being neglected: There was insufficient food, too much crowding, staff members were too busy. Simultaneously, administrative staff were preoccupied with an approaching hospital accreditation review which required attention to record keeping and administrative details. In the MFM many of these issues were raised for discussion. In two consecutive meetings family members had other commitments which required their departure before the end of the meeting. There was little interest in their absence on the part of the group members and connections made to ongoing tensions were discussed only by staff. Parents seemed bored. Nursing staff members began to complain of feeling unsupported in their work by parents and by administrative staff. An attempt to explore this issue in the MFM was met with seeming disinterest.

On the night of the disturbance (the eve of the accreditation visit), parents of four of the eight adolescents were visiting the unit until very late. Each parent perceived extraordinary tension in the adolescent group—no one mentioned it to nursing staff. All four sets of parents left the unit; some waited outside in their cars watching the windows, others sat by the telephone at home, waiting for the expected call. After the last one had left, the adolescents exploded in a short violent scene of confronting (but not injuring) staff, throwing food, and breaking furniture. No one was injured, and the damage was confined to the public living areas (including the kitchen and the living room—the site for the MFM). Parents were called, and an emergency MFM was held the next day in which staff presented to the group the task of coming to terms with their responsibility for both the physical damage and the possibly unsalvageable damage to working relationships with staff.

Although the disturbance was a complex, multidetermined event, it is possible to focus on the three regressive modes of interaction which emerged. The fight/flight dynamic is evident in the actions of the adolescents and in their discussion of them in the MFM. Their stated perception was that their actions were justifiable and that they represented the inevitable outcome of being forced to deal with incompetent, punitive staff. On this unlocked unit with voluntary participation, they paradoxically felt imprisoned and tormented by arbitrary, unsupportive treatment staff.

In their discussion of the disturbance in the MFM, parents joined the adolescents. Several parents elaborated a list of staff inadequacies and failures: Staff should have stricter rules, more athletic programs were needed, and communication should be better. The implications were that the staff was solely responsible for the adolescents' destructive behavior and that if they had been more perfect, it would not have happened. Many staff members struggled to contain angry responses to the perceived attack from the patient group.

Finally, one therapist, intervening, suggested that the parents' anger at the staff was an accurate reproduction of their usual feelings about themselves as parents when their children got into trouble. He suggested that their preoccupation with their own guilt and self-blame deprived their children of the help they needed in taking responsibility for their own behavior. The parents responded to the interpretation by recalling numerous examples of self-criticism and blame and were able to recognize in this discussion their unrealistic expectations of themselves. This understanding facilitated the parents' ability to be helpful to the adolescents in a subsequent meeting.

The dependency dynamic also emerged in the course of the disturbance. In the midst of the violence, one of the adolescents who was smashing furniture said to a nursing staff member, "If you wanted to, you could do something about this." In the MFM, several adolescents declared that the "staff could have prevented it." Several parents recounted their experience on the unit before the outburst, saying, "We knew there would be trouble, but who were we to interfere with the professionals?" Family members had felt helpless, unable to contribute any ideas. All sense of a shared responsibility had been lost.

In the staff meeting before the emergency MFM, staff members felt overwhelmed and tired. People spoke of insufficient sleep. Fantasies were expressed that the director would figure everything out, or that the administrator would decide which adolescents to expel. There was a shared difficulty in accepting and working with the experience of powerlessness and helplessness.

Finally, in the midst of the turmoil, there was evidence of the dynamic of hope. One father, after asking about his son's involvement in the tension, was assured by him that he had everything under control and that he would stay out of any trouble. Forgetting past experiences with his son and hopeful about this response, the father left the unit. In the MFM, this father and others clung to the idea that the boy's handing out weapons to other adolescents did not necessarily make him an active participant.

MULTIPLE FAMILY MEETING: AN EXAMPLE

In this second clinical example, we shall focus on a meeting in which the regressive tensions around fight/flight and dependency are illustrated. The meeting began with a focus of attention on one adolescent, Tom, whose parents were not present. Tom had had outbursts of rage before on the unit which frightened the adolescents and were preceded by headaches. As the meeting opened, Tom made an unusual request

335

to have a family friend present at the meeting. When the group failed to consider the meaning of this request in relation to the absence of Tom's parents, the friend was asked to leave. After some anger was expressed by the adolescents against the staff, Tom interrupted.

TOM: [Addressing staff] I have a headache, can I have an aspirin? [Silence] There wasn't time to get it before the meeting, and the staff was in a meeting anyway, so I'd like it now [silence]. [Speaking to nurse] Can I please have some aspirin?

NURSE: It would be best if we wait until after the meeting.

TOM: [Angrily speaking to administrator] What about it, Dr. X? Give me some aspirin now, I can't take it [all family members look at Dr. X].

DR. X: It is familiar to members of this group to feel on the verge of exploding, demanding and feeling the need for instant relief.

TOM: [Yelling] Damn it! Give me my aspirin, Dr. X! [Tom runs out of the room, shortly followed by the nurse who says "I'm going to talk with Tom."]

The adolescent knew that the nursing station was open during the MFM and that aspirin was available. His decision to present his request as part of the meeting may be understood as an attempt to communicate his angry sense of not being cared for by his absent parents. In this sequence, the adolescent may be seen as speaking for group members' experience of being frustrated and overwhelmed and demanding instant relief, implicitly threatening rage and retaliation if the demand is unmet. The group's watchful silence and their inability to help the adolescent manage his frustration and anxiety suggest an identification with this position of helplessness and rage. In addition to withstanding the demand for an action response to unbearable tension, the therapist interpretively calls attention to the group's identification with Tom and suggests the possibility that Tom may be speaking for everybody. Implicitly, he suggests that tension can be contained and examined rather than dispelled. Although staff members are shaken by the powerful scene, parents remain unruffled and, in Tom's absence, quiz the other adolescents about Tom's headache.

PAUL: [Another adolescent] [to parents] You haven't seen Tom when he gets bad. He's frightening. We've seen it—he needs something for his headaches.

SEVERAL PARENTS: [To staff] Why don't you give it to him?

At this point, parents and adolescents were united in an identification with the dependent, transference paradigm of the needy child who is being deprived by the cruel withholding parent, with treatment staff in the parental role. This is a scene which has been played out often within each family and within the parents' family of origin (E. R. Shapiro et al. 1975). Although parents know the experience of the staff in this interchange, they respond in the meeting in a regressive identification with the adolescent as though they had no understanding. Adolescents have recreated their struggle over nurturance with the staff. Parents have disavowed their own guilt and anxiety over their inability to provide and have projected these feelings onto the staff. With relief, they now experience the staff as cruel and withholding and themselves as calm observers. They watch to see how the staff will manage.

Recognizing the parental transference, staff members attempt to help family members put the experience into words.

DR. X: The question is, what's the matter with the staff here, withholding the treatment the adolescents feel is necessary?

MR. BLACK: Well, all right, since you mention it, why didn't you?

MRS. WHITE: [Quietly] I hope you know what you are doing [at this point, Tom quietly reenters the room, followed by the nurse, Carol. The group continues with five minutes of discussion without any notice taken of Tom's entrance].

MR. JONES: Did you get the aspirin?

TOM: Yes, Carol gave it to me.

MR. JONES: Is there a sign language?

MR. BLACK: There must be—Dr. X or Dr. Y gave Carol the high sign to give him the aspirin [Several parents nod in agreement].

DR. X: The staff must act together—efficiently and well. Apparently it's hard to consider the idea that Carol acted on her own.

In this interchange, both sides of the transference fantasy were revealed. Either the staff is cruel and withholding or it is omnipotent. The deprived and needy child, with whom the entire group is identified, must be in a relationship with a powerful, all-knowing parent (the wish is, "I hope you know what you're doing"). Such ideal parents (their expectations of themselves) must not be anxious, tentative, or susceptible to disagreement. Recognition of tensions or disagreements within the staff would compel family members to examine their own anxieties, failures, and impossible self-expectations. The interpretation encourages an examination of the transference fantasy, implicitly pointing it out as a fantasy and pointing to its defensive use. Dr. X implies that tension and uncertainty may exist in both family members and staff.

DR. Y: The group allows Tom to speak for all of its unbearable tensions as though people had no headaches of their own.

MR. BLACK: To me it seemed as if he wanted a crutch to lean on. Aspirin would not ease a headache this fast. I have been looking for crutches too.

MR. WHITE: Our family is not sure we'll be here next week. Sue doesn't want to stay.

DR. X: That's some headache.

MR. WHITE: Yes.

At this point, the externalization decreased and parents began to reintegrate their previously disavowed anxiety and helplessness. They now could begin to explore and work on elements of their own uncertainty. The exploration revealed that instead of magic, family members may have something realistic to offer each other.

MRS. WHITE: I have so many feelings. If someone has a hurt, you want it to go away. We are looking to the doctor for miracle cures. Sue does not want to be here. We feel guilty about having her here and are thinking about taking her home.

MR. WHITE: She feels we have abandoned her.

MR. SMITH: [A man whose seriously disturbed son, Frank, had made some gains after a five-month hospitalization] No, you would be abandoning her by taking her out of the program. At one time, I thought I was abandoning Frank here, but not now.

MR. WHITE: When we see the ups and downs. . . .

MR. SMITH: I've seen so many ups and downs over the months, Christ, ups and downs are all I see. You get your hopes up and then you're disappointed.

MR. WHITE: How much patience have you got?

MR. SMITH: There's no alternative—home is not good yet—it wasn't good for Frank. I don't know much about what Sue's done, but to take her home now would do no good. It would be giving up on her treatment.

MR. BROWN: How long have you had trouble?

MR. WHITE: We have been at it for a year but the troubles go back long before that.

MR. SMITH: You don't solve anything by leaving early.

Following a beginning recognition of shared tensions, parents acknowledged their own uncertainty and supported one another as they worked on their responsibilities as parents. As the meeting closed, staff members reminded the group of their regressive wishes for nurturance from the staff. Group members responded by reexperiencing and restating their earlier requests which were again interpreted by the therapists.

DR. X: Perhaps we could keep in mind the intensity of the struggle for aspirin.

TOM: My asking was bad, huh?

DR. X: Not bad—but intense.

DR. Y: I suspect Carol knows what a parent feels like—she experienced the same burden.

MRS. BROWN: Why didn't one of the doctors take the burden?

DR. Y: The wish is for the doctor to take the burden, as though Tom could pass it to Carol who could pass it to Dr. X and to me.

DR. X: If only someone could avoid being tense.

TOM: It's time for my Darvon. Can I have my Darvon now?

DR. X: It's time for us to stop.

In addition to the themes previously described, the excerpt above illustrates how staff members can sustain an interpretive stance in the face of extraordinary tension within the group, if a working alliance exists with family members. In such a setting, staff members can draw inferences from the group process about shared unconscious fantasies and invite group members to join in thinking about them.

It is important to note that although elements of the interpretive style in this meeting derive from the group relations work of Rice (1975), the MFM in this setting is not equivalent to Bion's stranger group. This meeting is supported by numerous formal and informal relationships in a complex treatment program. Staff members are known and familiar to patients in settings which have different tasks defined. Given the extent of regression in these patients, the group could not contain the frustration involved in this level of examination in the absence of the extended supports available within the program. In addition, the group consists of families who know each other and who work together over time. Evidence of strengths and anxieties in family members which emerge in other aspects of the program can be utilized in the MFM to provide the necessary modification of tension.

Conclusions

The hospitalization of a troubled adolescent occurs in the midst of a shared family regression. During his regression, family members develop complex responses to the treatment staff onto whom they have externalized troublesome aspects of themselves. The overlapping nature of family responses to treatment staff may be missed if the family is separated for treatment.

The MFM offers an opportunity to bring together all aspects of the treatment team in order to examine responses to staff on the part of both parents and adolescent. In this setting, the staff's capacity to recognize different needs of parent and child, to withstand the projection of hostility, and to maintain a capacity to observe provides family members with the opportunity to examine this shared family regression in the face of turmoil.

Using data from the Multiple Family Meeting we have described three dynamic themes around which this regression occurs. In the fight/flight mode, aspects of superego, unrealistic expectations, and punitive wishes are projected onto the staff. In the dependency mode, difficulties in accepting helplessness, powerlessness, and ambiguity are externalized. In the hope mode, excessive vulnerability to hopelessness and failure is disavowed. Through the use of clinical examples, we have illustrated how recognition and understanding of these dynamic tensions can allow for previously overwhelming experience to be put in perspective, facilitating the development of a working alliance with treatment staff in which family members can increase their capacity to be helpful to one another.

REFERENCES

Adler, G. 1973. Hospital treatment of borderline patients. *American Journal of Psychiatry* 130:32–36.

Berkowitz, D. A.; Shapiro, R. L.; Zinner, J.; and Shapiro, E. R. 1974. Family contributions to narcissistic disturbances in adolescents. *International Review of Psycho-Analysis* 1:353–362.

Bion, W. R. 1961. *Experiences in Groups*. London: Tavistock.

Boszormenyi-Nagy, I. 1972. Loyalty implications of the transference model in psychotherapy. *Archives of General Psychiatry* 27:374–380.

Greenson, R. R. 1965. The working alliance and the transference neurosis. *Psychoanalytic Quarterly* 34:155–181.

Johnson, A. M., and Szurek, S. A. 1952. The genesis of antisocial acting out in children and adults. *Psychoanalytic Quarterly* 21:323–343.

McGlashan, T. H., and Levy, S. T. 1977. Sealing-over in a therapeutic community. *Psychiatry* 40:55–65.

Rice, A. K. 1975. Learning from leadership. In A. D. Colman and W. Bexton, eds. *Group Relations Reader*. Sausalito, Calif.: Grex.

Rinsley, D. B., and Hall, D. D. 1962. Psychiatric hospital treatment of adolescents: parental resistances as expressed in casework metaphor. *Archives of General Psychiatry* 7:286–294.

Rinsley, D. B., and Inge, G. P. 1961. Psychiatric hospital treatment of adolescents: verbal and non-verbal resistance to treatment. *Bulletin of the Menninger Clinic* 25:249–263.

Shapiro, E. R. 1978. Research on family dynamics: clinical implications for the family of the borderline adolescent. *Adolescent Psychiatry* 6:360–376.

Shapiro, E. R.; Shapiro, R. L.; Zinner, J.; and Berkowitz, D. A. 1977. The borderline ego and the working alliance: indications for family and individual treatment in adolescence. *International Journal of Psycho-Analysis* 58:77–87.

Shapiro, E. R.; Zinner, J.; Shapiro, R. L.; and Berkowitz, D. A. 1975. The influence of family experience on borderline personality development. *International Review of Psycho-Analysis* 2:399–411.

Shapiro, R. L.; Zinner, J.; Berkowitz, D. A.; and Shapiro, E. R. 1975. The impact of group experiences on adolescent development. In M. Sugar, ed. *The Adolescent in Group and Family Therapy*. New York: Brunner-Mazel.

Sterba, R. 1934. The fate of the ego in analytic therapy. *International Journal of Psycho-Analysis* 15:117–126.

Zetzel, E. R. 1958. Therapeutic alliance in the analysis of hysteria. *The Capacity for Emotional Growth*. New York: International Universities Press.

Zinner, J., and Shapiro, R. L. 1972. Projective identification as a mode of perception and behavior in families of adolescents. *International Journal of Psycho-Analysis* 53:523–530.

Zinner, J., and Shapiro, R. L. 1974. The family group as a single psychic entity: implications for acting out in adolescence. *International Review of Psycho-Analysis* 1:179–186.

Zinner, J., and Shapiro, E. R. 1975. Splitting in families of borderline adolescents. In J. Mack, ed. *Borderline States in Psychiatry*. New York: Grune & Stratton.

22 THERAPEUTIC APPROACHES TO THE BORDERLINE ADOLESCENT

MAX SUGAR

Recent developmental studies have broadened our understanding of and led to modifications in the treatment of the borderline patient (Ekstein and Wallerstein 1954; Geleerd 1958; Kernberg 1975; Mahler 1972; Masterson 1972; Shapiro, Zinner, Shapiro, and Berkovitz 1975). According to Kernberg's formulations, the pathology derives from the failure to develop in the separation-individuation phase. Mahler, Pine, and Bergman (1975) and Settlage (1977) ascribe it more precisely to a failure of suitable development in the rapprochement subphase (fifteen to twenty-two months) which derails development of libidinal object constancy and the advance to utilizing repression as a phase-appropriate defense. Instead, splitting—which is normal for the practicing phase—continues and becomes a pathological defense.

This chapter will focus on some of the therapeutic approaches to borderline adolescents, used flexibly, concomitantly, and sequentially for changing conditions during a lengthy therapy. Rosenfeld and Sprince's remarks (1965) seem apt: "Working with borderline children appears to produce as many techniques as there are children and this figure can probably be multiplied by the number of therapists concerned."

According to Masterson (1972), hospitalization is required to treat seriously disturbed adolescents. Boyer and Giovacchini (1967) and Settlage (1977) feel that analysis is the treatment of choice. Kernberg (1975) suggested a structured arrangement, including hospitalization, using individual psychoanalytic psychotherapy for some borderlines and psychoanalysis for others.

Spotnitz (1976), in addition, uses group therapy; Williams (1975) adds family therapy when helpful; while Whitaker (1975) believes that family therapy is the treatment for all adolescents. Coughlin and Wimberger (1968) invited the parents of adolescents to the group therapy sessions and found confrontations between parents and adolescents useful. Having volunteer adolescents in adolescent group therapy (Fine, Knight-Webb, and Breau 1976) reminded the therapist of expectable behavior and function in nonpatient adolescents. This approach also provided the adolescent patients with modeling, reduced emotional distance, and improved the youngsters' attendance. Taylor (1969) observed that role playing in an institutional therapy group allowed adolescent patients to imitate the good (idealized) and the bad (devalued) aspects of their parents and staff, promoted social learning, and provided data about their past experiences.

Masterson (1972) recommended no contact between the adolescent and his family in the first phase of hospital treatment, as it led to more acting out or interfered with therapy. In the later stages of treatment, family sessions were combined with continuing hospitalization and individual sessions. Shapiro, Shapiro, Zinner, and Berkovitz (1977) found that family sessions combined with individual therapy in the hospital enhanced treatment.

For different patients, each of these approaches has merit. Instead of hospitalization for some selected youngsters (not the most seriously disturbed), I have used individual outpatient therapy and at times added other therapies, such as group, family, office network, the family home as mental hospital, and drugs. For outpatient therapy to be considered for such an adolescent, some primary requirements have to be met: the adolescent must have a certain minimal amount of motivation and controls, and the family must have stability and commitment sufficient to cooperate with bolstering and supporting the patient's wavering motivation, controls, and therapeutic alliance. The probability of success is increased when the family is intact.

Treating adolescents in groups is a useful way of helping them deal with ambivalence, hostility, or rebelliousness toward adults and authority figures. Therapy groups utilize the adolescents' natural tendency to form groupings, and they may feel less isolated and anxious, yet protected at the same time from retaliation for revelations by the presence of the other members of the group. For a youngster in individual therapy with an intense dependency, overidealized transference, or a transference psychosis, the addition of group therapy may dilute the intensity of these feelings, help him establish peer relationships, and thus enhance or initiate progress.

Family therapy may be the optimal treatment for the adolescent where problems center on separation, interpersonal conflict, communication blockages, and acting out (Offer and Vanderstoep 1975). In family therapy, features of the family members' pathology and health are displayed and may provide a better grasp of the dynamics and hence treatment success. Similarly, in office network therapy with an adolescent, particular aspects of the patient's personality, pathology, and strengths which are useful for therapy may be exposed in transactions with peers.

Office network therapy with adolescents or self-selected peer-group therapy is a useful adjunct for an adolescent who seems on the verge of disorganization and might otherwise need hospitalization, is suicidal, or is having massive resistances in therapy that are not responding to the usual therapeutic efforts (Sugar 1975). For this technique to be applicable, a sufficient amount of control and cooperation has to be available from the parents as well as from the patient.

When hospitalization is indicated but particular conditions militate against it, the young patient may be kept at home (Winnicott 1958a, 1965). The home then serves as a mental hospital, with the family acting as psychiatric nurses and attendants, and the psychiatrist providing therapy for the patient and guidance for the parents.

At times, the near-panic level of anxiety and the problem of modulation of stimuli and affects require that medication be used for a youngster, at least briefly. This provides another means to control impulsiveness and to decrease distress, which enhances the psychotherapeutic effort. Possibly, drugs might never be required if we were always able to be empathic and sympathetic in grasping the meaning of the patient's communication, thereby reducing the patient's anxiety with a propitious interpretation (Ekstein and Wallerstein 1954). However much we seek this ideal, we must recognize failures in our empathy and the consequences to the patient.

In any therapy with adolescents, countertransference may be especially difficult (Maltsberger and Buie 1974; Stierlin 1975; Winnicott 1958b), particularly if group, family, or network therapy is involved. The patient may stir up the therapist's unresolved separation or authority problems, which may lead the therapist to side with the adolescent and compete with the parents. He may inadvertently help the adolescent become the victim of the parents and thus fulfill the youngster's masochistic needs. This increases parental guilt feelings and leads the adolescent into becoming the victimizer by proving the parents' inadequacy.

The following case highlights some issues related to these treatment approaches.

Case Presentation

A fourteen-year-old girl from another town came for psychotherapy because of daily inebriation, truancy, suicide attempts, and impending academic failure. Her family viewed her request for psychiatric therapy the previous year as dramatics and part of her posturing, as they did her two suicide attempts five and six months later. When the parents wanted therapy for her after the suicide attempt, she refused it. Although the parents knew of her drinking, the psychiatric evaluation was arranged ambivalently by them and only after she appeared drunk to babysit at a neighbor's. The stimulus for her behavior, the patient and her parents felt, was her rejection by her best girl friend a year before.

The parents thought of their daughter as extremely bright, sensitive, and shy, passive socially, but very aggressive with them. She had not been dating or going to mixed parties and had stopped all socializing. At home she was silent or cried, isolating herself in her room and not participating with the family. In school she was quiet and withdrawn.

According to her mother, the patients' first words expressed gratitude in sentence form; she had no transitional object; and toilet training was completed by the age of two years. She had had childhood exanthema in the second and third grades and refused to go to school in the third grade.

After her only sibling, a brother, was born when she was two years old, she repeatedly hit him on the head. When the mother responded by including her more in everything and involving her more with the father and grandparents, she ceased hitting her baby brother. Afterward, she was a model child—"too good to be true"—and was very close to the father until the current symptoms began.

The youngster was fearfully ambivalent about seeing a psychiatrist and seemed to be depressed and in a dreamy state at times. She showed poor judgment and impulsivity, had poor tolerance of anxiety and displayed a transient loss of reality testing. She appeared deceptive, manipulative, grandiose, and extremely distrustful; she used splitting, denial, fantasy, and projective identification, but with a sublimatory channel.

Initially, she was treated for depression by means of individual therapy and an antidepressant. A month later, it was learned that three weeks earlier she had discontinued the medication and resumed drinking because of her fear of falling apart. She was about to be expelled from school and was eager to take disulfiram to control her drinking or go to a home for runaways, that is, anything to avoid therapy.

Since hospitalization could not be arranged, the home as a hospital was added to the therapy to maintain her at home. The parents became her supervisors and "nurses" around the clock, not allowing her to go anywhere alone, driving her to and from school, and allowing her few friends to visit her only at home. Guidance and support were given to the parents by phone or when they brought her to regular sessions.

Group therapy was soon provided to help her with peer relations and social anxieties, since she was generally isolated at this time from classmates. After several weeks in the therapy group, her anxiety increased, and she developed blocking along with paranoid delusions about me and the group members. The psychotic reaction may have been related to transference psychosis (feeling cornered by family and group) or additional strain elsewhere. A major tranquilizer was now prescribed.

In twelve group sessions, she was mostly quiet and dreamy but evasive when questioned. She had a need to sit and be accepted without exposing herself, not daring to risk rejection. Occasionally, when asked, she would talk briefly about her symptoms, family, friends, and school, but she quickly reversed it and started the other patient talking. The group members eventually commented angrily on this, but she smiled vapidly and retreated into fantasy. Thus, she was able to feel some acceptance and occasionally relate in an imitative fashion, but from a suspicious and deceptive stance. Although she did not experience rejection by the group members, as she had anticipated, this experience made no permanent rearrangements intrapsychically, which was no surprise.

In subsequent individual sessions, her anxiety seemed somewhat less, but she still manifested deceptiveness, manipulativeness, and grandiosity. She devalued her father as weak for trying to please her and being easily misled; she liked him better than her mother, however, whom she could not deceive readily, Individual therapy centered on the theme of her sense of self, her worthlessness, and her sensitivity to any hint of rejection. This led her to associate to stomach aches in the first grade when she felt alienated from her peers and used the symptom to avoid school. She now recalled that at menarche her mother had told her not to interfere in her mother and father's relationship; only as long as she followed that advice, would her mother be her friend and helper. This led to material about having been very close to her father, "his baby doll," before the threat.

About six months after the mental hospital at home was instituted, some controls were removed. Since parental supervision was being relaxed, her mother now became worried about the patient's dating and possible sexual activity.

Material in therapy now shifted to jealousy of her brother and mother. When resumption of drinking was discovered, the parents threatened her with commitment to the state hospital. It was learned ultimately that she had experienced a sense of loss about the group therapy sessions (she appeared for one after they were terminated) and wanted to increase the frequency of individual sessions. The mother told her, however, that this was not possible financially, although neither of them discussed it with me. The continued acting out seemed to be a rageful response to this deprivation and rejection. She now revealed much more in her individual therapy than previously about her hostile feelings and behavior toward her parents, including thefts of money and her father's whiskey. She slyly overdosed on the tranquilizer and enjoyed the panic that her symptoms caused her parents and pediatrician. She trusted me enough to tell me what she had done but refused to allow me to inform them of the facts, and, therefore, extensive medical testing was necessary. Thus, she forced her parents to pay for extra care anyway, which they had denied her in psychotherapy. She felt guilty and, fearful they would retaliate, was preparing to attack them again with some new misbehavior before they attacked her. Medication was now discontinued.

She claimed her mother called her paranoid, and she described her best girl friend as being jealous because she was not dating as much as the patient. The rage and lack of controls increased so that she was drinking more, although she now congratulated herself on not being truant—a deceptive grading for my approval. It seemed that her displacement of rage to the school was decreasing as she developed a negative transference attitude. She came into a session quite drunk, giddy, and seductive, explaining it on the basis of wanting to talk a lot with me and needing to relax first with liquor.

Her associations related to the question of the ownership of her body and suicidal notions as a way of inflicting pain on her mother. She felt her mother really owned her body, with me as part owner. Her drinking now was related to suicidal intent, based on wanting to anger and hurt me in the same way that slashing her wrists had inflicted pain on her mother.

At the next week's session, she described her date as embarrassed and angry due to her drunkenness. This upset her so much that the following evening, after he had not called all day, she took an overdose of tranquilizers to help her sleep. This behavior may have been related to her readiness to feel annihilated, based on guilt about sexual wishes; but her suicidal ideas, drinking, and school problems continued, indicating further disorganization.

Office network therapy was now offered to help control her continuing disorganization, and she eagerly accepted it, especially since she "would have to face the idea of changing psychiatrists" if she went to a state hospital. She added that she had wanted her best friend to come in with her for a long time and had recently requested this of her mother, who refused to allow it. Her notion was that talking with her friend would help give me ideas about her which would help her therapy.

She had four office network therapy sessions over the next ten weeks, interspersed with individual sessions or family sessions to which she brought her father, mother, or brother. In the network sessions she discussed dating, other friends, her drinking, and her suicidal behavior. Her friends showed their caring acceptance of her with shocked anger at her self-destructiveness. They also indicated awareness of the patient's dramatic devices, which only created social distance for her and forced her to confront her other behavior. It was apparent that she used her friends as maternal substitutes and to provide directions and restraints. In one of the sessions, she whispered with them in retaliation for an interpretation during the previous session.

In her sessions with the whole family, she was mostly silent; but with individual family members, she was voluble. From these conversations there developed further clarification, as well as confirmation, by the parents of many of the patient's accusations. The mother attested to being argumentative, competitive, and unfair and to feeling hurt if the patient did not agree with her; she also admitted to warning her daughter away from her father at menarche. The father expressed his double bind clearly through his expectation (as a passive listener) that the patient should talk to him like his wife and mother did. He added that when the patient was withdrawn he felt she was deliberately trying to hurt him. He would not allow her in the living room, however, since he anticipated that she would mess it up with food. When made aware of these contradictions, the parents accepted them. Later, they felt humiliated and projected blame ("you're mixing me up") and confusion.

When the office network sessions ended, the patient entered another adolescent therapy group and had thirty-nine sessions and an occasional individual session. She was eager to be in the group since improved ability to relate to her peers had been demonstrated in the network therapy. At this time, about one and a half years after beginning therapy, she was not suicidal, was better controlled with regard to her other symptoms, and was functioning fairly well in school. The self-selected peer group therapy had helped her with some further outside controls from peers who were also schoolmates. She now felt more accepted and worthwhile. The parents were no longer supervising her twenty-four hours a day; she attended school on her own, drove alone, and held a part-time job.

In the group sessions her primitive, rageful, and retaliatory feelings to her mother emerged, especially in connection with the mother's current (at times sadistic) behavior toward the patient.

The patient felt abandoned for awhile when her father's job promotion involved his regular absences from home. This feeling increased when her paternal grandmother visited for several months, during which the patient had to give up her room to the grandmother and sleep with her brother. These arrangements forced her into greater defensiveness. Her mother was also fearful that the grandmother would learn of the patient's psychiatric therapy, feeling that it would reflect shamefully upon her as a poor mother. The girl threatened to inform the grandmother to hurt her mother.

After the grandmother left, the patient vacillated between rages and plans to avenge herself by hurting her mother in some way; yet she complained when her mother left her at home alone. When her separation anxiety and guilt about hostile omnipotent wishes to the mother were interpreted, confirmatory material became more manifest in the transference, and she wished to discontinue therapy, and hurt or embarrass me. Her hostility was not confined to the transference, and she reported that she had provoked her mother over a minor item to the point where her mother had hit her, to which she responded in kind along with profuse profanity. She was now going through an open hostile separation from a sometimes sadistic, confining parental nest.

There followed acting out of the transference in and out of the sessions, with missed sessions and claims of being forced to attend group therapy. The group consensus was that she was not ready to discontinue therapy, even though she was more in control of herself, was not destructive, and was functioning satisfactorily with the family. She had a part-time job, was doing well in school, and behaved better with peers. Her acting out seemed to be a negative therapeutic reaction or a transference need to separate from me since she could not leave home yet. We agreed on a three-month vacation from therapy followed by a reevaluation of her therapy needs.

When she returned for the assessment, she felt comfortable with herself and her peers (and her steady boy friend), and she was achieving well academically, even getting prizes. But she complained that both her parents were drinking nightly before and after dinner. She had completely stopped drinking about the time her therapy vacation began when she realized she could not have just one drink but had to go on and on.

She looked forward to going to the college of her choice in the next year, but her parents opposed her leaving and wanted her to enter college in their hometown instead. She was able to discuss this with them instead of withdrawing. She was able to clarify some past misperceptions in thinking they were uninterested in her and now felt that sometimes they simply disagreed with her and did not want to hear her complaints about them or her different opinions.

She spontaneously went on to detail the onset of her illness, her feeling of being disorganized, her parents' refusal to obtain therapy for her, her increased symptoms and their subsequent determination to get therapy for her, and her positive response to therapy followed by a plateau at the time of her therapy vacation. This resistance, which was now dealt with, was connected to the use of the home as a substitute mental hospital, from which she feared she could be sent off to the state hospital anytime I chose; she therefore had intense rage toward, and fear of, me as her jailer. She had never been officially discharged from that situation and was still worried that I would send her off on a whim or revengefully as she had expected of her mother. Then she described an empathic inadequacy on my part some six months before which was related to a negative paternal transference reaction that involved her feeling abandoned by her father, unprotected from her mother's sadism, and unable to manipulate her mother when his traveling increased. This was also related to the feeling of abandonment she had gotten in the group because of my involvement with the other group members instead of solely with her.

The parents now requested a joint session with her about their refusal to have her apply to the college of her choice. Their fears about her being in college away from home led to an interpretation about their separation anxiety. The parents' subsequent reaction to her being accepted by that college was to discontinue her therapy, "unless she was in a completely overwrought state," since if she was "mature enough to go to college, she [didn't] need therapy." In her two truncated termination sessions, she explained that they felt that she was too attached to me and that they did not want her to continue therapy with anyone who disagreed with them. This may have been a distortion exaggerated due to her anger about the loss.

Discussion

Winnicott's (1958c, 1960, 1969) ideas about a holding environment are significant contributions to the understanding of the mutuality needed for integration of "good" and "bad" self-objects. If a mother survives her child's instinctual assaults without retaliation or withdrawal, the child is able to develop a relationship with her as a real object rather than as a projective entity. However, if the mother retaliates or withdraws from his demands, she confirms his fear of the power of his aggressively tinged self- and object representations. Responding to the retaliation and withdrawal, the infant generates increased rage and greater demands, thus intensifying his need for defensive splitting and projection (Shapiro et al. 1975). These developments in the rapprochement phase would leave the youngster vulnerable to their resurgence and to a regression occurring in adolescence, given that the same features are operating in the parents at both crisis periods.

If we assume a similar development for this girl, when her mother was pregnant with and after she delivered her brother, then one can see that at subsequent periods of crisis the vulnerability became exposed. This apparently occurred in the early grades with evidences of separation anxiety; again at puberty as a response to her mother's use of projective identification to primitively express the oedipal theme and its consequences to the patient with projective retaliation; and yet again when her girl friend rejected her and withdrew. The mother's continued projective identification with retaliatory actions further compromised the girl, leading to an escalation of rage and culminating in her attack on the bad object—her body (which belongs to mother but is not mother)—while sparing the good object, her mother (Laufer 1968).

Neither parent allowed the patient to be a dependent child, but at times they wanted her to be their supportive, nurturing parent—the father wanted her to amuse him as she had in the past when she was his baby doll. Her mother would not allow the girl to show any aggression yet expected that she fully accept the mother's own.

They did not allow her to separate or individuate, but if she accepted the mother's aggression she reversed roles with the mother and could not be dependent. If she talked to (fed) the father, as the paternal grandmother had done, she became his mother and could manipulate him. A role reversal was operating in both parents which furthered her bind. The mother's background included a family game of frequent argumentativeness and angry competition, apparently a defense against affectionate intimacy, sharing, and mutuality.

The mother's projective identification with the girl's revived oedipal conflict and her threat to the girl at menarche was experienced as a severe trauma, interfering with her ordinary development. It tended to promote merging with, instead of separating from, the mother. Apparently, she was able to defend against this by displacement to her erstwhile girl friend. When the relationship ended, she developed symptoms.

The patient was a model child who sacrificed her autonomy and self-regulation to maintain her relationship with her mother. Her use of imitation and "as if" behavior was long standing. Projection and splitting along with her use of objects at the need-satisfying level were evident through most of her treatment. She imitated in her relations with peers and was easily led but was unable to commit herself or initiate.

She used alcohol in an effort to reduce her anxiety and isolation, since intoxication allowed her to attend class and to feel less isolated, inhibited, and anxious and more witty and outgoing. She longed for and feared intimacy and used alcohol in an attempt to achieve it. The dissociation evident in this behavior prevented her from using the experiences for her growth and was obvious when she said she wanted to talk with me but needed to reduce her inhibitions first by becoming intoxicated. She was submissive to her teachers as new editions of her mother in grade school, but in adolescence her anger turned against her teachers, who were seen as unreliable and rejecting as her mother. At the same time, she hoped they would still accept and care for her. Whether she stole to supply her own needs never became clear from her material.

In individual sessions, she was quiet for long periods. If her silence was accepted and communication continued empathically in spite of her silence, she was able to maintain contact. If my countertransference interfered and led to unempathic reactions, she fled into fantasy or a dreamy state and became unavailable for therapeutic alliance and any productive work. Then I was seen as the demanding father who wished to be nurtured by her or as the demanding, overcontrolling, competitive, nongiving mother whom she could not please except by submission. Part of her reaction was based on transferences that were contaminated at times by countertransferences. A working transference developed slowly due to her distrust and her defensive splitting.

Early in therapy she felt I was omniscient and that she could be omniscient too through imitation. She was jealous of this attribution and anxious to attain it for herself through the attendance of sessions and her own professional attainments. This seemed similar to the symbiotic and acting-out relationship she had with her mother.

GROUP THERAPY

In the first therapy group, she imitated me and acted as an auxiliary therapist. Using projective identification, the patient irritated and disappointed her father when she imitated him in her efforts to prompt others to talk to her to show her that they cared. She also imitated her mother's behavior when she tried to control and organize others; gave little of her affects and experiences; and behaved as a smiling, low-key sergeant marshaling his troops. Her object was to stave off an attack from me, whom she saw alternately as part father, who demanded she talk to keep him comfortable, and part mother, who demanded she listen and do the right thing. By behaving in therapy as she did, she placated the parental aspects of her self which were in conflict yet simultaneously retaliated against them.

Similarly, in her attitude toward certain school subjects, she barely met scholastic requirements. In some courses she was outstanding, that is, in those that met her own needs; while in other, less meaningful subjects she was vengeful and retaliated by doing poorly. She would leave school and miss classes rather than be confronted by an angry teacher (mother) for whom her performance was unsatisfactory. Instead of being passive and rejected, she became aggressive and rejected the mother (teacher).

In the group she showed no curiosity about my personal life like the other teenagers did and rarely volunteered material. She remained passive, ready to be fed by me and the group members, thus maintaining her need-satisfaction level of object relations and her control of the situation. In her simultaneous individual therapy, however, she was able to expose more personal material.

Showing up for group therapy when no group session was scheduled indicated her reaction to separation with magic, wishful behavior—if she were present, there would be a change in schedule and the group would meet. In response to reality and the embarrassment of lacking omnipotence, she increased her drinking and suicidal behavior. She also had death wishes toward me for disappointing her, which were turned around on her body as a dissociated part (Laufer 1968).

HOME AS A MENTAL HOSPITAL: FAMILY AND NETWORK THERAPY

While her superego functioning was faulty and she had a need for real objects to control her function (Rosenfeld and Sprince 1963), the use of the family as a mental hospital provided improved superego function and controls for the youngster. The increased and focused contact with objects involved in the family setting provided need satisfaction and ego support, that is, a holding environment which partly undid the abandonment-rejection experiences, allowed treatment to continue, and protected the youngster from harm. Similarly, network therapy supplied protection, support, some controls, and peer-group superego. Her attitude about network therapy reflected her need to feel cared for in a symbiotic way, and though there was evidence of some therapeutic alliance, it was partly compliance and partly alliance.

Although support and guidance were given freely to the parents early in her treatment, especially during the time when home was used as a mental hospital, they had a most difficult task, as Winnicott (1965) observed. For example, they could not have a day or night off from their "nursing." When this was discussed, I empathized with their position and offered them guidance. Possibly, some residual anger about this restrictive task was involved in their resistance to the girl's interest in increasing the frequency of sessions, in retaliatory comments in the later family sessions, and in their response that the girl's separation from them required her separation from therapy.

The parents' use of projective identification against her dependency needs was unclear and was slowly discerned through family therapy. When their confounding and contradictory double-bind communications were deciphered, the mother felt attacked and retaliated, while the father projected further and attacked me for confusing him. When their dependency needs were threatened by her maturation and separation efforts, they burdened her by promoting the guilt to conform and meet their dependency wishes and by treating her as a two-year-old. When she was able soberly to plan leaving home for college, their separation anxiety surfaced, but therapy led to separating her anxiety from theirs. Their hostile response to her phase-appropriate autonomous strivings conforms to observations made by Shapiro and his associates (1975) about the parents of borderline adolescents. This was in keeping with their inability to meet the phase-appropriate dependency needs of their daughter at puberty and at earlier critical periods in her life, which were so intertwined with their use of projective identification and splitting that they denied their own dependency needs.

TREATMENT EFFECTS AND CHANGES

With a borderline patient, increased trust is an outcome of, not a prerequisite for, a therapeutic alliance, while attribution and projection of omniscience and omnipotence to the therapist allows therapy to start.

This patient's independence was furthered by unintrusive, empathic, interpretive work and by understanding and sympathy for her silences, her manipulative behavior, and her need for control. Identification led to internalization, to overcoming her regression in object-relations development, and to moving on by termination time to the phallic-oedipal level. This was fostered by the gradual process of treatment at the patient's rate of, and ability for, communication. This eventually decreased her need for clinging (which at times seemed like torture by her) and controlling the therapy thru silence or acting out at home or against the self (mother); acting out at school (where teacher equaled mother); or acting out in the therapy by walking out or not showing up and remaining in the car outside until it was time to go home. Eventually, there was a decreased tendency toward splitting. With increased repressive capacity developing, her creative and other sublimatory avenues were supported.

When her identification with me helped her attain progressive ego structure and function, she was able to separate from her mother, which became evident in the network and family therapy. When her own alloplastic symptoms left, she reported that her brother began stealing and her mother started drinking heavily and regularly when alone in the day time. This may have been exaggerated and distorted data, but it also reflected her having unconsciously acted out for the mother (Giffin, Litin, and Johnson 1954).

At the time of the therapeutic assessment after her therapy vacation, it emerged that the patient felt like a prisoner in her own home as a result of using the home as a mental hospital. Since she was never officially discharged from the home as hospital, she still felt threatened by psychiatric hospitalization. In reality, this had been quite clearly stated and observed previously since she could drive, date, etc.; but due to her own distrust, she wanted approval of change of status that she was discharged from past therapy, free from the threat of disorganization, able to leave the parents, and could engage now in a different therapy—analysis.

By the end of her therapy, splitting and projective identification were less evident. Although she continued using some projection and denial, there was increased capacity for repression and sublimation, with a decrease of rage, retaliation, and separation anxiety. Her artistic, creative interests and abstract thinking abilities continued to serve her well as sublimations. In the past she could pursue them only privately, but now she was able to share them and obtain secondary narcissistic gratification.

Events prior to her trial separation from therapy were stormy and appeared to have been a reflection of the resistance involving transference, with libidinal and aggressive feelings as well as punishment for my empathic failure. For borderlines, the development of a new relationship implies an aggressive one since they cannot conceive of the possibility of a safe relationship (Rosenfeld and Sprince 1965). This may have been another factor in her need to break off treatment for three months, allowing her further time to integrate what she had obtained from therapy and to assess the safety of being involved further in treatment. After she resumed therapy voluntarily, the parents intruded with their own separation anxieties. She clearly indicated her wish to separate from them saying, "Once I get to college, I'm never going home," and wished to get on with further therapy. Their separation anxieties were projected onto her in the guise of worries about sexual behavior. Their fantasy was accurate possibly in predicting that she was ready to find a heterosexual object following her separation from them. Her parents' retaliatory pattern was obvious when they discontinued her therapy at the point where she was highly motivated, and it recapitulated their earlier behavior.

Conclusions

Diverse opinions exist about treatment approaches to the borderline adolescent. For some selected borderline adolescents, individual outpatient psychotherapy along with other modalities during lengthy treatment may be optimal. These may include chemotherapy; group, family, and office network therapy; and using the home as a mental hospital. A case is presented to highlight some of these considerations and the vicissitudes encountered in the therapy.

Chemotherapy helped to decrease anxiety and promote the psychotherapeutic effort. Group therapy provided peer support and insight over a lengthy period. Individual therapy allowed the development of insight and identification and the working through of splitting, distortions, and transference. The use of the family as a mental hospital at home supplied a holding environment. Office network therapy provided support during an acute crisis of threats of disintegration and suicide. Family therapy was very helpful in exposing mutual regressive phenomena operating in the parents and the patient, the understanding of which were helpful to separate the youngster's needs from theirs and to promote individuation.

REFERENCES

Boyer, L. B., and Giovacchini, P. L. 1967. *Psychoanalytic Treatment of Characterological and Schizophrenic Disorders*. New York: Science House.

Coughlin, F., and Wimberger, H. D. 1968. Group family therapy. *Family Process* 7:37–49.

Ekstein, R., and Wallerstein, J. 1954. Observations on the psychology of borderline and psychotic children. *Psychoanalytic Study of the Child* 9:344–369.

Fine, S; Knight-Webb, G; and Breau, K. 1976. Volunteer adolescents in adolescent group therapy: effects on patients and volunteers. *British Journal of Psychiatry* 129:407–413.

Geleerd, E. R. 1958. Borderline states in childhood and adolescence. *Psychoanalytic Study of the Child* 13:279–295.

Giffin, A; Litin, M; and Johnson, A. 1954. Specific factors determining antisocial acting-out. *American Journal of Orthopsychiatry* 24:668–684.

Kernberg, O. 1975. *Borderline Conditions and Pathological Narcissism*. New York: Aronson.

Laufer, M. 1968. The body image, the function of masturbation and adolescence. *Psychoanalytic Study of the Child* 3:114–137.

Mahler, M. 1972. The rapprochement subphase of the separation-individuation process. *Psychoanalytic Quarterly* 41:487–506.

Mahler, M.; Pine, F.; and Bergman, A. 1975. *The Psychological Birth of the Human Infant*. New York: Basic.

Maltsberger, J. T., and Buie, D. H. 1974. Countertransference hate in the treatment of suicidal patients. *Archives of General Psychiatry* 30:625–633.

Masterson, J. F. 1972. *Treatment of the Borderline Adolescent*. New York: Wiley Interscience.

Offer, D., and Vanderstoep, E. 1975. Indications and contraindications for family therapy. In M. Sugar, ed. *The Adolescent in Group and Family Therapy*, New York: Brunner/Mazel.

Rosenfeld, S. K., and Sprince, M. P. 1963. An attempt to formulate the meaning of the concept ''borderline.'' *Psychoanalytic Study of the Child* 18:603–635.

Rosenfeld, S. K., and Sprince, M. P. 1965. Some thoughts on the technical handling of borderline children. *Psychoanalytic Study of the Child* 20:495–517.

Settlage, C. F. 1977. The psychoanalytic understanding of narcissistic and borderline personality disorders: advances in developmental theory. *Journal of the American Psychoanalytic Association* 25:805–834.

Shapiro, E. R.; Shapiro, R. L.; Zinner, J.; and Berkowitz, D. A. 1977. The borderline ego and the working alliance: indications for family and individual treatment in adolescence. *International Journal of Psycho-Analysis* 58:77–87.

Shapiro, E. R.; Zinner, J.; Shapiro, R. L.; and Berkowitz, D. A. 1975. The influence of family experience on borderline personality development. *International Review of Psycho-Analysis* 2:399–411.

Spotnitz, H. 1976. *Psychotherapy of Preoedipal Conditions*. New York: Aronson.

Stierlin, H. 1975. Countertransference in family therapy with adolescents. In M. Sugar, ed. *The Adolescent in Group and Family Therapy*. New York: Brunner/Mazel.

Sugar, M. 1975. Office network therapy with adolescents. In M. Sugar, ed. *The Adolescent in Group and Family Therapy*. New York: Brunner/Mazel.

Taylor, J. F. 1069. Role playing with borderline and mildly retarded adolescents in an institution. *Exceptional Child* 36:206–208.

Whitaker, C. A. 1975. The symptomatic adolescent: an AWOL family member. In M. Sugar, ed. *The Adolescent in Group and Family Therapy*. New York: Brunner/Mazel.

Williams, F. 1975. Family therapy: its role in adolescent psychiatry. In M. Sugar, ed. *The Adolescent in Group and Family Therapy*. New York: Brunner/Mazel.

Winnicott, D. W. 1958a. A case managed at home. In *Collected Papers: Through Paediatrics to Psychoanalysis*. New York: Basic.

Winnicott, D. W. 1958b. Hate in the countertransference. In *Collected Papers: Through Paediatrics to Psychoanalysis*. New York: Basic.

Winnicott, D. W. 1958c. The depressive position in normal emotional development. In *Collected Papers: Through Paediatrics to Psychoanalysis*. New York: Basic.

Winnicott, D. W. 1960. The theory of the parent-infant relationship. *International Journal of Psycho-Analysis* 41:585–594.

Winnicott, D. W. 1965. A child psychiatry case illustrating delayed reaction to loss. In M. Schur, ed. *Drives, Affect and Behavior*. New York: International Universities Press.

Winnicott, D. W. 1969. The use of an object. *International Journal of Psycho-Analysis* 50:711–716.

23 ADOLESCENTS AND FAMILIES: AN OVERVIEW

JOHN L. SCHIMEL

There are fads and fashions in the practice of child and adolescent psychiatry. A historical survey of child-rearing practices indicates that there has been a pendulum swing from the extremes of rigidity (let them cry it out) to indulgence (demand feeding, etc.) and back that takes an average of twenty years, or one generation, to complete. Bruch (1970) reported that the mother of a patient, when asked about the child-rearing practices she had followed, replied, "I really don't remember, but you can be sure it was the latest thing at the time."

On a broader scale, there have been swings of the pendulum concerning the nature of man, and hence the way the emerging human being is viewed, since antiquity. The ancient Greek ideal of beauty and serenity has been in conflict with the Judeo-Christian ideal of purity for millennia and is reflected in, among other things, alternations in psychiatric theory and practice.

Rousseau's noble savage and Thoreau's natural man were visions of the nature of man in which there is a corruption of the innocent by the repressive and irrational (i.e., the unnatural) in society. Theirs was a reaction against the then prevalent and continuing notion that man is born in sin and must be carefully scrutinized and punished for any sign of his evil nature, reflected in the "let them cry it out" attitude. Freud seemed to follow the notion of natural man in his early theories and to view the developing individual as if he lived in a cocoon, a neutral environment in which the vicissitudes of internal forces determined the fate of the individual. The violence of World War I, during which Freud lost a son, seems to have moved him to consider aggression as a primary drive, along with sexuality, and inclined him toward his theory of the death instinct, an echo of the notion of man's evil nature, along with a pessimistic or even cataclysmic view of man's fate. Other analytic theorists, such as Jung, Adler, Aichhorn, Fromm, Horney, and Sullivan, clung to a more sanguine view of the nature of man. Their views were also reflected in clinical practice with adolescents.

The earliest adolescent services borrowed heavily from child psychiatry. Basically, in the psychiatric practices of twenty years ago, this meant the virtual ostracism of the parents. The prevailing child and adolescent psychiatric practices then rested heavily on two notions. The psychiatric notion was explicit: Emotional problems were seen as intrapsychic and required parents only for the arranging of ongoing meetings of child and therapist. The mother had to be involved since she had to deliver the child to the therapist. With the older child or adolescent, the mother and/or father had to be involved, if for nothing else, in order to pay the bills. In a word, the therapist and his patient were sequestered in the treatment from the parents. In some clinics, the primary patient was seen (and still is seen) by the psychiatrist and the mother by the social worker. As early as 1955, Fine and Schimel (1955) reported good results when the father as well as the mother were required to participate in the treatment program. The parents, although seen therapeutically, were, nevertheless, sequestered from the therapy of the index patient.

The second notion upon which clinic practices were based was implicit or even denied. This was the concept that the parents were to blame for the difficulties of their children. This was the era of the schizophrenogenic mother, the parent so masterfully endowed that she was able to produce schizophrenia in her offspring. This paranoid view of parents led Mead (1972) to observe that the most characteristic thing about psychiatrists was their hatred of parents. Such attitudes toward parents are still common. Searles (1975) has reported his dawning recognition of the fact that parents, especially fathers, who were willing and could afford to send their offspring to a treatment center must, after all, have some positive attributes.

Family therapy, which has proliferated in recent years, began in the contributions of interpersonal, interactional, or transactional theories of human development and behavior, chiefly attributable to the seminal works of Sullivan (1953). Sullivan's theories focused on the genesis of character and personality (and psychopathology) as derived from the earliest transactions of the infant and significant others and as being reflected and maintained in continuing and parallel experiences. Sullivan's work inspired that of Jackson, Bateson, Reusch, Ackerman, Minuchin, Wynne, and others who studied patterns of communication and behavior in disturbed families.

The disturbed child or adolescent came to be viewed by family therapists as an integral part of an ongoing system of family transactions. His disturbance is considered to be essential to the maintenance of family equilibrium. This is an important concept, although it may be difficult for the uninitiated to see the principle of equilibrium operating in some of the chaotic families we study. The thrust of this concept may, in fact, tend to lead to the neglect of the effect of the social forces impinging on the patient and his family. It may, further, tend to neglect or minimize the powerful role of peer relationships in adolescent development. Sugar (1971) has reported on the logical extension of these considerations by his use of network therapy which brings together members of the extended family, neighbors, peers, etc., in addition to the adolescent, his parents, and his siblings.

I am not altogether persuaded by the rationale of family therapy for adolescents, particularly as a mindless passenger on a pendulum. One now sees adolescents routinely referred to family institutes or clinics in which family therapy is the sole or primary modality. When everyone undergoes family therapy, painful and unfortunate experiences can result. I was recently consulted by a father whose son had been hospitalized for the fourth time. He and his wife had been told they would have to take part in family therapy sessions. The couple had already spent six years in family therapy. The wife would cry herself to sleep the night of each session and the husband would drink. They were apparently the victims of the repetition-compulsion of the clinician.

The notion of the need for the restructuring of family dynamics as a primary operation to prepare the adolescent for the final stages of separation and individuation is an interesting but unproven notion. Twenty years hence, our experiences with family therapy for adolescents may be more valued for their focusing of attention on the importance of the kinds of transactions engaged in by the various members of the family system than for their therapeutic successes.

There are numerous ways to engage parents of adolescent patients constructively without routinely resorting to family therapy. Viewing the adolescent who comes into treatment as the index patient may be considered obsolete by some, but it is a concept that is not without its own virtues. The adolescent, for example, may be self-referred, with or without the parents' knowledge. Sometimes he is self-referred with prior agreement with the parents that they will not be involved in the treatment process. Sometimes this kind of referral has followed a prior experience with family therapy.

Goals of Treatment

In general, the goal of the treatment of the adolescent patient is to foster his maturation. How this is approached depends on a number of factors, including age, diagnosis, degree of pathology, socioeconomic and other situational factors, physical health, previous experiences with therapy, school adjustment, intelligence, sex, parental and family psychopathology, etc. If one does not subscribe to the notion that one must facilitate the growth of the adolescent by the prior rehabilitation of the family, the primary goal is to foster a therapeutic alliance with the adolescent patient in which his growth and welfare become a shared project for patient and therapist.

An equally important task may be the facilitation of a working alliance with the parents. More often than not, one of the parents contacts the therapist to arrange consultation. It may be well to spend sufficient time on the telephone to ascertain the nature of the problem and, more important, to determine whether it is the wish of the parents to meet alone with the therapist to discuss the situation. It is well to respect this wish when it is present. The possibility that this might lead to subsequent difficulties with the adolescent patient can be handled later.

There are a number of tasks to be accomplished in the initial contacts with parents. The goal of obtaining information is relatively unimportant compared with the primary task of achieving a state of rapport and trust between parents and therapist and developing a working alliance. There are a number of crucial matters to be attended to. Let us start with a point emphasized by Sullivan (1953). An interview is at least a two-way process. The therapist is not merely an observer; he is also being studied very carefully. Sometimes the parents or the adolescent may be at least as perceptive as the therapist in this regard. In one referral, the therapist reported the mother to be a hostile and controlling personality. The mother reported the therapist to be passive-aggressive, stubborn and inflexible, and afraid of women.

The time taken on the telephone by the therapist to get some idea of the problem and his willingness to meet with the parents, alone if they wish, may be reassuring to them. How they are greeted at the beginning of the interview, the tone and demeanor of the therapist, and his attention to their comfort are important in establishing rapport. The therapist as scientist coolly eliciting facts can be but a thin veneer, more likely to be maintained where there are plenty of referrals or a clinic population to be dealt with. One mother told me she "wouldn't put up with that smug, supercilious, tight-assed bastard. Who does he think he is?" The psychiatrist can rationalize that no one could get along with that particular lady, but that is not necessarily true. I have published the opinion that if some of my patients had been able to adhere to at least minimal standards of courtesy they would not need me. Why not the psychiatrist? Grotjahn (1960) suggested that "scientific" Americans have never understood the way psychoanalysis was practiced in Europe. For example, he noted that an analyst would welcome a woman patient in his native Hungary in the traditional manner, kissing her hand in greeting and helping her remove her coat and overshoes. After that, "the hour" would begin. Freud reported that after a psychoanalytic session he might press advice on the patient who was leaving.

The parents arrive in an anxious state, apprehensive and fearful that they will be judged as inadequate or hurtful parents by the therapist, a judgment which they, more or less consciously, have made about themselves. Perhaps the parents are defensive and blame their troubles on the adolescent's companions, the child himself, the school, the community, or each other. As in individual psychotherapy, one of the first tasks is to soften the harsh superego judgments under which patients are laboring. Their connection with the rest of humanity needs to be reestablished, they can be told of the frequency of the kind of problems they are experiencing, and they can be helped to become more optimistic by a realistic statement of the fact that many troubled adolescents do somehow pull through. It often takes such support to elicit the parents' concerns about the child and their own possible role in the creation of the problem. Taking the time and the trouble to provide a respectful climate in order to note the commonality of the parents' concerns with those of other parents about problem children may seem like a small issue, but is really a significantly different procedure than eliciting such concerns in a vacuum. In the latter case, parents often feel alienated from the problems of ordinary people and judged harshly by the therapist.

It is well to conduct the interview with the parents in a manner that is relatively easy for them to follow and that seems natural. This usually means starting with a statement of the chief complaints, as in regular medical practice. The developmental history can be deferred to later in the interview or to a later interview. I have seen a number of parents with pressing concerns who had not been provided with sufficient time to talk through the presenting complaints in an initial interview. A number of therapists have noted an increasing compassion for parents and what they need to talk about—as contrasted with what the therapist thinks he needs to know—when their own children become adolescents.

The therapist may note for the parents, in addition to statements that may indicate the possibility of a favorable outcome, the possibility that there may be exacerbations of the adolescent's difficulties while he is in treatment, although not necessarily caused by it. The therapist may also note the possibility of unreported concerns by parents, such as the possibility of drug busts, pregnancy, or suicide. This may open the door to a plethora of serious worries by the parents, often kept secret from each other and, often enough, representing justified fears.

There are a number of other matters to be considered with parents. These include issues of confidentiality, the subsequent availability of the therapist to the parents, possible changes of behavior expected of parents, the question of further joint sessions with or without the adolescent patient, and the matter of hours and fees.

The issue of confidentiality seems to be a problem with therapists dealing with adolescents. There are references in the literature to the normal paranoia of adolescents in treatment, particularly with regard to their parents. I suggest that some of this is iatrogenic, a kind of self-fulfilling prophecy. Parents are told that what is learned in interviews with them may be helpful to the therapist in his work with the adolescent and will be used by the therapist when indicated. An occasional parent may reveal something he wishes kept from the adolescent. This is rarely a matter of consequence to the treatment, and confidentiality can be promised. The parents are also told, however, that the conversations between therapist and adolescent will not be discussed with them. They are warned that an angered adolescent may tell them that his therapist thinks they are "wrong, stupid, rigid, and old fashioned.'' There is often a paradoxical consequence of this warning. When the adolescent accuses the parents of being rigid or stupid and that his therapist thinks so too, the parents tend not to overreact to the adolescent's statement, even if he is reporting his therapist's opinion accurately, and to respond more objectively.

The adolescent is also informed of this double standard: his interviews are confidential; those of his parents are not. He is usually delighted with the arrangement. In addition, he is asked what he would like his parents to be told and what he would not like them to be told. The response is frequently revealing and may open numerous possibilities for subsequent therapeutic interactions. Generally, the issue of confidentiality is smoothly resolved in this way, and the trust usually present in adolescents which needs to be expressed and reciprocated, even with grownups, is fostered.

Parents are encouraged to keep in touch with the therapist, particularly if they are concerned about the adolescent's activities. They are also assured that they will be called by the therapist if the adolescent is engaged in activities that they should know about. The effect of offering parents access to the therapist is once again, more often than not, paradoxical. The availability of communication not only seems to discourage telephoned appeals to the therapist but also to lessen the anxiety or even desperation parents feel about the child and the therapeutic situation.

Parents frequently beseech the therapist for advice about handling the adolescent. They want to know whether and how they should change their own behavior. Unless some remarkably destructive behavior on their part is discovered, they are advised not to change anything, that one of the tasks of the treatment process is to study the situation exactly as it is. The thrust of this statement is to establish the fact that there are no treatment expectations for the parents. This is important in establishing the working alliance. Clinical judgment may subsequently incline the therapist in the direction of specific suggestions to the parents. The caveat is not to offer suggestions of an ambiguous nature. Any advice to parents should be within their capacities and not such as to lead to further failures on their part.

The therapist should permit himself sufficient time to make a thoroughgoing survey of the presenting complaints, the plight of the adolescent, the psychological and economic resources of the parents, and the variety of situational factors that may be relevant before deciding on a treatment strategy. Naturally, having a plan that works for all situations can obviate the effort and expense indicated by the foregoing. After my first few years of practice, I reviewed all the consultations I had done. I realized that, after considerable pondering in each instance, I had, nevertheless, recommended individual psychotherapy for every one. This led to a sobering thought: Who needed me? I could have made such stock recommendations over the telephone.

Generally speaking, family interviews or family therapy is reserved for younger adolescents or for extremely immature or severely disturbed adolescents who are so immersed in the family system that there is practically no opening to the age-appropriate tasks of the adolescent. If the adolescent is further along in his psychosexual development, individual treatment may be supplemented by group therapy, particularly for shy, isolated, or schizoid adolescents who are nevertheless functioning reasonably well at home and/or in school. Ongoing regular contact with parents may be more frequent with younger adolescents, those who are engaged in dangerous activities, or those whose parents are extremely anxious. There are a number of other useful variations, such as occasional meetings of the adolescent and one of his parents or periodic meetings with parents while seeing the adolescent individually. The variation is determined by circumstances and is, ideally, a reflection of the clinical judgment of the therapist.

Conclusions

In this chapter, I have provided a brief overview of the attitudes, theories, and practices of psychiatrists who deal with adolescent patients. I have also suggested that potentially useful modalities of treatment appear from time to time but are supported by such fervor that clinical judgment and the resourcefulness required to operate optimally in such a complex field as human relations may be suspended. A rationale for the flexible selection of appropriate treatment strategies is offered for dealing with families in which the adolescent is the index patient. Suggestions are given for enlisting the parents in a collaborative effort designed to foster the optimal development of the adolescent.

369

REFERENCES

Bruch, H. 1970. Personal communication.

Fine, A., and Schimel, J. 1955. Including fathers in a child guidance clinic. Paper presented at the annual Meeting of the American Orthopsychiatric Association, March.

Grotjahn, M. 1960. Personal communication.

Mead, M. 1972. Personal communication.

Searles, H. 1975. Personal communication.

Sugar, M. 1971. Network psychotherapy of an adolescent. *Adolescent Psychiatry* 1:464–478.

Sullivan, H. S. 1953. *The Interpersonal Theory of Psychiatry*. New York: Norton.

PERSPECTIVES ON PSYCHOPHARMACOLOGY AND THE ADOLESCENT

24 PSYCHOPHARMACOLOGY AND THE ADOLESCENT: AN INTRODUCTION

ARTHUR D. SOROSKY

Psychopharmacology as an adjunctive measure in the treatment of adolescents has been seriously neglected. Reliable information is scarce, and the prevailing thought on the subject is filled with unproven ideas and misconceptions. Neither the childhood nor the adult psychopharmacologic literature has addressed directly the unique problems of prescribing for the teenager. With these concerns in mind, the Southern California Society for Adolescent Psychiatry sponsored a program entitled, "Psychopharmacology and the Adolescent—an Update." Each of the participants dealt with a specific area of pharmacologic concern, and their papers have been revised for inclusion in this special section.

These chapters will review the use of various medications in the treatment of adolescent psychological problems, including stimulant medications, minor tranquilizers, major tranquilizers, antidepressants, and lithium carbonate. The authors have gone beyond a chemical review of the various drug properties and have concerned themselves with the particular management problems, side effects, and unique concerns of using these drugs with adolescent patients.

The major tranquilizers, used in the treatment of schizophrenia, are probably the most widely accepted of the psychopharmacologic agents used for adolescents. The minor tranquilizers, especially diazepam, are frequently prescribed for adolescents by nonpsychiatric physicians, but most psychiatrists seem reluctant to use these drugs for their young patients. Either they are under the impression that the minor tranquilizers are not effective in countering the anxiety experienced in adolescence or they are concerned that covering up the patient's symptoms will be counterproductive to their psychotherapeutic efforts. In actuality, judicious use of these minor tranquilizers can expedite the work of the psychotherapist.

Most psychiatrists are also under the impression that antidepressants are ineffective in a patient who is not fully grown. This is not true, and these medications can be extremely helpful in treating an endogenous depression or the behavioral equivalents of depression. Likewise, few psychiatrists are attuned to the possibility that their adolescent patient is suffering from a first episode of manic-depressive illness which would benefit from treatment with lithium carbonate. Finally, the prevailing myth that hyperkinetic children outgrow their illness, along with a therapeutic response to amphetamines or methylphenidate (Ritalin), has been disproven. Many of these youngsters will show a positive response to the stimulant medications until the age of eighteen or beyond.

It is important to emphasize that many psychiatrists are reluctant to prescribe psychopharmacologic agents for adolescents, sometimes with good reason. Some psychotherapists feel that giving tranquilizers to young patients is merely teaching them to avoid the introspective process and the painful feelings that are likely to arise. There is also an understandable concern about accentuating the typical adolescent dependency/independency conflicts by putting the patient into a submissive relationship to the prescribing therapist. This may lead to an uncomfortable sense of infantilization or to a counterphobic attempt at resisting or sabotaging the treatment program.

Adolescents are particularly sensitive to the development of medication side effects. They are very much concerned about feeling out of control, overly sedated, or artificially stimulated. The phenothiazines are particularly prone to inducing frightening side effects such as extrapyramidal symptoms, weight gain, retarded ejaculation, etc. These side effects, combined with the usual mistrust of adults, make adolescent psychopharmacology a delicate art. At no time is the establishment of a therapeutic alliance of greater importance and the empathy of the adolescent psychiatrist more challenged than in using psychotropic drugs to enhance psychotherapy.

25 USE OF STIMULANT MEDICATION WITH PSYCHIATRICALLY DISORDERED ADOLESCENTS

DENNIS P. CANTWELL

The use of psychopharmacologic agents has had a major impact on both research and clinical aspects of psychiatric practice with adults in the United States. The development of phenothiazine medications allowed many chronic schizophrenic patients who previously had to be treated on the back wards of state hospitals to be managed in out-patient clinics. The introduction of the tricyclic antidepressants and the MAO inhibitors has made a major difference in the treatments of patients with major depressive disorders. Moreover, the biological action of these drugs is somehow involved in the genesis of depressive disorders in adults. The study of central monoamine neurotransmitters is now one of the major biological research areas in adult psychiatry.

The development of lithium carbonate has produced a drug which not only is apparently effective in the active manic phase of manic-depressive disorder but which may also have a prophylactic effect on the development of subsequent manic and depressive episodes. Lithium may be also effective in the depressive phases of patients with bipolar affective disorder.

The field of childhood psychopharmacology actually precedes these developments if one begins its history with Bradley's (1937) use of stimulants. While the use of psychopharmacological agents in child psychiatry has not produced any theoretical or practical breakthrough comparable to that in adult psychiatry, the use of stimulants with hyperactive children is the best documented of all psychophar-macologic treatments of psychiatric disorders of childhood (Cantwell and Carlson 1978). A growing body of biological research suggests that at least some hyperactive children have disorders of monoamine metabolism (Shaywitz, Cohen, and Shaywitz 1978), and neurophysiologic theories have been developed to explain the seemingly paradoxical clinical effect of stimulant medication on such children (Satterfield, Cantwell, and Satterfield 1974).

However, compared to the voluminous adult psychopharmacologic literature and the growing literature of childhood psychopharmacology, literature on the psychopharmacologic treatment of adolescent populations is scarce. There are probably several reasons why this is so. First of all, in psychiatry as in medicine, adolescents are a somewhat in-between group. Just as many adolescents are medically "lost" between pediatricians and internists, there are adolescents who become lost between child psychiatrists and adult psychiatrists, particularly in psychopharmacologic research. Second, though there are societies for adolescent psychiatry in the United States, it is not a formal subspecialty. Moreover, there is some question whether there is an adequate amount of training of both a didactic and experimental nature both in general and child psychiatric training programs and in the psychopharmacologic treatment of adolescent disorders.

The diagnosis of adolescent psychiatric disorders is not as clear-cut as the diagnosis of adult disorders. There are accepted research criteria, such as the Feighner Criteria (Feighner, Robins, Guze, Woodruff, Winokur, and Munoz 1972) and the Research Diagnostic Criteria (RDC) (Spitzer, Endicott, Robins, Kuriansky, and Gurland 1975) which are reliable in classifying psychiatric disorders in adults. Hudgens (1974) and others have shown that there are adolescent patients with psychiatric disorders who can be adequately described and classified according to these criteria. However, there are also many adolescent patients who do not fulfill any specific diagnostic criteria. This means that diagnostic indications for psychopharmacologic intervention developed on the basis of studies of psychiatrically disordered adults cannot automatically be applied to adolescents. The same is true of diagnostic indications developed from studies of psychiatric disorders of childhood, especially in the use of stimulants. As will be discussed, the diagnostic category in childhood which is the most unique indication for the use of stimulant medication is the hyperactive child syndrome, or attentional deficit disorder with hyperactivity. As might be expected, as hyperactive children grow they lose many of their initial clinical characteristics, and they may be misdiagnosed in adolescence. The same applies to other psychiatric disorders beginning in childhood. Finally, many clinicians are reluctant to prescribe a potentially addicting drug to a psychiatrically disordered adolescent.

Clinical Actions

Like all psychoactive drugs, central nervous system stimulants affect many bodily systems and functions. These include physiological effects on the central nervous system, the cardiovascular system, the musculoskeletal system, the smooth muscle and renal systems, the gastrointestinal tract, and the metabolic system (Cantwell and Carlson 1978). From the practicing clinician's standpoint, the most important effects of the stimulants are those on behavior, activity level, cognitive functioning, academic achievement, mood, and personality. The evidence for stimulant effects on these various clinical functions comes mainly from studies of children, primarily those with the disorder characterized by the symptom pattern of hyperactivity, short attention span, and impulsive behavior. Whether or not the same functions are affected in exactly the same way in adolescents with this disorder or in adolescents with other disorders cannot be stated with certainty.

There are a number of sound, well-controlled studies indicating that stimulants have a consistently positive effect on disruptive, socially inappropriate behavior (Barkley 1977; Gittelman-Klein 1975). There is no clear evidence that stimulants positively affect neurotic symptoms such as fears, phobias, and anxiety. However, experienced clinicians and researchers, such as Fish (1971) and Conners (Conners and Werry 1978) reported positive effects on these types of symptoms in some of their patients.

With regard to activity level, the literature on stimulant effects seems at first glance to be confusing and contradictory. Cantwell and Carlson (1978) explain that this problem is at least partly due to different usages of the term "hyperactivity." In some cases hyperactivity means activity level, while in others it means disruptive behavior. Moreover different measures have been used to quantify activity level. Thus different results can be expected if rating-scale data are compared with data collected by recording instruments. Finally, the situations in which activity level has been measured very often differ from study to study.

Stimulants seem to have a different effect on free field activities, such as those exhibited on the playground, than on activity manifested during performance of vigilance tasks in a laboratory setting.

Stimulants probably affect the quality of motor activity, at least as much as the quantity of motor activity. Stimulants can produce an increase or a decrease in activity level, depending upon the type of motor activity being measured, the type of instrument used to quantify it, and the situation under which the child is tested. However, in the usual clinical situation the effect of stimulant medications on motor activity is a desired one.

While there is no clear evidence that stimulants improve performance on general cognitive measures, such as concept learning, language skills, reading achievement, and measured intelligence, there is a solid body of evidence reporting a consistent positive effect when more specific laboratory measures are used.

The effects of stimulants upon cognitive functioning may be summarized as follows: there is a reduction in errors of omission in laboratory settings where sustained performance is the required response (Campbell, Douglas, and Morgenstern 1971); there is an increase in accuracy of performance in laboratory tasks which require vigilance and in tests requiring immediate and delayed perceptual judgments (Campbell et al. 1971; Werry and Aman 1975); in reaction-time tests where the expected response is a rapid one, stimulants reduce latency and increase speed of reaction time (Sykes, Douglas, Weiss, and Minde 1971; Sykes, Douglas, and Morgenstern 1972); in reaction-time tests where the desired response is one of less impulsive responding, stimulants lead to a more deliberate response (Campbell et al. 1971); finally, on both simple and choice reaction-time tests, stimulants positively affect performance and reduce variability in these reaction-time tasks (Sroufe 1975). In short, a review of the effects of stimulants on cognitive functioning suggests that those tasks that are improved by stimulant medication are those in which sustained attention is required. This is verified by Barkley's (1977) review of stimulant medication with hyperactive children in which inattentiveness was found to be the best predictor of response.

It might be hypothesized, since there is such a solid body of evidence indicating a positive effect of stimulants on certain cognitive functions, that academic achievement is likewise improved. Evidence for this view is distinctly lacking (Barkley and Cunningham 1977), but this does not mean that academic achievement is not improved by the use of stimulant medication, since a proper study evaluating the effect of stimulant medication alone on academic achievement has not yet been carried out.

The effect of stimulants on mood with children and adolescents has also been inadequately studied. Often the general statement is made that stimulants do not produce euphoria in children. There are isolated clinical studies and case reports suggesting the opposite (Conners, Eisenberg, and Sharpe 1965). However, there is also clinical evidence to suggest that the chronic use of stimulant medication may lead to depression as a side effect, necessitating discontinuation of the medication (Barkley 1977).

Finally, stimulant effect on the personality structure of children and adolescents has been inadequately investigated. In younger children the effect of stimulants on personality can be negative, with parents making statements such as "he's not my child," or "I don't know what it is but I don't like him this way." Such effects on personality are at times significant enough to cause a discontinuation of the medication even though the other effects are positive.

Clinical Syndromes

In the author's opinion there is only one definitely established indication for the use of stimulant medication: the disorder called Attentional Deficit Disorder with Hyperactivity (DSM III [1978]) or, in DSM II (1968), the hyperkinetic reaction of childhood. Unofficially it has been called the hyperactive child syndrome, hyperkinetic syndrome, and minimal brain dysfunction. This disorder is characterized by a chronic symptom pattern of attentional difficulties, activity level which is greater than expected for the patient's age, and impulsive behavior. Barkley's (1977) review of stimulant drug research with this disorder found an overall improvement rate of about 75 percent with all three of the major stimulants: amphetamines, methylphenidate, and magnesium pemoline.

One of the myths about this syndrome was that it is a disorder of childhood only, which disappears with maturation. The assumption was that once neurophysiologic maturity had occurred, treatment with stimulant medication would no longer be necessary. The Freedman report (1971) stated unequivocally that stimulants were useful for younger children with this disorder but should not be used with adolescent patients beginning about age eleven or twelve. Now, however, an extensive amount of evidence from prospective and retrospective follow-up studies (Cantwell 1978) indicates that in fact this disorder is not "outgrown," but that its clinical manifestations change, particularly the activity level symptoms. Moreover, secondary problems such as learning disabilities, antisocial behavior, depression, and low self-esteem become predominant and obscure the original clinical picture.

There is no evidence in the literature that the adolescent patient with this disorder exhibits a stimulation reaction to stimulant medication as he grows older. Moreover, there is also no evidence that adolescents with this disorder stop responding. A study by Mackay, Beck, and Taylor (1973) indicates the exact opposite. They studied ten adolescents, aged thirteen to eighteen, all of whom had manifested the clinical picture of the hyperactive child syndrome. All ten showed some improvement in the capacity to learn, integrate, and remember when they were placed on methylphenidate with an average does of 30 mg and a maximum dose of 60 mg per day. There was not only clinical improvement, but there was an improvement in the electroencephalogram and in certain psychological tests. Moreover there was no evidence of tendency toward addiction in any of these adolescents as a result of their use of methylphenidate.

An increasing body of evidence from clinical studies and systematic controlled studies (Wood, Reimherr, Wender, and Johnson 1976) suggests that adults who are "grown-up hyperactive children" still have a positive response to stimulant medication. Thus, when a clinician is faced with an adolescent patient who manifested the classical clinical picture of the attentional deficit disorder with hyperactivity when younger and who is still manifesting psychiatric difficulties, even though he no longer has the classical picture, a trial of stimulant medication would seem to be indicated.

What other conditions are there in adolescence in which a trial of stimulant medication might be indicated? Based on the above review of the clinical functions which are affected by the stimulants and on what we know about their effect on children, some possible indications may include: those children who manifest an attentional deficit disorder without hyperactivity; those who manifest conduct disorders; and those who manifest specific learning disabilities associated with difficulty in attention and impulsivity.

The attentional deficit disorder without hyperactivity is a new diagnostic category in DSM III (1978). Since it has been shown that inattentiveness is the clinical symptom most strongly associated with a positive response to stimulants, and since there are clinical reports of children, particularly girls, with attentional disorder without excess motor activity, it makes theoretical sense that such adolescents may also respond positively to stimulants. However, there are few clinical studies to support this view, and there are no definite controlled studies to date.

Since conduct-disordered adolescents are considered addiction prone, the use of an addicting drug with such adolescents is controversial, and might seem to some to be countertherapeutic. However, there are investigators (Eisenberg, Lackman, and Molling 1963; Maletsky 1974) who have found stimulants to be effective for delinquent teenagers. Maletsky studied fourteen pairs of delinquent teenagers and documented a significant positive effect with dexedrine as compared with placebo, particularly in those conduct-disordered adolescents who had an earlier history of the hyperactive child syndrome. None of the adolescents in Maletsky's study developed tolerance, showed withdrawal, reported effects of euphoria, or gave any sign of becoming addicted to the drug. Conduct-disordered adolescents are extremely difficult to treat and often are placed in correctional institutions, such as juvenile halls and reform schools, rather than therapeutically oriented institutions. The work of Lewis and Balla (1976) also suggests that a significant proportion of delinquent adolescents are grown-up hyperactive children.

As noted, there is no definitive evidence to suggest that stimulant medication positively affects classroom academic achievement. A review of the clinical functions affected by stimulant medications, however, suggests that a trial of stimulants might be indicated in underachieving adolescents. There is abundant evidence that certain laboratory measures of learning are positively affected by the use of stimulants. Second, there is a good deal of evidence to suggest that academic underachievers often have problems with inattention and impulsive behavior which lead to academic difficulties (Ross 1976). A properly conducted study of such adolescents who are being treated with stimulant medication would seem to be a fruitful area for research.

Finally, there are other disorders in adolescents, such as mental retardation and organic brain syndromes, which in selected cases may benefit from stimulants. While stimulants have no positive effect on the core symptoms of either mental retardation or any of the organic brain disorders, many of these adolescents have problems with inattentiveness, impulsivity, and hyperactivity which can be positively affected by the use of stimulants.

On the other hand, stimulants are considered to be contraindicated in adolescents with anorexia nervosa, Gilles de la Tourettes disease, all types of schizophrenia, and primary affective disorders. There are also medical contraindications, such as hypertension, which would preclude the use of any medications with sympathomimetic activity.

Clinical Use of Stimulants

The use of stimulants with psychiatric disordered adolescents is not an either/or proposition; either stimulants or psychotherapy or stimulants or special education. It is likely that, whatever the disorder being treated, some other therapeutic intervention—individual psychotherapy, family therapy, or behavior modification—will have to be used along with stimulants. Nor are stimulants to be construed as inferior therapeutic interventions. There is often an unspoken feeling in the United States that use of any psychopharmacologic agent is only to be considered as a last resort after psychotherapy or other therapeutic interventions have been found wanting. Such a view is based on ignorance of the true use of any psychopharmacologic agent. The goal of treatment for psychiatrically disordered adolescents is to promote maturation and development. Any therapeutic intervention which will aid in doing this should be used.

While an exhaustive treatment of the monitoring of stimulant medication is beyond the scope of this chapter, some discussion of the clinical usage of stimulants with adolescents is in order. After a comprehensive diagnostic evaluation determines whether the adolescent has any psychiatric disorder and the nature of that disorder, the clinician must further determine whether the disorder is one which meets the criteria as likely to respond to stimulants. Psychiatric diagnosis in adolescents, as in adults and children, is essentially based on the presence of a specific clinical picture. The clinical picture is developed from interviews with parents and significant others in the adolescent's environment, interviews with the adolescent, and information obtained from school. The physical examination, neurological examination, laboratory studies, and psychological tests may offer little to the determination of whether or not stimulant medication should be used, but these studies are necessary to rule in or rule out certain conditions, such as a specific learning disability or some medical or neurological disorder, presenting with psychiatric symptomatology.

For any adolescent placed on stimulant medication a baseline blood count and a screening battery are recommended. Blood tests should only be performed if there is a clear clinical indication of specific physical, neurological, or toxic effects.

As part of the initial diagnostic evaluation it is important to obtain proper baseline assessment of all the clinical symptoms and functions that are likely to be affected by the stimulants. The Conners Parent Rating Scale and the Conners Teacher Rating Scale are quite useful for this purpose, as are the physician rating scales based on interviews with the adolescent (Guy 1976).

Once the decision has been made to use stimulant medication, the next step is to involve the adolescent and his parents in the treatment process. Adolescents in general do not like to take psychoactive medication. Because body-image issues are so important at this age, the taking of any medication confirms that they are somehow different, deviant, or defective; these feelings must be worked with therapeutically. Too often stimulants are given to the parents to give to the adolescent without any attempt made to involve the adolescent himself in the process. It is important to help him understand the nature of his difficulty and how the use of the stimulants is aimed at helping him overcome his specific problems.

Likewise parents should be fully involved in the treatment process from the very beginning. It is likely that either the dosage or type of stimulant will have to be changed in order to obtain the proper effect. Parents should be told in great detail about the positive and negative effects of the medication, and should be encouraged to observe their child carefully for the development of any side effects.

Contact with school personnel is also mandatory in order to monitor properly the clinical effect of the medication. Stimulants are often prescribed so that they are effective only throughout the school day, and thus parents may never see the adolescent while he is on an effective dose of medication. Moreover the parents generally see the adolescent only in a home situation which may not bring out the difficulties for which the child is being treated. The school setting is much more likely to make demands for attention and vigilance which the stimulants are likely to positively affect. Relying solely on reports from parents or only on observations and reports of the adolescent is likely to lead to underestimation of both positive and negative effects of stimulants.

As to which stimulant to use, there are three primary groups: amphetamines, methylphenidate, and magnesium pemoline. Properly controlled clinical studies have failed to demonstrate significant positive clinical effects for either deanol or caffeine (Cantwell and Carlson 1978). Published studies indicate, at least with children with attentional problems and hyperactivity, that methylphenidate, the amphetamines, and magnesium pemoline are about equally effective. However, as a general rule, an older drug which has been in use for a number of years should be used before a newer drug like magnesium pemoline, unless there is overwhelming evidence of the latter's clinical superiority. Thus methylphenidate and the amphetamines should be given a thorough trial before considering the use of pemoline.

With regard to clinical monitoring, the smallest available dosage should be the starting dose. The duration of action of the stimulant is the most important factor in determining how often to prescribe the medication. Pemoline is different from methylphenidate and from the short-acting forms of the amphetamines; its duration of action is longer and it tends to build up significant blood levels. The short-acting forms of the amphetamines and methylphenidate have a duration of action of about four hours, do not build up significant blood levels, and are given at least twice a day to get the adolescent through the school day and possibly three times a day if there are certain aspects of behavior which require control beyond the school period.

There are only very rough guidelines that one can use for optimal dosage of individual stimulant drugs on a milligram per kilogram basis of body weight. This is a controversial area, and we suggest the physician start with a low dose and titrate the dosage upward until either a clinical improvement is noticed or side effects occur which necessitate discontinuation of the drug. Some adolescents may require a great deal more medication than would be expected on the basis of their body weight. There are at times large individual differences in blood levels of medication per comparable dosage of the same stimulant in patients with the same body weight (Cantwell and Carlson 1978). Other studies indicate that stimulants may continue to have a positive effect on learning up to a certain dosage and then have a negative effect as the dosage is increased, however, behavior continues to improve with increasing dosage. Thus it is important to have some measure of learning as an indication of the effectiveness of stimulants so that learning is not impaired at the expense of better behavioral control (Sprague and Sleator 1975). If improvement occurs initially but disappears, there are two possibilities: (1) the initial effect was a placebo effect, or (2) tolerance has developed and the dosage may have to be increased. We have found the need to increase medication, particularly with adolescents, to be idiosyncratic. Many adolescents remain on the same dosage of stimulants for a year before requiring any increase, others require increases at three or six months. We follow adolescents on stimulant medication with at least monthly visits, obtaining parent and teacher behavior rating scales at that time as well as making systematic observations in the office. If there is a negative response to one of the stimulants, it is worthwhile trying another. While many adolescents respond equally well to methylphenidate, the amphetamines, and magnesium pemoline, there are certain adolescents who respond positively to one and not as well to another.

There are few published reports of significant side effects in children and adolescents on stimulant medication, which is indirect evidence that they are probably relatively uncommon. The common short-term side effects include insomnia, anorexia, stomach aches, headaches, and moodiness. These short-term side effects generally subside with time. Only rarely do they lead to discontinuation of medication. The one long-term side effect which has caused the greatest concern is possible height and weight suppression. Stimulants do have an inhibiting effect on both height and weight in the first year or two of therapy. However, after the second year this suppression seems to be completely overcome with no permanent effect.

Adolescents who are on chronic stimulant medication need to be given a drug-free trial at some time during the course of the year to determine whether or not medication should be continued. An ideal technique is to substitute a placebo for the active medication with the parents' knowledge but without patient or teacher knowing. Ratings of behavior can then be obtained and if there is a deterioration in performance, either in behavior or in academic tasks, it can be assumed that the medication is still needed. If a placebo is not available, the adolescent will simply have to be taken off the medication with the knowledge of both parent and child. However, blind ratings can still be obtained from teachers, and if objective psychological measures, such as a continuous-performance task or paired-associate learning tasks, reveal a deterioration in performance, the medication should be resumed.

Conclusions

Adolescents often ask how long they will have to be on medication. The answer is that for an individual patient clinical judgment is the only way one can determine when stimulant medication can be stopped completely. Stimulants should be stopped only when the clinical picture indicates that they are no longer needed, not because a certain age is reached. There is considerable evidence (Huessey 1978; Wood et al. 1976) to indicate that some grown-up hyperactive children still respond to stimulant medication well into adulthood.

REFERENCES

Barkley, R. 1977. A review of stimulant drug research with hyperactive children. *Journal of Child Psychology and Psychiatry* 18:137–165.
Barkley, R., and Cunningham, C. 1978. Do stimulant drugs improve academic performance of hyperkinetic children? A review of outcome research. *Clinical Pediatrics* 17(1):85–92.
Bradley, C. 1937. The behavior of children receiving benzedrine. *American Journal of Orthopsychiatry* 94:577–585.
Campbell, S.; Douglas, V.; and Morgenstern, G. 1971. Cognitive styles in hyperactive children and the effect of methylphenidate. *Journal of Child Psychology and Psychiatry* 12:55–67.
Cantwell, D. P. 1978. Drug treatment of the hyperactive child syndrome. In M. E. Jarvik, ed. *Psychopharmacology in the Practice of Medicine*. New York: Appleton-Century-Crofts.
Cantwell, D. P., and Carlson, G. A. 1978. Stimulants. In J. S. Werry, ed. *Pediatric Psychopharmacology—the Use of Behavior Modifying Drugs in Children*. New York: Brunner/Mazel.
Conners, C.; Eisenberg, L.; and Sharpe, L. 1965. A controlled study of the differential application of outpatient psychiatric treatment for children. *Japanese Journal of Child Psychiatry* 6:125–132.
Conners, C., and Werry, J. 1978. Pharmacotherapy of psychopathol-

ogy of childhood. In H. Quay and J. Werry, eds. *Psychopathological Disorders of Childhood*. 2d ed. New York: Wiley.

DSM-II. 1968. *Diagnostic and Statistical Manual of Mental Disorders*. Washington, D.C.: American Psychiatric Association.

DSM-III. 1978. *Diagnostic and Statistical Manual of Mental Disorders*. 3d ed. draft. Washington, D.C.: American Psychiatric Association.

Eisenberg, L.; Lackman, R.; and Molling, P. A. 1963. A psychopharmacologic experiment in a training school for delinquent boys: methods, problems, findings. *American Journal of Orthopsychiatry* 33:431–447.

Feighner, J. P.; Robins, E.; Guze, S. B.; Woodruff, R. A.; Winokur, G.; and Munoz, R. 1972. Diagnostic criteria for use in psychiatric research. *Archives of General Psychiatry* 26:57–63.

Fish, B. 1971. The "one child, one drug" myth of stimulants in hyperkinesis. *Archives of General Psychiatry* 25:193–203.

Freedman, D. 1971. Report of the conference on the use of stimulant drugs in the treatment of behaviorally disturbed young school children. *Psychopharmacology Bulletin* 7:23–29.

Gittelman-Klein, R. 1975. Stimulant drug treatment of hyperkinesis. In D. Klein and R. Gittelman-Klein, eds. *Progress in Psychiatric Drug Treatment*. Vol. 1. New York: Brunner/Mazel.

Guy, W. 1976. ECDEU assessment manual for psychopharmacology, revised. Kensington, Md.: Biometric Laboratory, George Washington University.

Hudgens, R. W. 1974. *Psychiatric Disorders in Adolescents*. Baltimore: Williams & Wilkins.

Huessey, H. R. 1978. Clinical explorations of adult MBD. Paper presented at the Conference on Minimal Brain Dysfunction in Adults, Scottsdale, Arizona.

Lewis, D. O., and Balla, D. A. 1976. *Delinquency and Psychopathology*. New York: Grune & Stratton.

Mackay, M. C.; Beck, L.; and Taylor, R. 1973. Methylphenidate for adolescents with minimal brain dysfunction. *New York Journal of Medicine* 73(4):550–554.

Maletsky, B. 1974. d-Amphetamine and delinquency: hyperkinesis persisting? *Diseases of the Nervous System* 35:543–547.

Ross, A. O. 1976. *Psychological Aspects of Learning Disability and Reading Disorders*. New York: McGraw-Hill.

Satterfield, J.; Cantwell, D. P.; and Satterfield, B. 1974. Pathophysiology of the hyperactive child syndrome. *Archives of General Psychiatry* 31:839–844.

Shaywitz, S. E.; Cohen, D. J.; and Shaywitz, B. A. 1978. The biochemical basis of minimal brain dysfunction. *Journal of Pediatrics* 92(2):179–187.

Spitzer, R. L.; Endicott, J.; Robins, E.; Kuriansky, J.; and Gurland, B. 1975. Preliminary report of the reliability of research diagnostic criteria applied to psychiatric case records. In A. Sudilovsky, S. Gershon, and B. Beer, eds. *Predictability in Psychopharmacology: Preclinical and Clinical Correlations*. New York: Raven.

Sprague, R., and Sleator, E. 1975. What is the proper dose of stimulant drugs in children? *Pediatric Clinics of North America* 20:719–735.

Sroufe, L. 1975. Drug treatment of children with behavior problems. In F. Horowitz, ed. *Review of Child Development Research*. Vol. 4. Chicago: University of Chicago Press.

Sykes, D.; Douglas, V.; and Morgenstern, G. 1972. The effect of methylphenidate (Ritalin) on sustained attention in hyperactive children. *Psychopharmacologia* (Berlin) 25:262–274.

Sykes, D.; Douglas, V.; Weiss, G.; and Minde, K. 1971. Attention in hyperactive children and the effect of methylphenidate (Ritalin). *Journal of Child Psychology and Psychiatry* 12:129–139.

Werry, J., and Aman, M. 1975. Methylphenidate and haloperidol in children: effects on attention, memory and activity. *Archives of General Psychiatry* 32:790–795.

Wood, D. R.; Reimherr, W. F.; Wender, P. H.; and Johnson, G. E. 1976. Diagnosis and treatment of minimal brain dysfunction in adults. *Archives of General Psychiatry* 33:1453–1460.

THEODORE VAN PUTTEN

If the adolescent's first exposure to an antipsychotic drug is a dysphoric or frightening experience, he is likely to be drug reluctant for years to come. Minimizing dysphoric subjective responses without compromising the desired antipsychotic effect is the art of pharmacotherapy. In this chapter, I offer guidelines which come from clinical experience, from our laboratory, and from controlled studies in adults, there being no reported controlled studies of antipsychotic drugs in adolescents.

The Right Diagnosis

Since lithium is the treatment of choice for bipolar manic-depressive illness, and since most manic-depressive patients have very dysphoric responses to antipsychotic drugs, it is important to begin by ruling out manic-depressive illness. This can be very difficult. Kraepelin (1921) pointed out that the first episode of manic or mixed manic-depressive illness can resemble closely the first break of schizophrenia. Wellner and Marstal (1964), in a study of 279 manic episodes, found that only 30 percent of the patients had the three cardinal symptoms of mania: elevated mood, flight of ideas, and psychomotor overactivity. Forty percent of the patients were atypical in that they had delusions not in harmony with the basic deviation of mood, or showed transient autism, ideas of influence, or thought derailment. Still others experienced rapid mood swings and showed a mixture of hebephrenic- and paranoid-like symptoms. The recent literature (Abrams, Taylor, and Gaztanaga

1974; Carlson and Goodwin 1973; Lipkin, Dyrud, and Meyer 1970; Morrison 1973; Taylor and Abrams 1972; Van Putten 1975) documents that manic-depressive illness is not infrequently misdiagnosed as either paranoid or catatonic schizophrenia, the former being the more usual misdiagnosis. The fashionable practice of aggressively administering antipsychotic drugs as soon as the patient enters the hospital will obscure the telltale manic intrusiveness, the expansive-irritable mood, and the hyperactivity (Van Putten 1975).

The Right Dosage

If a baseline observation period confirms the diagnosis of schizophrenia, the adolescent should be given a trial of treatment with one of the antipsychotic drugs. Choice of antipsychotic drug is much less important than achieving optimal dosage with whatever drug is most familiar to the practitioner. Except for the management of severe psychotic excitement, there is little to be gained by the immediate administration of high doses, either oral or parenteral. The fact that it takes time—six to seven weeks—to achieve a peak drug effect (Cole and Davis 1969) is often forgotten. For example, one study demonstrated that a moderate dose of fluphenazine (30 mg) over an increased period of time was more effective than a high dose (1,200 mg) in young nonchronic treatment failures (Quitkin, Rifkin, and Klein 1975). Aside from such general guidelines, derived from controlled studies in adults, the practitioner has to prescribe for the individual adolescent. And in the individual patient, the physician should be guided by side effects and the subjective response. The latter can be evaluated by asking: "How does the medication agree with you?" (Van Putten and May 1978a).

Subjective Response

No matter how much a patient improves behaviorally, in the end we have to ask him how he feels. Surprisingly, there is virtually no systematic investigation of the schizophrenic's subjective response to antipsychotic drugs. We do know that substantial numbers of schizophrenics do not like to take their medications, and that these drugs are not agreeable to normals (Henninger, DiMascio, and Klerman 1965; Safer and Allen 1971). In an interesting experiment, Belmaker and Wald (1977) administered haloperidol, 5 mg intravenously, to themselves and described the effect as follows: ". . . a marked slowing of thinking and movement developed, along with profound inner restlessness. Neither subject could continue work, and each left work for over 36 hours. Each subject complained of a paralysis of volition, a lack of physical and psychic energy. The subjects felt unable to read, telephone or perform household tasks of their own will, but could perform these tasks if demanded to do so. There was no sleepiness or sedation; on the contrary, both subjects complained of severe anxiety." The problem is that roughly a third of patients with clear-cut schizophrenia have a dysphoric response akin to that of normals on conventional doses of antipsychotic medications (Van Putten and May 1978a).

Dysphoric responses are especially common in active adolescent boys, as work with normal subjects would suggest. Working with healthy male student volunteers, Henninger et al. (1965) found that in those who were notably extroverted and athletic, 200 mg of chlorpromazine had a considerable disturbing and anxiety-provoking effect, whereas those who were introverted and introspective became more tranquil and indifferent to their surroundings.

A dysphoric response should be a danger signal to the physician. First, dysphoric responders tend not to accommodate the medication (at least not at conventional dosages) and, naturally enough, tend not to take it on their own (Van Putten 1974). Second, even if we can persuade dysphoric responders to continue with medication, the prognosis for further treatment is likely to be poor (Singh 1976; Van Putten and May 1978a).

The importance of the subjective response to drug treatment was first pointed out by Sarwer-Foner (1960, 1961, 1963), who emphasized that drug response must be understood in terms of the patient's expectations and fears, the philosophy of the treatment setting, and both the patient's and the doctor's transferences. In this psychodynamic view, dysphoric responses occur because the pharmacologic action of the drug has particular emotional meaning and significance to the subject. For example, the sedation and psychomotor retardation produced by chlorpromazine may be especially threatening to those adolescents who use activity as a defense against repressed and unacceptable passive-feminine identifications. Removal of this defense may precipitate marked anxiety, further psychotic deterioration, body-image changes, increased somatization, and preoccupation with guilt, punishment, and fear of death (Sarwer-Foner 1960, 1961, 1963; Nevins 1977).

In practice, dysphoric responses to antipsychotic medication are difficult to correct. Some patients with a dysphoric response to conventional doses of antipsychotic drugs do well, both subjectively and objectively, when the medication is decreased to very low doses. For example, one or two milligrams of fluphenazine (Prolixin) may suffice. Not infrequently, dysphoric responses are extrapyramidally based, with the degree of dysphoria depending on the emotional meaning and significance that the adolescent attaches to the extrapyramidal symptoms (EPS). The two EPS that have the most far-reaching impact on the patient's mental life are akinesia (absence or diminution of voluntary motion) and akathisia (inner restlessness).

Detection of Akinesia and Akathisia

Physicians differ considerably in their detection of extrapyramidal symptoms. For example, in a survey of long-acting fluphenazine studies, the reported incidence of EPS with the enanthate ester ranged from 0 percent to 100 percent (Groves and Mandel 1975). Since the dosages in these studies were conventional, these marked differences in reporting suggests that physicians differ greatly in their ability to detect the EPS of akinesia and akathisia: presumably everybody would record such readily obserable EPS as tremor, dyskinesia, rigidity, or dystonia. Or it could be that clinicians regard a mild akinesia as therapeutic. Freyhan (1975), for example, believed that akinesia is "a regular effect of neuroleptic drugs, part and parcel of their therapeutic action, which in many instances makes it seem arbitrary to define borderlines between therapeutic quanta of hypomotility and early signs of Parkinsonism." More likely, however, physicians mistake the mental representations of the milder akinesias and akathisias for the vicissitudes of schizophrenia.

The Subclinical Akinesias

In its grosser form, akinesia manifests such easily observable akinetic manifestations as slowed movement, shuffling gait, absence of spontaneous muscular movement, and lifeless appearance. A double-blind procedure in which patients received biperiden (Akineton), 5 mg intramuscularly, alternating with placebo (or vice versa) and in later trials an oral test dose of 4 mg of trihexyphenidyl (Artane) alternating with placebo has enabled us to confirm subtler or subclinical akinesias. Objectively these milder akinesias, as noted by Rifkin, Quitkin, and Klein (1975), are evident mostly as a "behavioral state of diminished spontaneity characterized by few gestures, unspontaneous speech, and, particularly, apathy and difficulty with initiating usual activities."

Subjectively, these patients may complain of feeling listless and fatigued, lack interest, or deny any feelings at all. In adolescent males an akinetic weakness can heighten feelings of passivity or helplessness, and not infrequently, it is elaborated into increased concerns about masculinity and homosexual fears (Nevins 1977; Sarwer-Foner 1960, 1963). Others will become somatically preoccupied and importune for frequent medical examinations. In the overtly psychotic, an akinesia can be elaborated into delusions of bodily destruction (Quitkin et al. 1975; Van Putten, Mutalipassi, and Malkin 1974). Thus, one woman with smoldering nihilistic delusions interpreted a mild akinesia as evidence that "rigor mortis" was setting in. Another thought she had "swine flu" and started to drink copious amounts of red wine "to nourish the red blood corpuscles."

Akinesia is insidious, and only half of the patients with a mild akinesia complain of this subjective state. The remainder seem to accept it, and it does appear that both doctor and patient can get used to it. Indeed, it is not always easy to distinguish between a mild akinesia and blunted affect, schizophrenic apathy, or non-drug-related psychomotor retardation. It is therefore helpful to know that there is a high association between akinesia and both objectively rated sedative effect ($r = +.71$, $P < .0005$) and ratings of subjectively experienced sedative effect ($r = +.70$) (Van Putten and May 1978b). Thus, an akinesia is not likely if the patient does not look or feel at least somewhat drowsy.

Akinetic Depression

Although "intense despair" (Mayer-Gross 1920) and "melancholic symptoms" (Bleuler 1950) occurring in the wake of a psychotic experience were observed in the preneuroleptic era, reports of postpsychotic depression have multiplied during the past twenty years, the reported incidence varying from 0 percent to 50 percent with an average of about 25 percent (McGlashan and Carpenter 1976). This raises the possibility that some of these depressions may be a side effect of antipsychotic drugs, but there is no agreement on a causal relationship, let alone a mechanism or treatment (Floru, Heinrich, and Wiltek 1975).

Schizophrenic patients with postpsychotic depression have been described as "wooden" in appearance (Steinberg, Green, and Durell 1967); motorically inactive or retarded, and lacking initiative to perform routine tasks (Wildroe 1966); experiencing overwhelming fatigue and neurasthenic symptoms (Kayton 1973); and "hypersommic" and "emotionally withdrawn" (Stern, Pillsbury, and Sonnenberg 1972). Nearly all reports comment on the patient's disinclination to speak (McGlashan and Carpenter 1976). All of these symptoms, however, can be manifestations of antipsychotic-drug-induced akinesia (Rifkin et al. 1975).

If postpsychotic depression is indeed related to akinesia, schizophrenic populations treated with high doses of antipsychotic drugs should, by and large, experience more of it. Unfortunately, most of the reports reviewed by McGlashan and Carpenter (1976) make no exact mention of dosage, and, in any event, dosage was not controlled.

A review of the controlled dosage comparison studies in the English literature indicate that higher doses in chronically hospitalized schizophrenics do not result in increased depression. But these results may not generalize to more acute, younger patients (Van Putten and May 1978b).

Indeed, the findings for the three controlled-dose comparison studies in more acute patients are rather different. Wijsenbeck, Steiner, and Goldberg (1974) compared trifluoperazine (Stelazine), 60 mg and 600 mg, in newly admitted schizophrenics and noted no significant differences in either side effects or clinical ratings. Both Goldstein, Rodnick, Evans, May, and Steinberg (1978) and Quitkin, Rifkin, and Klein (1975), however, report increased depression in subgroups of the high dosage patients. Goldstein et al. (1978) compared fluphenazine enanthate, 25 mg and 6 mg every fourteen days, in acute schizophrenics in their early twenties. The males on the higher dose became significantly more anxious and depressed (no side effect records kept). Quitkin et al. (1975) compared oral fluphenazine HCl, 30 mg and 1,200 mg, in non-chronic treatment failures between the ages of sixteen and thirty-seven and found increased depression in a subgroup who developed akinesia.

A recent study (Van Putten and May 1978b) investigated the consequences of an akinesia by comparing one group of schizophrenics who, by virture of individual sensitivity, developed an akinesia with a very similar group who, although identically treated, never developed EPS. Those who developed akinesia became less psychotic, but they also experienced a significant, although modest, increase in depression ratings. Successful treatment of the akinesia resulted in significant ($P =$ .013 − .000) improvements in depression, somatic concern, anxiety, emotional withdrawal, blunted affect, and motor retardation on both physicians' and nurses' ratings. A high association between akinesia and both objectively rated and subjectively experienced sedative effect indicates that an akinetic depression is not likely if the patient does not look or feel at least somewhat drowsy. The thirty-two nonakinetic patients also became less psychotic, but not more depressed.

An unrecognized akinesia might be responsible for the observation that "suicidal ideation often develops after the patient discovers that he is too anergic to function as he did before he first fell ill and therefore assumes that he is permanently impaired" (Detre and Jarecki 1971). Patients with akinetic depression do not tell us that they are depressed because of the akinesia. They speak of loss, of personal failure and humiliations, of personal inadequacy and lack of meaning—in short, the psychodynamics of postpsychotic depression (McGlashan and Carpenter 1976). We are not saying that the patient's assessment of his situation is wrong; we can only say that a patient whose akinesia has been corrected no longer speaks this way.

Akathisia

Akathisia is an emotional state which refers, not to any type or pattern of movement, but rather to a subjective need or desire to move (Crane and Naranjo 1971). This urge to move is always accompanied by affective distress and, objectively, is manifested by restless pacing, inability to sit still, and continuous alterations in posture. With the subtler akathisias,[1] the patient may not use the word "restless," but complains instead of "jitteriness," inability to feel "comfortable," "impatience," "irritability," feeling "keyed up" or "wired," or being a "bundle of nerves" (Van Putten 1975). Many experience a vague sense of dread, and most will not tolerate an akathisia for very long. In our experience, patients who claim to be "allergic" to antipsychotic drugs often mean that they were tormented by an akathisia. Hodge (1959) stated that akathisia "may appear like an anxiety state . . . in which real anxiety can be neither recognized nor verbalized." Kalinowsky (1958) remarked that akathisia can be "more difficult to endure than any of the symptoms for which [the patient] was originally treated."

Other characteristics are: Akathisia is nearly always experienced as ego-alien. The inner agitation and restlessness are difficult to articulate, and the patient feels better when moving about. Once the patient has gained relief from an antiparkinson drug he will seek relief from the next episode. The subtler akathisias often go unrecognized by the physician—but not by the patient! Even a mild akathisia can preclude sitting through the dinner hour, a movie, a therapy session, or a sedentary job. Akathisia can be experienced as a "foreign force driving one to move" even in a normal subject (Kendler 1976), and it is therefore not surprising that akathisia can be associated with dramatic exacerbations of psychosis (Van Putten 1974).

Treatment of Extrapyramidal Symptoms

It is often difficult to distinguish between a subtle akathisia or akinesia and the disease for which the patient is being treated. The inaccessible and floridly disorganized cannot articulate the subtler akinesias and akathisias, which are primarily feeling states. Even in the more reconstituted articulate patient it can be very difficult to distinguish between akathisia and psychotic agitation, between schizophrenic apathy and akinetic lethargy. A short course of treatment with high doses of an antiparkinson drug—for example, trihexyphenidyl (Artane), 4 mg two or three times daily, or benztropine (Cogentin), 4 mg twice daily—will usually supply the answer. We have observed that trihexyphenidyl exerts mild euphoriant properties and for this reason tend to prefer it. However, some akinesias can be stubbornly resistant to conventional therapy, and in such cases a trial of amantadine (Symmetrel), an antiparkinson drug with dopamine agonist properties, may be worthwhile (DiMascio, Bernardo, and Greenblatt 1976).

Maintenance Treatment

It has been established that discharged adult schizophrenics do better on maintenance antipsychotic drugs than on placebos (Hogarty, Goldberg, et al. 1973, 1974; Davis 1975). Much less is known, however, about the utility of maintenance treatment in those schizophrenics who have never been hospitalized and whose illness is therefore presumably of lesser severity. Even in the once hospitalized, 20 percent of those maintained on placebo did not relapse over a two-year period, and these placebo survivors were, if anything, better adjusted than the surviving drug patients (Hogarty et al. 1974). Since we have no way of prospectively identifying which schizophrenic does just as well or better without drugs (May and Goldberg 1978), every adolescent should have a trial period off antipsychotic drugs. A good time to try drug withdrawal is about six months after the acute episode.

Regarding maintenance dosage, there is agreement that it should be taken at bedtime and that "drug holidays" (never on Saturday or Sunday) are feasible. But, even in adult schizophrenics, there is very little knowledge about the smallest effective dose. The recently completed study by Goldstein et al. (1978) shows that many young schizophrenics can be maintained on surprisingly small doses of fluphenazine (Prolixin) decanoate, 6 mg every two weeks, as long as they receive supportive family therapy. Experienced clinicians (e.g., Bann and Lehmann 1977) find that patients can be maintained on 50–200 mg of chlorpromazine (Thorazine) or its equivalent. Finding the lowest maintenance dose is important, not only because it supposedly lowers the risk for developing tardive dyskinesia (which can be very severe and disabling in the young), but also because higher doses may interfere with spontaneity and drive.

Conclusions

There is an art to the pharmacotherapy of schizophrenia, for the guidelines to optimal dosage are few. Finding the right dose for each patient requires patience and considerable knowledge of the psychic state. This is particularly true in treating an adolescent, who already has to cope with multiple changes. If in addition he is overmedicated or medicated too aggressively, the intrapsychic changes brought about by the chemical effects of the drug may result in a disorganizing unfamiliarity (Nevins 1977). Complaints of "feeling not myself," or having "no feelings at all," of feeling "strange," "changed," or "unreal" may represent a drug effect and should stimulate a search for side effects. With such an individualized approach it may be possible to establish a working alliance in which the adolescent himself participates in the selection of the optimal dosage.

NOTE

1. In order for a particular emotional state to be scored as akathisia, the following test had to be passed: disappearance or marked improvement after intramuscular administration of 5 mg biperiden (Akineton), and no improvement after a placebo injection (double blind).

REFERENCES

Abrams, R.; Taylor, M. A.; and Gaztanaga, P. 1974. Manic-depressive illness and paranoid schizophrenia. *Archives of General Psychiatry* 31:640–642.

Bann, T. A., and Lehmann, H. E. 1977. Myths, theories, and treatment of schizophrenia. *Diseases of the Nervous System* 38:665–671.

Belmaker, R. H., and Wald, D. 1977. Haloperidol in normals. *British Journal of Psychiatry* 131:222–223.

Bleuler, E. 1950. *Dementia Praecox or the Group of Schizophrenias*. New York: International Universities Press.

Carlson, G. A., and Goodwin, F. K. 1973. The stages of mania. *Archives of General Psychiatry* 28:221–228.

Cole, J. O., and Davis, J. M. 1969. Anti-psychotic drugs. In L. Bellak and L. Loeb, eds. *The Schizophrenic Syndrome*. New York: Grune & Stratton.

Crane, G. E., and Naranjo, E. R. 1971. Motor disorders induced by neuroleptics. *Archives of General Psychiatry* 24:179–184.

Davis, J. M. 1975. Overview: maintenance therapy in psychiatry: schizophrenia. *American Journal of Psychiatry* 132:1237–1245.

Detre, T. P., and Jarecki, H. G. 1971. *Modern Psychiatric Treatment*. Philadelphia: Lippincott.

DiMascio, A.; Bernardo, D. L.; and Greenblatt, D. J. 1976. A controlled trial of amantadine in drug-induced extrapyramidal disorder. *Archives of General Psychiatry* 33:599–602.

Floru, L.; Heinrich, K.; and Wiltek, F. 1975. The problem of postpsychotic schizophrenic depressions and their pharmacological induction. *International Pharmacopsychiatry* 10:230–239.

Freyhan, F. A. 1957. Psychomotility and parkinsonism in treatment with neuroleptic drugs. *Archives of Neurology and Psychiatry* 78:465–471.

Goldstein, M. J.; Rodnick, E. H.; Evans, J. R.; May, P. R. A.; and Steinberg, M. 1978. Drug and family therapy in the aftercare treatment of acute schizophrenia. *Archives of General Psychiatry*, in press.

Groves, J. E., and Mandel, M. R. 1975. The long acting phenothiazines. *Archives of General Psychiatry* 32:893–900.

Henninger, G.; DiMascio, A.; and Klerman, G. L. 1965. Personality factors in variability of response to phenothiazines. *American Journal of Psychiatry* 121:1091–1094.

Hodge, J. R. 1959. Akathisia: the syndrome of motor restlessness. *American Journal of Psychiatry* 116:337–338.

Hogarty, G. E.; Goldberg, S. C.; and the Collaborative Study Group. 1973. Drug and sociotherapy in the aftercare of schizophrenic patients. *Archives of General Psychiatry* 28:54–64.

Hogarty, G. E.; Goldberg, S. C.; Schooler, N. R.; Ulrich, R. F.; and the Collaborative Study Group. 1974. Drug and sociotherapy in the aftercare of schizophrenic patients. II. Two-year relapse rates. *Archives of General Psychiatry* 31:603–608.

Hogarty, G. E.; Goldberg, S. C.; Schooler, N. R.; and the Collaborative Study Group. 1974. Drug and sociotherapy in the aftercare of schizophrenic patients. III. Adjustment of nonrelapsed patients. *Archives of General Psychiatry* 31:609–618.

Kalinowsky, L. B. 1958. Appraisal of the "tranquilizers" and their influence on other somatic treatments in psychiatry. *American Journal of Psychiatry* 115:294–300.

Kayton, L. 1973. Good outcome in young adult schizophrenia. *Archives of General Psychiatry* 29:103–110.

Kendler, K. S. 1976. A medical student's experience with akathisia. *American Journal of Psychiatry* 133:454–455.

Kraepelin, E. 1921. *Manic-Depressive Insanity and Paranoia*. Edinburgh: Livingstone.

Lipkin, K. M.; Dyrud, J.; and Meyer, G. G. 1970. The many faces of mania. *Archives of General Psychiatry* 22:262–267.

McGlashan, T. H., and Carpenter, W. T., Jr. 1976. Postpsychotic depression in schizophrenia. *Archives of General Psychiatry* 33:231–239.

May, P. R. A., and Goldberg, S. C. 1978. Prediction of schizophrenic patients' response to pharmacotherapy. *Archives of General Psychiatry*, in press.

Mayer-Gross, W. 1920. Uber die Stellungsnahme auf abgelaufenen akuten psychose. *Zeitschrift fur die gesamte Neurologie und Psychiatrie* 60:160–212.

Morrison, J. R. 1973. Catatonia. *Archives of General Psychiatry* 28:39–41.

Nevins, D. B. 1977. Adverse response to neuroleptics in schizophrenia. *International Journal of Psychoanalytic Psychotherapy* 6:227–241.

Quitkin, F.; Rifkin, A.; and Klein, D. F. 1975. Very high dosage vs. standard dosage fluphenazine in schizophrenia. *Archives of General Psychiatry* 32:1276–1281.

Rifkin, A.; Quitkin, F.; and Klein, D. F. 1975. Akinesia. *Archives of General Psychiatry* 32:672–674.

Safer, D. J., and Allen, R. P. 1971. The effect of fluphenazine in psychologically normal volunteers: some temporal, performance, and biochemical relationships. *Biological Psychiatry* 3:237–249.

Sarwer-Foner, G. J. 1960. The role of neuroleptic medication in psychotherapeutic interaction. *Comprehensive Psychiatry* 1:291–300.

Sarwer-Foner, G. J. 1961. Some comments on the psychodynamic aspects of the extrapyramidal reactions. *Revue Canadienne de Biologie* 20:623–629.

Sarwer-Foner, G. J. 1963. On the mechanisms of action of neuroleptic drugs: a theoretical psychodynamic explanation. *Recent Advances in Biological Psychiatry* 6:217–232.

Singh, M. M. 1976. Dysphoric response to neuroleptic treatment in schizophrenia and its prognostic significance. *Diseases of the Nervous System* 37:191–196.

Steinberg, H. R.; Green, R.; and Durell, J. 1967. Depression occurring during the course of recovery from schizophrenic symptoms. *American Journal of Psychiatry* 124:699–702.

Stern, M. J.; Pillsbury, J. A.; and Sonnenberg, S. M. 1972. Postpsychotic depression in schizophrenics. *Comprehensive Psychiatry* 13:519–598.

Taylor, M. A., and Abrams, R. 1972. The phenomenology of mania: a new look at some old patients. *Archives of General Psychiatry* 29:520–522.

Van Putten, T. 1974. Why do schizophrenic patients refuse to take their drugs? *Archives of General Psychiatry* 31:67–72.

Van Putten, T. 1975. The many faces of akathisia. *Comprehensive Psychiatry* 16:43–47.

Van Putten, T., and May, P. R. A. 1978a. Subjective response as a predictor of outcome in pharmacotherapy. *Archives of General Psychiatry* 35:477–480.

Van Putten, T., and May, P. R. A. 1978b. "Akinetic depression" in schizophrenia. *Archives of General Psychiatry* 35:1101–1107.

Van Putten, T.; Mutalipassi, L. R.; and Malkin, M. D. 1974. Phenothiazine-induced decompensation. *Archives of General Psychiatry* 30:102–105.

Van Putten, T., and Sanders, D. G. 1975. Lithium in treatment failures. *Journal of Nervous and Mental Diseases* 161:255–264.

Wellner, J., and Marstal, M. B. 1964. Symptoms in mania, an analysis of 279 attacks of manic-depressive elation. *Acta Psychiatrica Scandinavica* 40(180):S175–S176.

Wijsenbeck, H.; Steiner, M.; and Goldberg, S. C. 1974. Trifluoperazine: a comparison between regular and high doses. *Psychopharmacologia* 36:147–150.

Wildroe, H. J. 1966. Depression following acute schizophrenic psychosis. *Journal of Hillside Hospital* 15:114–122.

27 MINOR TRANQUILIZER USE IN ADOLESCENTS

SAMUEL BLACK

The extent and quality of research that has been performed on the utilization of antianxiety medications in adolescents is markedly deficient, and many examiners appear to take a dim view of their use. White (1977, p. 58) states that "while the chief use of diazepam in adults is to control anxiety, it is not used for this purpose in children or adolescents." Some investigators feel that these medications are actually contraindicated. This view is held by Shaffer (1977), who concludes that minor tranquilizers may not only be ineffective in childhood, but also may produce unwanted behavior changes. Shaffer bases his conclusions on a study by Lucas and Pasley (1969) on the use of haloperidol and diazepam in children. This study, however, while stressing that tranquilizing medication is not of value with the younger child and early adolescent, does indicate that in older adolescents tranquilizers can be quite useful by diminishing anxiety. Patterson and Pruitt (1977, p. 176) also write that "there is no absolute documentation of benefit for the use of sedatives and minor tranquilizers in children."

Rothman (1968), in *Current Pediatric Therapy*, while discussing the treatment of vomiting associated with anxiety, asserts that it is wrong to prescribe medication. His approach is to "tell the child that the same manifestation has been described as occurring in men and women who have performed tasks requiring incredible courage" (p. 1029). However, in the same volume, Gallagher (1968) recommends the use of phenothiazines for mild neurosis and anxiety. Kanner (1972), in discussing the treatment of anxiety attacks, makes no mention of using medication; and, finally, Work (1968) suggests the benefit of "sedation"

© 1979 by The University of Chicago. 0-226-24052-5/79/1979-0010$00.81

in treating acute anxiety attacks, without delineating the type of medication or dosage.

These attitudes represent the general conclusions of researchers concerning the use of tranquilizers for treatment of anxiety in the adolescent. While there are reports of positive responses to antianxiety medications, these are largely reports of individual clinical cases or that include an undetermined number of adolescents grouped with adult patients, which does not allow the specific response of the adolescent patients to be determined. The clinician, then, is in a difficult position in his consideration of the use of minor tranquilizers for his adolescent patients. He may conclude that the literature has not shown any clear indication for the utilization of minor tranquilizers in the treatment of anxiety in the adolescent, or he may choose to focus on inconclusive studies and individual case reports which indicate positive benefits. That this dilemma has been solved outside the United States is suggested by Simon (1974) in a sampling study of thirty-four foreign countries. The respondents in this study showed the highest agreement in their use of diazepam in treating anxiety in children (adolescents were not specifically indicated).

The Selection of Tranquilizers

In discussing antianxiety medication, the benzodiazepines will be considered the drugs of choice. However, several other anxiolytics may be considered: barbituates, meprobamate, hydroxyzine, and diphenhydramine. Diphenhydramine (Benadryl) is often used to reduce anxiety in very young children but drops in effectiveness at puberty. After ten to eleven years of age, children tend to respond to diphenhydramine like adults. Thus, in the adolescent the medication produces drowsiness and can be useful as a bedtime sedative rather than in the treatment of anxiety (Fish 1968a, 1968b). Available studies comparing these medications (almost exclusively in adult patients) conclude that the benzodiazepines are the antianxiety agents of choice, considering the spectrum of currently available drugs (Greenblatt and Shader 1974).

The confusion over the use of minor tranquilizers for adolescents is underscored by a review of the prescribing indications recommended by the drug companies. Diazepam (Valium) is indicated to be safe for use after the age of six months, while chlordiazepoxide (Librium) is indicated for use only after six years of age. Chlorazepate monopotassium (Azene), prazepam (Verstran), and chlorazepate dipotassium (Tranxene) are not recommended for use under the age of eighteen. Finally, oxazepam (Serax) is not indicated for use under six years of age, and the absolute dosage has not been established in ages six to twelve, but it may be used in children over twelve years of age.

A Proposed Treatment Philosophy

There can be no doubt that more controlled research is needed to determine the effectiveness of minor tranquilizers in treating adolescents. The child is more vulnerable than the adult but is also more flexible. Evaluation of the effect of a given therapy requires that all variables which might influence the clinical picture be kept as constant as possible. This last requirement, the standardization of the research setting, is even more difficult to accomplish with children than with adults (Van Praag 1969).

I would like to suggest that the individual therapist adopt an empirical approach to this treatment dilemma. The judicious use of minor tranquilizers by the individual therapist may provide him with the data he needs to determine, for himself, the efficacy of the use of minor tranquilizers for the treatment of anxiety. This would serve a dual purpose, in that it would provide the therapist with specific data on which to base his own conclusions, as well as adding to the general consensus in this area.

The manifest expressions of anxiety in the adolescent include somatic symptoms, aggression toward the producer of the anxiety, phobic symptoms, obsessional behavior, and hysterical conversion symptoms, as well as the overt expression of anxiety itself. While sleeping and eating disturbances are often considered separately, anxiety is often the main cause of these conditions. In addition, anxiety may result in learning disorders secondary to interference with concentration.

The defense system of the adolescent is in a constant state of flux. At times it shows an amazing degree of resistance in dealing with conflicts, while at other times it is overwhelmed to the point of leaving the adolescent in a state of intense anxiety or resulting in the formation of neurotic symptoms in an attempt to bind the anxiety. Psychotherapy is, of course, a consideration for the adolescent whose behavior indicates that there are not sufficient internal resources available to deal with the anxiety or its manifestations. The use of medication at such times may serve the same purpose as psychotherapy, or it may be used in conjunction with therapy. "The two methods are both sound and should be regarded as complementary" (Van Praag 1969, p. 139).

There is, of course, the danger that the therapist will use a tranquilizer as a means of avoiding an evaluation of the patient's psychic life and fail to delineate the underlying causes of the anxiety. These medications should be reserved only for those situations in which the adolescent is being overwhelmed by anxiety, whether in or out of psychotherapy, and is in need of a palliative treatment to prevent his suffering undue psychic damage.

The Resistance of Therapists

It is possible that the reluctance of therapists to use anxiolytic medication with adolescents is secondary to the many necessary dynamic considerations. It is sometimes enough for a therapist to hear about a problem or side effect that resulted from the use of medication to cause him abruptly to stop prescribing medication. It is important to keep in mind that, as with any treatment approach, the inherent problems associated with that treatment must be carefully weighed against the obvious advantages.

The system involved when an adolescent is given any medication includes patient, parents, and therapist. The manner in which the patient reacts to the idea of medication must be explored by the therapist. Any fantasies, expectations, and resistance must be verbalized and dealt with. If a therapist does not wish to spend the time and energy necessary to clarify the introduction of medication, or if the resistance in either the patient or the parents is too great, the use of medication should not be attempted. The expectation of the results of the medication, as well as any change in how the therapist conceives of the therapeutic process, are important considerations which the individual therapist must evaluate.

Side Effects and Abuse of the Medication

Monitoring the compliance with the medication prescription, which includes the handling of any side effects, presents the next obligation of the therapist. I have found that adolescent patients with marked obsessive features, even though they have agreed to take medication, are reluctant actually to use it due to a concern that it will alter their "feelings"; thus, it is seen as a threat to their ability to remain in control. To encourage the continuation of medication in the face of this resistance can only be detrimental. With the benzodiazepines, which make up the most important group of antianxiety medications, a single dosage at bedtime appears to minimize any side effects, produces adequate blood levels, and helps to increase compliance.

It is my practice to make contact with the patient two or three days after he starts a new medication, either by office visit or phone, in order to review the effects of the medication, including the side effects. Any dosage changes can be made at this time, rather than waiting for the next office visit or relying on the adolescent to call to report problems.

Medication abuse is often felt to be a marked contraindication to giving the adolescent antianxiety medication. White (1977) indicates that the benzodiazepines have a significant abuse potential and concludes that they should not be used in the disturbed adolescent, although he does indicate that diazepam has a place in the treatment of adolescents with sleep disorders. It is my experience that the benzodiazepines are seldom abused in a primary fashion. It is not uncommon to see diazepam used secondarily by adolescents to modify the effects of self-administered amphetamine or psychedelic drugs. To my knowledge, there has been no clear correlation between the therapeutic use of antianxiety medication and future drug abuse.

The lethality of the benzodiazepines has been found to be extremely low, with large doses of benzodiazepines rarely producing serious or fatal poisoning when taken alone. In the medical literature there are no reported cases of fatal overdosage due to benzodiazepines alone, and serious sequelae of overdosage are much less common than with any other sedative-hypnotics (Greenblatt and Shader 1974, 1975).

Dosage and Prescribing Recommendations

The dosage of antianxiety agents will vary; their plasma levels are highly unpredictable. In addition, therapeutic effects and plasma levels are only roughly correlatable. Because the benzodiazepines are slowly excreted, it may take from seven to ten days until a steady state is reached, and there will be a cumulative effect from steady usage and residual effects after discontinuation (Goodwin 1975). One difference between adults and children is that the peak blood level of diazepam occurs earlier in children, although the plasma half-life is similar in both age groups (Patterson and Pruitt 1977).

There is no consistent evidence that any one benzodiazepine is clinically superior to the others. However, diazepam is the only one that is approved for use in young children as well as adolescents. By starting with a daily dosage of five milligrams of diazepam, it is possible to adjust the dosage up or down depending on the response. While an individual dosage as needed may be helpful, best results are obtained by daily use for a minimum of seven days. Discontinuance can then be considered, depending upon the therapist's judgment of the clinical picture. The typical side effects are similar to those found with adults. With careful dosage monitoring, and by utilizing a single nighttime dosage, these side effects are minimized and rarely need result in a discontinuation of the medication.

The effect of the minor tranquilizers on school performance must be constantly monitored. If excessive anxiety is contributing to poor performance in school, it would be expected that successful reduction in anxiety would directly correlate with improved school performance. However, school performance is influenced by many factors and cannot always be understood in a direct cause and effect manner. Nonetheless, the adolescent's behavior in school must be followed and the medication adjusted accordingly. With a single dosage at bedtime, no medication need be taken during school hours.

Conclusions

Fish (1968a, 1968b) reviews and discusses methodology in child psychopharmacology, emphasizing the problems presented by the lack of definition of the initial pretreatment state and the assessment of change. She concludes that generalizing whether a child will respond to a given drug, and in what manner, can be accomplished only if clear operational definitions are developed for both the initial state and the specific types of change. While this advice appears to apply to the research study of medication, it may also be pertinent to the clinical use of antianxiety agents with adolescents. The clinician must first clarify the psychodynamic aspects of the patient. If an excessive degree of anxiety can be defined, and if the therapist believes that the anxiety cannot be adequately dealt with by traditional psychotherapeutic means in sufficient time to prevent the development of overwhelming anxiety, then the utilization of anxiolytic medication is indicated. Judicious use of medication in treating anxiety in the adolescent can facilitate the therapeutic process by providing the careful therapist with yet another tool.

REFERENCES

Cleckly, H. 1965. Use of diazepam as adjunctive therapy in psychiatric disorders. *Journal of the South Carolina Medical Association* 61:1–4.

Fish, B. 1968a. Drug therapy in children's psychiatric disorders. In F. Freyhan, ed. *Modern Problems of Psychopharmacology*. Basel, N.Y.: Kringer.

Fish, B. 1968b. Methodology in child psychopharmacology. In D. Efron, ed. *Pharmacology: Review of Progress, 1957–1967*. Washington, D.C.: Public Health Publications.

Gallagher, W. 1968. Emotional problems of the adolescent. In S. Gellis and B. Kagan, eds. *Current Pediatric Therapy*. Philadelphia: Saunders.

Goodwin, D. 1975. Psychopharmacology. *Psychiatric Digest* 5:41.

Greenblatt, D., and Shader, R. 1974. *Benzodiazepines in Clinical Practice*. New York: Raven.

Greenblatt, D., and Shader, R. 1975. Benzodiazepines. *New England Journal of Medicine* 291:19.

Kanner, L. 1972. *Child Psychiatry*. New York: Thomas.

Lucas, A., and Pasley, F. 1969. Psychoactive drugs in the treatment of emotionally disturbed children: haloperidol and diazepam. *Comprehensive Psychiatry* 10:376–386.

Patterson, J., and Pruitt, A. 1977. Treatment of mild symptomatic anxiety states. In J. Wiener, ed. *Psychopharmacology in Childhood and Adolescence*. New York: Basic.

Rothman, P. 1968. Vomiting. In S. Gellis and B. Kagan, eds. *Current Pediatric Therapy*. Philadelphia: Saunders.

Shaffer, D. 1977. Drug treatment. In M. Rutter and L. Hersou, eds. *Child Psychiatry*. Oxford: Blackwell.

Simon, J. 1974. Pediatric psychopharmacology outside the U.S.A. *Diseases of the Nervous System* 35:37.

Van Praag, H. 1969. Psychotropic drugs in child psychiatry. *International Pharmacopsychiatry* 3:139.

White, J. 1977. *Pediatric Psychopharmacology*. Baltimore: Williams & Wilkins.

Work, F. 1968. Psychiatric emergencies. In C. Varga, ed. *Handbook of Pediatric Medicine*. New York: Mosby.

28 LITHIUM CARBONATE USE IN ADOLESCENTS: CLINICAL INDICATIONS AND MANAGEMENT

GABRIELLE A. CARLSON

The use of lithium carbonate for the treatment and prophylaxis of bipolar manic-depressive illness (MDI) has become increasingly widespread and accepted over the past twenty-five years. Numerous double-blind studies have demonstrated the undeniable therapeutic efficacy of lithium in patients with this disorder (Fieve 1975). Furthermore, attempts to ascertain the specific effects lithium is having on a spectrum of psychopathological illnesses have revealed variable successes in other conditions, notably recurrent unipolar depressions (Prien and Caffey 1976), aggression (Marnini and Sheard 1977), and personality disorders in which there is a pronounced mood component (Rifkin, Quitkin, Carillo, Blumberg, and Klein 1972).

Lithium has been used clinically in children and adolescents (Annell 1969; Brumback and Weinberg 1977; Carlson and Strober 1978; Feinstein and Wolpert 1973; Horowitz 1977; Schou 1971; Van Krevelen and Van Voorst 1959). To this author's knowledge, however, double-blind studies comparable to those done on adults have not yet been published (Youngerman and Canino 1978). However, those few studies which have been published suggest that lithium is as effective in adolescents as in adults. The major reason for the paucity of systematic investigations seems to be the hesitation of clinicians to identify and diagnose MDI in teenagers.

Diagnostic and Clinical Considerations

There are three important points to remember in using lithium in adolescents. The first is that the major indication for its use in this age group, as in adults, is in the treatment and prophylaxis of bipolar MDI. While this fact may not be surprising, the frequency of occurrence of this disorder beginning in adolescence may be. Twenty-eight persons, fully one-quarter of the bipolar patients admitted with mania to the National Institutes of Mental Health, noted their first episode of illness before the age of nineteen (Carlson, Davenport, and Jamison 1977). Some of those patients were obviously manic-depressive at the onset, but most of them had their first episodes misdiagnosed as adjustment reactions, schizophrenia, school phobia, hyperactivity, or anorexia nervosa. Rarely did the first episode lead to hospitalization. It should be emphasized, then, that MDI in adolescence is more common than most people think.

A case history will illustrate the importance of making the proper diagnosis:

Janet, a previously pleasant and friendly girl, was brought to the psychiatric outpatient department at age twelve by her mother because she had recently become withdrawn, tearful, and had expressed the wish that she were dead. This had followed a two-week period of uncharacteristic hyperactivity, excessive talking, staying up all night, and being generally uncontrollable. The combined stress of family problems and beginning junior high school led the admitting psychiatrist to diagnose her illness as an adjustment reaction. She was treated in group therapy and her symptoms gradually remitted. Exactly one year after her first presentation, Janet was again very withdrawn, lethargic, confused, crying, and complaining of nightmares. She was verbally and behaviorally slowed down and was sleeping all of the time. She was also quite paranoid, saying that she was a sinner and that others were accusing her of bad things. Though she looked depressed, her delusions and the occasional hallucinated voice telling her she should die prompted the diagnosis of schizophrenia. Phenothiazines were not helpful. Again, Janet's symptoms remitted gradually: first the psychotic symptoms, then the depressive symptoms. She was discharged, followed as an outpatient, and was generally well until one and one-half years later when she again began to feel "hyper," became very active, was up all night, hyperverbal, irritable, euphoric, hypersexual, paranoid, and seen as "obnoxious" by her family and friends. She was clearly manic and was admitted for lithium treatment. In retrospect, she had been hypomanic, mildly depressed, and psychotically depressed earlier. She has been on lithium since and followed in psychotherapy for the past two years with no further episodes of illness. Both by her admission and by her therapist's observation, her normal mood state has allowed her to profit from psychotherapy, for which she had previously been considered a poor candidate. She recently was able to handle the stress of beginning college and another recrudescence of family problems.

I have seen a total of six young adolescents with diagnosed MDI (mean onset age, fifteen) at UCLA's Neuropsychiatric Institute over the past three years. Their symptoms are summarized in table 1. It is important to recognize that patients are not always good observers of their affective state and do not always present the clinician with classical histories (Carlson and Strober 1978). The second point, then, is that it is imperative that a history be obtained from family members as well as the patient and that mood, cognition, and psychomotor and vegetative symptoms be investigated systematically. The presence of psychotic symptoms, especially in very deep depressions or very severe mania, is not uncommon and does not preclude the diagnosis of MDI (Carlson and Strober 1978; Horowitz 1977).

Of the six patients noted in table 1, three have responded well to lithium. One patient has been intermittently unreliable about continuing her medication and has had many family and interpersonal problems. Since she left home, however, medication compliance has been less problematic, and for the past year she has been normothymic. Two patients have had recurrences of mania despite therapeutic lithium levels, but when the medication was discontinued recently both became acutely manic, suggesting that some episodes were being aborted by the lithium.

The third point, then, is that lithium is not always a panacea. In dealing with people at this important phase of their lives it is necessary to treat their entire situation. It is often difficult to separate affective symptoms from core problems. After a few months of mood stabilization, one has a much clearer picture of what needs to be dealt with psychotherapeutically—and frequently one has a more psychologically available patient.

As with adults, lithium should be used on those adolescents with a

TABLE 1

AFFECTIVE SYMPTOMS DURING THE COURSE OF
ILLNESS IN SIX ADOLESCENT PATIENTS

A. AFFECTIVE REACTIONS

Symptom	Patients with Symptom	
	No.	%
Mania:		
Euphoric or expansive	6	100
Irritable or aggressive	5	83
Grandiose	4	66
Distractible	5	83
Sleep loss	4	66
Hyperactivity	6	100
Pressure of speech	6	100
Hypersexual	6	100
Flight of ideas	3	50
Bizarre dress	2	33
Depression:		
Dysphoric mood	6	100
Psychomotor retardation	6	100
Impaired concentration	6	100
Agitation	5	83
Loss of interest	6	100
Thoughts of death or suicide	5	83
Self reproach or guilty thoughts	6	100
Loss of weight or appetite	3	50

B. PSYCHOTIC SYMPTOMS

Symptom	Patients with Symptom			
	Depression		Mania	
	No.	%	No.	%
Delusions:				
Somatic, sexual, guilt	3	50	0	...
Persecution or reference	5	83	4	66
Grandiose	0	...	3	50
Auditory hallucinations	3	50	1	17
Catatonia or mannerisms	3	50	0	...
Confusion	5	83	0	...
Regressive behavior or nudity	0	...	3	50

history of acute mania or severe mood swings. These may be disrupting their lives, though hospitalization is not necessarily required. Adolescent manic-depressive patients seem to respond as well and as frequently to lithium as adults (Carlson and Strober 1978; Horowitz 1977; Schou 1971; Youngerman and Canino 1978). In patients presenting with acute depression, one should inquire about a previous history of hypomania and a family history of MDI. Although lithium is not the first treatment of choice for depression, it may act as an antidepressant in the depressive phase of bipolar MDI (Goodwin and Ebert 1977).

Clinical Management

Although medical problems are not usually present in this age group, a good medical history should be taken and cardiac and renal disease excluded. Since lithium excretion falls when salt intake is lowered, patients treated with diuretics or salt-free diets require electrolyte monitoring as well. Because of the thyroid-suppressant effects of lithium, a baseline T4 should be drawn. Patients with low normal thyroid function should have another T4 a few months later and annually after lithium treatment begins, and if below normal, thyroid supplement should be given (Maletsky and Blachly 1971).

Lithium is a drug where blood level is the major determinant of dose. The general therapeutic range of lithium carbonate is 0.8–1.4 meq/L. Below that level it is generally ineffective; above it the likelihood of toxicity increases. Some patients can tolerate higher doses, while others have a much narrower therapeutic range. Adolescents excrete lithium easily and often need a higher dosage of medication to maintain therapeutic levels (Schou 1971). The average dosage I have prescribed for adolescents is 1,500 milligrams, with a range between 900 milligrams and 2,700 milligrams. Patients in a manic phase usually require a higher dosage to maintain therapeutic levels than patients in a depressed or normothymic phase.

Lithium is well absorbed by the gastrointestinal tract, peaks in approximately two hours after ingestion, and is almost entirely excreted by the kidneys. Lithium half-life in adolescents is eighteen to twenty-four hours. Lithium levels should be drawn twelve hours after the last dose because it takes that long to reach equilibrium. Usually the morning dose is held until after blood is drawn. Generally it takes a week after beginning lithium treatment before that dose has generally stabilized. Although lithium is given in divided doses, a twice-a-day schedule is sufficient (Schou 1973). More frequent doses are necessary only when the patient suffers immediate gastrointestinal distress secondary to lithium ingestion. Lithium levels should be measured weekly until stable and thereafter if the clinician fears noncompliance or toxicity, or if the patient develops symptoms of mania or depression. Subsequently, the lithium levels need to be drawn only every four to six weeks. Manic patients usually respond within two weeks of reaching a therapeutic lithium level, but antidepressant effects are less dramatic; the prophylactic effects generally take several months of treatment to become apparent (Goodwin and Ebert 1977).

Table 2 summarizes the unwanted side effects of lithium. The medication has surprisingly few side effects. Adolescents are no more or less likely to have these side effects than anyone else. Nausea is usually secondary to local gastrointestinal irritation which can be treated symptomatically. The fine tremor is not Parkinsonian in nature but is frequently diminished by lowering the dosage slightly. Polyuria and polydipsia are secondary to the lithium, which induces nephrogenic diabetes insipidus. These side effects are more troublesome at night because of the nocturia. Weight gain is not infrequent and may be due to water retention, improved appetite, or less manic motor activity

TABLE 2

DIFFERENT TYPES OF SIDE EFFECT WHICH
MAY OCCUR DURING LITHIUM TREATMENT

Side Effect	Initial, Harmless	Persistent, Harmless	Prodromes of Intoxication
Nausea, loose stools	+	+	−
Vomiting, diarrhea	−	−	+
Fine tremor of the hands	+	+	−
Coarse tremor of the hands	−	−	+
Polyuria and polydipsia	+	+	−
Weight gain	−	+	−
Edema	−	+	−
Sluggishness, sleepiness	−	−	+
Vertigo	−	−	+
Dysarthria	−	−	+

SOURCE.—Schou and Shaw (1973).

415

(Maletsky and Blachly 1971). Signs of toxicity, both neurological and gastrointestinal, are confirmed by an elevated lithium level.

Lithium has been used in conjunction with tranquilizers and antidepressants, and no adverse drug interactions have been satisfactorily demonstrated. Also, long-term, irreversible effects have not been reported in any reliable way. However, there are reports of reactions which are not often clearly related to the drug itself (Ayd 1975). Lithium is generally contraindicated in pregnancy as there is some suggestion that it may cause fetal anomalies (Goldfield and Weinstein 1971). On the other hand, I was asked to see one rapidly cycling manic-depressive, pregnant eighteen-year-old who became suicidal when depressed and indiscriminately promiscuous when manic (resulting in her pregnancy). For her, in my opinion, the mood swings were much more dangerous to her and to the baby than was the careful use of lithium. The same considerations should be given to patients with impaired renal function or other complicating problems.

Other Indications for Lithium

There are several other psychiatric conditions in which lithium has been used. In general, the more the problem resembles MDI the more likely lithium is to help. It has been useful in treating some episodic behavior problems, especially in patients who have a family history of MDI (Annell 1969; Greenhill, Rieder, Wender, Buchsbaum, and Zahn 1973). It has also been reported to be useful in treating severe premenstrual depression when started about ten days before the onset of menses and discontinued with the first day of flow (Maletsky and Blachly 1971). It has been used with some success in calming aggressive, mentally retarded adolescents, affecting the mood-irritability component similar to manic irritability. Even in very aggressive prisoners the number of fights and impulsive behavior are significantly diminished by lithium. The mechanism for this is unclear (Marnini and Sheard 1977). Lithium seems to be a mood stabilizer in adolescents and young adults, especially emotionally labile women, who have what used to be called emotionally unstable character disorders. In these people, highs and lows last for hours rather than days or weeks, and some authors consider this condition closely allied to the affective disorders (Rifkin et al. 1972).

Conclusions

Adolescents develop MDI, and lithium carbonate treatment is indicated as in adults. Lithium is also worth trying, though experimentally, in patients displaying episodic psychiatric problems with a mood component, in patients with severe aggression, and in women with severe premenstrual depression. It should be used cautiously in persons with potential electrolyte problems and avoided in pregnancy unless absolutely necessary. Serum lithium levels provide dosage guidelines. The frequency of response and side effects is similar to that in adults. Although lithium should be used cautiously, as should any medication, it need not be feared. Good clinical judgment is the foundation of its use, alone or in combination with other modalities, in adolescents and in adults.

REFERENCES

Annell, A. L. 1969. Lithium in the treatment of children and adolescents. *Acta Psychiatrica Scandinavia* 207 (Suppl.): 19–23.

Ayd, F. J. 1975. Lithium-haloperidol for mania. Is it safe or hazardous? *International Drug Therapy Newsletter* 10:29–36.

Brumback, R. A., and Weinberg, W. A. 1977. Mania in childhood. A therapeutic trial of lithium carbonate and a further description of manic-depressive illness in children. *American Journal of Diseases in Children* 131:1122–1126.

Carlson, G. A.; Davenport, Y. B.; and Jamison, K. 1977. A comparison of outcome in adolescent and late onset bipolar manic-depression illness. *American Journal of Psychiatry* 134:919–922.

Carlson, G., and Strober, M. 1978. Bipolar manic-depressive illness in early adolescence. *Journal of the American Academy of Child Psychiatry* 17:138–153.

Feinstein, S. C., and Wolpert, E. A. 1973. Juvenile manic-depressive illness: clinical and therapeutic considerations. *Journal of the American Academy of Child Psychiatry* 12:286–290.

Fieve, R. R. 1975. Lithium therapy. In A. F. Friedman, H. I. Kaplan, and B. J. Sadock, eds. *Comprehensive Textbook of Psychiatry.* Baltimore: Williams & Wilkins.

Goldfield, M., and Weinstein, M. 1971. Lithium therapy in pregnancy: a review with recommendations. *American Journal of Psychiatry* 127:888–893.

Goodwin, F., and Ebert, M. 1977. Specific antimanic and antidepressant drugs. In M. E. Jarik, ed. *Psychopharmacology in the Practice of Medicine*. New York: Appleton-Century-Croft.

Greenhill, L. I.; Rieder, R. O.; Wender, P. H.; Buchsbaum, M.; and Zahn, T. P. 1973. Lithium carbonate in the treatment of hyperactive children. *Archives of General Psychiatry* 28:636–640.

Horowitz, H. A. 1977. Lithium in the treatment of adolescent manic-depressive illness. *Diseases of the Nervous System* 38:480–483.

Maletsky, B., and Blachly, P. H. 1971. *The Use of Lithium in Psychiatry*. London: Butterworths.

Marnini, J. L., and Sheard, M. H. 1977. Anti-aggressive effect of lithium ion in man. *Acta Psychiatrica Scandinavia* 55:269–286.

Prien, R. F., and Caffey, E. M. 1976. Relationship between dosage and response to lithium prophylaxis in recurrent depression. *American Journal of Psychiatry* 133:567–569.

Rifkin, A.; Quitkin, F.; Carillo, C.; Blumberg, A. G.; and Klein, D. F. 1972. Lithium carbonate in emotionally unstable character disorder. *Archives of General Psychiatry* 27:519–523.

Schou, M. 1971. Lithium in psychiatric therapy and prophylaxis: a review with special regard to its use in children. In A. L. Annell, ed. *Depressive States in Childhood and Adolescence*. Proceedings 4th United States Psychiatric Congress. Stockholm: Almquist & Wiksell.

Schou, M. 1973. Practical problems of lithium maintenance treatment. *Journal of Psychiatry, Neurology, and Neurochemistry* 76:511–522.

Schou, M., and Shaw, D. M. 1973. Lithium in recurrent manic-depressive disorders. *Practitioner* 210:105–111.

Van Krevelen, D. A., and Van Voorst, J. A. 1959. Lithium in the treatment of cryptogenic psychosis in a juvenile. *Acta Paedopsychiatrica* 26:148–152.

Youngerman, J., and Canino, I. A. 1978. Lithium carbonate in the use of children and adolescents. *Archives of General Psychiatry* 35:216–224.

PART V

LEGAL AND PSYCHIATRIC PERSPECTIVES ON DELINQUENCY AND ACTING OUT

EDITORS' INTRODUCTION

Man's classic struggle with himself and others consists to a large extent of a problem with communication. Born only with tension outlets, man begins almost at once to develop ways of transferring messages, and observers are beginning to recognize interactive capacities that appear shortly after birth. On the other hand, these interactive patterns are very primitive, and the main modality of communication is through action. In infancy action becomes the main pathway to reduce tension, and throughout life it remains a remnant of an old adaptation: immediately available but regressive and potentially destructive to man's quest for higher levels of communication.

Behaviors that are distressing to society show direct evidence of man's primitive drives. In adolescence sexual and aggressive drives emerge as requiring renegotiation of the sublimative defensive operations of the developing ego. During this remodeling process, regression naturally appears and action again becomes a most important communication resource. It is these disorders of action that society rejects and begs its behavioral scientists to "cure."

These action disorders can be mastered, however, and eventually give way to superior communication devices. Can science find a way to encourage development and avoid the wasteful price society must pay for the use of action rather than verbal forms of communication? This special section is devoted to exploring the psychodynamic dilemmas that delinquency, acting out, violence, and aggression present to individuals, families, schools, and the justice systems of society.

Richard C. Marohn presents an overview of juvenile delinquency as a Special Editor. He focuses on the psychiatric aspects of delinquency and acting out and characterizes delinquents as pseudoautonomous and counterdependent persons who express their emotional problems in behavioral action symptoms rather than diagnosable psychiatric illness. Marohn emphasizes that it is in the nature of the adolescent to externalize, to act, and any intelligent assessment of the teenage delinquent must account for this propensity. Further research and an extension of therapeutic programs will provide more insight into the causes of this extensive problem.

Judge Noah Weinstein traces the history of the interrelationship of legal and psychological determinants of guilt and behavior. He reviews critical court cases that have gradually defined the responsibility of the psychiatrist to the patient and summarizes the current legal status of children in regards to their rights in relationship to institutionalization.

Carl P. Malmquist examines the consequences to adolescents of coming before a court. Charged with a serious offense, an adolescent may remain within the juvenile system or be prosecuted as an adult. The laws, rationales, and historical development of the juvenile court movement are reviewed. The question of treatability or presence of adequate treatment programs as a criterion for transfer is debated. The ambivalence in society around treatability versus retribution is noted.

Jonas Robitscher characterizes our current psychosocial period as an ''age of antiauthority.'' He views the rise of consumerism and the questioning of authority as causing a fundamental shift from a parental transference framework to a concept of mutuality and egalitarianism. The newer relationship of the therapist and patient is of coadventurers on a mutual exploration. These notions are particularly conflictual when parents and psychiatrists are forced to commit a child and deprive him of his liberty or to request a young person's informed consent. The current legal and psychiatric positions on these issues are discussed. Robitscher concludes that while increased rights for adolescents are inevitable, society will have to recognize their special vulnerabilities.

Richard Marohn, Daniel Offer, Eric Ostrov, and Jaime Trujillo report that they were able to identify four psychodynamic types among a group of carefully selected, hospitalized delinquent adolescents. They describe these types as an impulsive delinquent, a narcissistic delinquent, a depressed delinquent, and a borderline delinquent. The authors believe that by highlighting the psychological instead of demographic factors, the therapeutic approach to delinquents will be enhanced.

Meyer Sonis retraces the development of concepts of acting out in delinquent behavior beginning with August Aichhorn, William Healy, and Sheldon and Eleanor Glueck. Using these concepts, he studied a group of seriously acting-out adolescents referred to a juvenile court. He concluded that this group would be representative of court populations in general and manifests in large measure: poverty, minority status, early and middle adolescence, history of aggression, thievery, and running away. Surprisingly, most were first offenders, reacting to a developmental crisis; manifesting emotional, cognitive, or central nervous system defects; and requiring special services. Sonis recommends an approach which recognizes the need for a broad range of human services rather than simplistic solutions.

Michael Kalogerakis is concerned about the deprivation of rights of juveniles through the unjustifiable application of adversary procedure to a child or adolescent. He believes that the minor's dependency; incomplete biological, emotional, and cognitive development; and normal rebellion against parental figures creates a dilemma for the average attorney. He conceptualizes the development of a new type of professional to represent children, the clinician-advocate, and outlines the type of training and background for this position as well as how this concept might operate.

In sharp contrast to previous patterns, girls now constitute up to 30 percent of cases in some juvenile court jurisdictions. There has been, in addition, a considerable change in the nature of their delinquent activities. This qualitative and quantitative shift in girls' delinquency has accompanied the great changes that have occurred in our culture and social institutions during the past generation. In an introduction to a meeting on delinquency in girls Donald Hayes Russell pointed these facts out and concluded that the loosening of social mores and sanctions may have enlarged the female arena and elevated the threshold of adolescent self-expression.

Perihan A. Rosenthal studied a group of delinquent girls who in her opinion manifested evidences of a new emerging role for women. They, like boys, expressed their conflicts by delinquency, suicide, depression, running away, and identity confusion. All suffering from early deprivation, these girls struggle with their preoedipal ties, but the ambiguity of new roles creates new complex identity problems for young women. Therapeutically the author found two developmental types which required different approaches: one, struggling with separation-individuation, was treated with individual approaches; the other, still held by symbiotic ties, required family approaches to effect separation before individual therapy could be utilized.

Bret Burquest discusses the therapeutic approaches to families with severely delinquent girls. Classifying these families as of three types, collusive, intolerant, and permissive, he reviews the techniques to be used with each example and concludes that helping families deal with their child's aggression will lead to more effective resolution.

Elissa Benedek also approaches the issue of female delinquency and categorizes three types: psychological, sociological, and organic. She concludes that little is known about the etiology of female delinquency and advises an extension of research and treatment opportunities.

29 A PSYCHIATRIC OVERVIEW OF JUVENILE DELINQUENCY

RICHARD C. MAROHN

In 1974, there were reportedly over 6,100,000 arrests in the United States for serious crimes such as criminal homicide, forcible rape, robbery, aggravated assault, and arson; of these, 1,700,000, or just over 27 percent, were committed by persons under eighteen years of age (Mann 1976). Juveniles commit 10 percent of all the murders, 19 percent of all the forcible rapes, 32 percent of all the robberies, 17 percent of all the aggravated assaults, and 58 percent of all the arsons. When burglary, larceny, and motor vehicle thefts are added to this list, more than half of all the serious crimes in the United States are found to be committed by youths from ten to seventeen ("Youth Crime Plague," 1977). An exhaustive survey of youth in Illinois conducted by the Institute for Juvenile Research (Schwartz and Puntil 1972) demonstrated that from 25 percent to 94 percent of Illinois youth were involved in violent acts, varying with gender, race, age, socioeconomic status, and community size.

A serious deficiency of these data is the fact that much delinquency goes undetected or unreported, and yet is serious. Many affluent teenagers are handled, not by the juvenile justice system, but either by the mental health system or not at all. Many psychiatrists see these young people in their offices, and there they are called "behavioral disorders." And, of course, true to the biases of our society, if these teenagers are ever brought to the attention of the juvenile justice system, people are surprised because they come from such good homes and good neighborhoods. This is consistent with society's preoccupation with teenage unemployment, racism, poor schools, and poverty as being factors primarily responsible for juvenile delinquency. Similarly, high-level debate about deinstitutionalization and institutionalization is not based on research, or even on theoretical bias, but rather is determined primarily by political winds and the condition of the state treasury.

The *Task Force Report: Juvenile Delinquency and Youth Crime*, presented to the President's Commission on Law Enforcement and the Administration of Justice (1967), contains thirty-eight recommendations, most of which had to do with improving the quality of life and of communities, schools, employment, and the juvenile justice system. Three related to treatment. The Task Force (which included no psychiatrists) recommended that private and public efforts should be intensified to "make counseling and therapy easily obtainable." The Task Force acknowledged that despite the best of community circumstances, some families need help. "Counseling and therapy provide one promising method of dealing with complex emotional and psychological relationships within the family." Nothing was said about individual psychology and psychopathology.

A second recommendation was to intensify public and private efforts to "provide community residential centers." "Small residential centers have proved successful in a number of communities in steering youth away from incipient trouble by providing more supervision than they get at home, yet in an atmosphere that is not institutional or coercive."

The final treatment-oriented recommendation was that, with particular reference to the "slum child," private and public efforts should be expended to "deal better with behavior problems." Unfortunately, this appears to be an issue outside of the slum as well. The Task Force explained that "it is also important that schools learn to understand and control the child who arrives at school accustomed to autonomy, and averse to assertions of authority. New methods of dealing with behavior problems are needed that avoid labeling the child a troublemaker, excluding him from his group, and reinforcing misbehavior patterns." Our own work suggests that most of our delinquents exhibit pseudoautonomy and counterdependency; this is not limited to the poor or the slum dweller.

And so we hear a good deal about housing and recreation, family planning and religion, inner-city life and job placement, new job opportunities and the training of police, but nothing in essence uniquely psychiatric. If we know one thing about adolescence, we know that many teenagers express their emotional problems in behavioral symptoms and not necessarily in diagnosable psychiatric illness. It is in the nature of the adolescent to externalize, to act. An intelligent assessment of the teenage delinquent must account for this propensity.

The Rand Report (Mann 1976), *Intervening with Convicted Serious Juvenile Offenders*, was quite thoughtful and focused on a multiplicity of viewpoints and approaches, although in too cursory a manner. Yet it pointed up the significant need for solid research and the development of programs for the serious offender. Indeed, there are many contributing factors to the final common pathway of delinquent behavior. And though psychopathology is culturally expressed in a variety of ways, it cannot be ignored. Society needs to address itself to this aspect of adolescent mental health, as do more and more psychiatrists.

The Psychodynamics of Delinquency

All behavior has psychological meaning, and the delinquent act can be understood psychodynamically. Following upon Freud's (1905) finding that certain character disorders and perversions are the reverse of the psychoneuroses, a number of investigators have attempted to formulate juvenile delinquency and adolescent behavior disorders from a psychodynamic point of view. Aichhorn (1925) utilized the classical transference situation in an attempt to get to and modify the delinquent's neurotic conflict, but with a certain kind of delinquent he had first to establish a relationship and then work with the narcissistic transference. Alexander and Staub (1931) observed that certain criminals acted out of a sense of guilt which they hoped to expiate by being caught and punished. In this tradition, Friedlander (1960) postulated that it was important to convert delinquent character disorders to neuroses by blocking the avenues for acting out discharge and creating an internalized conflict which could then be worked with psychotherapeutically.

Anna Freud (1958, 1965) viewed delinquency as a failure of the socialization process, but also noted that some delinquency develops because of the chance availability of delinquent peer groups onto whom the adolescent separating from his parents displaces his investments. The focus here is on delinquent value systems, as are also emphasized in the work of Johnson and Szurek (1952) who described a number of children responding to the unconsciously transmitted delinquent urges of their seemingly upright parents. Glover (1950) distinguished two kinds of delinquents: the structural, who gives evidence before and after adolescence of significant psychopathology, and the functional, whose delinquent behavior is a result of the temporary psychic imbalances of the adolescent maturation process. Blos (1966, 1967, 1971) has offered a variety of psychodynamic explanations including separation struggles, precocious development, the propensity for action language, and delinquency as a symbolic communication. Redl's (1966) emphasis has been on the vicissitudes of ego development and ego functioning, and has underlined the importance of a psychodynamic understanding of the delinquency in an attempt to engage the child therapeutically.

Our own work (Marohn 1974, 1977; Marohn, Dalle-Molle, and Offer 1973; Offer, Marohn, and Ostrov 1975; Ostrov, Offer, and Marohn 1976) has demonstrated that some delinquents act out violently when they are overstimulated not by angry or hostile feelings, but by strong affectionate longings and emotions; that contagion or riot in a group has many causes and results from the participation of many systems, the psychological and intrapsychic system among them; that violence escalates from verbal violence and threats, to damage to property, to personal assault; that newer ideas on narcissism and the self can enrich our understanding of delinquent behavior; that we can predict the likelihood of violent behavior from psychological test data; and that we can identify four statistically and psychologically meaningful subtypes or formulations of delinquency, excluding the psychotic and brain damaged: the impulsive, the narcissistic, the depressed borderline, and the empty borderline. We have developed ways of working with delinquent adolescents in a tightly controlled, highly structured, long-term hospital treatment program involving one to two years of hospitalization, integrating individual psychotherapy and milieu therapy, and attempting to achieve internal psychological change and character restructuring (Offer, Marohn, and Ostrov 1979).

Others, too, are attempting to understand delinquents psychologically. Warren (1977) acknowledged that a significant number of delinquents "act out internal conflicts, identity struggles, or family crises." She developed a system of classifying youth psychodynamically which points to specific treatment goals, treatment strategies, and treatment modalities. She demonstrated that matching the counselor or therapist with specific kinds of delinquents results in more favorable prognoses, and questions the idea that a good therapist has a full range of "talents, sensitivities, and interests" which enable him to deal effectively with whatever type of client comes his way. Yet even these sophisticated studies are challenged by Martinson (1974), who raises questions about the "normality" of criminality in our society and points up the serious problems in doing competent efficacy research.

Lewis and Balla (1976) have noted that the juvenile justice system is a "repository for large numbers of seriously impaired children" with central nervous system dysfunction and psychotic symptoms.

The American Society for Adolescent Psychiatry has brought together prominent psychiatrists and other professionals to focus on such issues as institutionalization and deinstitutionalization; individual, family, and group psychotherapy of the delinquent; the juvenile court and the rights of the delinquent; the violent delinquent; female delinquency, its apparent increase and frequency in severity; and new research in delinquency in each of its national meetings. I do not mean to propose that psychiatry has the final answer, and I believe I can understand the problem that Wilson (1977) confronts when he talks about the "frightful expense" of intensive milieu therapy. Yet I contend that such frightful expense is justified because from it we can learn much, develop less expensive forms of treatment, and confront the issue that there is no ready or easy solution to our problem. It is facile to say that broken homes cause delinquency. Yet, it is only through studying intact families in which delinquency occurs that we can begin understanding, for example, those kinds of family constellations and communications which might promote or precipitate delinquency. And, of course, it may very well be that the same factors that cause the home to break may also be responsible for the delinquency. I do not mean to depreciate sociological research, but I hope to underline the importance of psychological and psychiatric research. An outstanding example of how psychoanalytic and sociological data can be integrated, correlated, and enrich each other, rather than compete or negate each other, is contained in the studies of a Chicago gang described by Baittle and Kobrin (1964).

Conclusions

But what must now be done?

There must be longitudinal studies of delinquents who are treated, as well as those who are not treated. Short-term and long-term modalities must be compared, as must family therapy and individual therapy, as must institutional programs and deinstitutional programs. Perhaps then we can decide which treatment works best for whom. We must determine whether delinquency, particularly violent delinquency, is increasing or decreasing. And we must learn whether there are more female delinquents and in what ways these girls are different.

Working with adolescents and delinquents must become part of the core training of every psychiatrist, and we psychiatrists must not only take the lead in developing model diagnostic and treatment programs for delinquent teenagers, but also spearhead the training of other professionals in a psychodynamic appreciation of the delinquent.

We need to learn more about the idealizing transference and the role of deidealization in the therapy of the delinquent. We must understand more about the negative transference, and not confuse it with the absence of a working or therapeutic relationship or alliance. As psychiatrists, we must be willing to hospitalize character disorders or behavioral disorders, and we must insist that third-party payers and insurance companies support such treatment. We must revise our commitment laws so that disordered development and the need for hospitalization become the criteria for commitment to a psychiatric program designed specifically for teenagers, not proven or demonstrable violence. Therapy of the delinquent and the behaviorally disordered adolescent is a clinical, not legal, issue.

Countertransference, frustration, and resistance will, of course, express themselves in new and modern disguises. We are tempted to explain away or deny psychopathology as economic problems, organicity, or political unrest. Or we might return to theories of moral degeneracy.

The problem is vast, but not hopeless. As Winnicott (1958, 1972) taught us, the delinquent is continually reaching out for his lost object; the mother once possessed but later lost, whom the delinquent hopes to recapture through his behavior. We know that the delinquent is still searching, has not given up, and may, indeed, include the therapist in his search.

REFERENCES

Aichhorn, A. 1925. *Wayward Youth.* New York: Meridian Books, 1960.
Alexander, F., and Staub, H. 1931. *The Criminal, the Judge and the Public.* New York: Collier Books, 1956.

Baittle, B., and Kobrin, S. 1964. On the relationship of a characterological type of delinquent to the milieu. *Psychiatry* 27:6–16.

Blos, P. 1966. *A Developmental Approach to Problems of Acting Out.* New York: International Universities Press.

Blos, P. 1967. The second individuation process of adolescence. *Psychoanalytic Study of the Child* 22:162–185.

Blos, P. 1971. Adolescent concretization: a contribution to the theory of delinquency. In I. M. Marcus, ed. *Currents in Psychoanalysis.* New York: International Universities Press.

Freud, A. 1958. Adolescence. *Psychoanalytic Study of the Child.* 13:255–278.

Freud, A. 1965. *Normality and Pathology in Childhood: Assessments of Development.* New York: International Universities Press.

Freud, S. 1905. Three essays on sexuality. *Standard Edition* 7:123–243. London: Hogarth, 1953.

Friedlander, K. 1960. *The Psychoanalytic Approach to Juvenile Delinquency.* New York: International Universities Press.

Glover, E. 1950. On the desirability of isolating a "functional" group delinquent disorder. *British Journal of Delinquency* 1:104–112.

Johnson, A., and Szurek, S. A. 1952. The genesis of antisocial acting out in children and adults. *Psychoanalytic Quarterly* 21:323–343.

Lewis, D. O., and Balla, D. A. 1976. *Delinquency and Psychopathology.* New York: Grune & Stratton.

Mann, D. 1976. *Intervening with Convicted Serious Juvenile Offenders.* Santa Monica, Calif.: Rand Corp.

Marohn, R. C. 1974. Trauma and the delinquent. *Adolescent Psychiatry* 3:354–361.

Marohn, R. C. 1977. The juvenile imposter: some thoughts on narcissism and the delinquent. *Adolescent Psychiatry* 5:186–212.

Marohn, R. C.; Dalle-Molle, D.; and Offer, D. 1973. A hospital riot: its determinants and implications for treatment. *American Journal of Psychiatry* 130:631–636.

Martinson, R. 1974. What works?—questions and answers about prison reform. *Public Interest* 35:22–54.

Offer, D.; Marohn, R. C.; and Ostrov, E. 1975. Violence among hospitalized delinquents. *Archives of General Psychiatry* 32:1180–1186.

Offer, D.; Marohn, R. C.; and Ostrov, E. 1979. *The Psychological World of the Juvenile Delinquent.* New York: Basic.

Ostrov, E.; Offer, D.; and Marohn, R. C. 1976. Hostility and impulsivity in normal and delinquent Rorschach responses. *Mental Health in Children* 2:479–492.

The President's Commission on Law Enforcement and Administration of Justice. 1967. *Task Force Report: Juvenile Delinquency and Youth Crime*. Washington, D.C.: Government Printing Office.

Redl, F. 1966. *When We Deal with Children*. New York: Free Press.

Schwartz, G., and Puntil, J. E. 1972. Summary and policy implications of the youth and society in Illinois reports. Chicago: Institute for Juvenile Research.

Warren, M. Q. 1977. Measuring the impact of specific therapist-patient matches in work with juvenile delinquents. Paper presented to the Society for Psychotherapy Research, Madison, Wis., June 1977.

Wilson, J. C. 1977. *Thinking about Crime*. New York: Vintage.

Winnicott, D. W. 1958. The antisocial tendency. In *Collected Papers*. New York: Basic.

Winnicott, D. W. 1972. Delinquency as a sign of hope. *Adolescent Psychiatry* 2:363–372.

Youth crime plague. 1977. *Time* (July 11), pp. 18–28.

30 LIBERTY AND MENTAL HEALTH: A PHILOSOPHICAL CONFLICT

NOAH WEINSTEIN

For one whose professional life span has covered much of the period of the infusion of the behavioral sciences into the legal system of our nation, I must confess that at this moment there is a great deal of confusion as to their proper place in the complex scheme which comprises a system of justice.

Law has a historical background of influence by moral metaphysical elements. The use of hot coals and submerging in water to determine guilt/innocence was brought to an abrupt end in 1215 by virtue of a papal decree which forbade participation by clergy in the ritual which lay courts relied upon to decide cases brought before it. But the reluctance of the legal system to devise its own and distinct system of determining guilt has continued in varying degrees throughout its history to the present time. In its effort to read the minds of men to determine moral guilt, we find a variety of experiments by the legal system. The 1843 M'Naughten test was criticized by psychiatrists because it forced them to testify specifically on whether or not the accused knew right from wrong. Such testimony in effect determined the ultimate issue which should be left to the jury.

The *Durham* case (*Durham* v. *United States* 1954) was an attempt to restore to the jury its traditional function and, at the same time, to bring into the trial whatever knowledge psychiatrists had about behavior. But, after almost two decades of use, *Durham* failed to take the issue of criminal responsibility away from the experts. Psychiatrists continued to testify to their conclusions instead of providing information to enable the jury to determine the issue of criminal responsibility.

Durham was abandoned in 1972 in favor of a different approach to end the domination of juries by psychiatrists in determining the ultimate issue: whether the accused can be justly held responsible. The new principle announced in *Brawner* (*United States* v. *Brawner* 1969) was intended to provide the jury with a broad range of information concerning the accused. Other disciplines with special skill in the area of behavior thus could be called upon to show the relevance of their data.

The use of the insanity defense, as exemplified by *M'Naughten* and its progeny, represents a digression by the legal system into matters which it is not equipped to handle—in fact, matters which are incompatible with its proper basic tenets. Law, during its early development, had its experience with measuring the wrath of God and delving into the metaphysical. By today's standards that historical segment of jurisprudence developed sanctions for crime that would be considered cruel, unusual, and inhumane.

This revulsion against the excesses that were then practiced resulted in the appearance, in the eighteenth century, of a system of criminology which became known as classical or utilitarian. This movement proposed a definite and uniform scheme for the application of penalties, thus avoiding the impossible task, for a lay court, of attempting to determine the quantum of moral guilt and applying punishment commensurate with the imponderables there involved. However, it had little effect on the development of Anglo-American jurisprudence which became involved, almost to the point of obsession, with what was going on in the mind of the criminal when he was committing his criminal act. It appears that the law was seeking justification for acts which organized society had decreed violated accepted norms and accordingly were subject to punishment. The deterministic philosophy, developed in the latter half of the nineteenth century by Lombroso, Ferri, Garofolo, and others, seemed to satisfy the law's reluctance to accept bare physical facts, was readily adaptable into the developing legal system, and provided a receptive environment for the burgeoning psychiatric and sociological schools of thought.

The chronology of what I describe may not fit neatly into each compartment, and I do not suggest that the developing legal system was preplanned and systematically adopted. However, analytically, the foundation existed that was receptive to a system that became captivated with a concern for the effect of mental disorder upon culpability and the concept of guilt and resulted in the creation of complex problems that now appear nearly insolvable.

The psychopathological concept of crime has been attributed to the writing of Alexander and Staub (1929). They divided criminals into two types: normal and neurotic. The normal could properly be subjected to "retaliative" penology. The "neurotic criminal" should be exempted from all forms of punishment and turned over to a psychoanalyst for treatment. Theirs was the advocacy of the principle that the law should not punish the act but the actor by transferring the control over the deviant from the government to the psychiatrist. This is probably the beginning of the development of the current phase of confusion of law with psychiatry, resulting in institutional or coercive psychiatry. And this is the point where the improper use of forensic psychiatry has resulted in the imposition of severe restrictions upon the right of psychiatry to treat its patients.

If the legal system had defined crime as the single element of the prohibited physical act, instead of a combination of a physical act and a nonphysical or subjective element, requiring an inquiry into the state of mind of the actor (criminal intent), we would not be confronted with the many problems arising today between psychiatry and the law. This is not to say that psychiatry has no place in the system of justice. It does have an appropriate function to perform, but it arises not during the trial of criminal cases, where it is accused of usurping the functions of the judge and jury, but after a determination of guilt. It then can discharge a valuable function in the determination of disposition, or treatment, if you prefer. Would this mean that prisons would become psychiatric hospitals for the involuntary patient or psychiatric hospitals would become prisons for the involuntary committed patient? This is purely a matter of linguistics; for the person who is confined in either there is no difference.

The problem confronting psychiatry today is a particularly puzzling one to the psychiatrist in his involvement with the patient who is about to be or who is involuntarily committed.

The limits placed upon the confinement of patients against their will has been announced in many lower-court decisions. This evidences a growing concern that too many people are deprived of their liberty without due process of law; that definitions of mental illness are too vague and unscientific to justify involuntary confinement and treatment. And, from the psychiatrist's point of view, it raises questions about competing values of mental health and liberty. It is said that by valuing liberty so highly we may find ourselves in an antihumanistic position; "that the value of mental health encompasses the values of survival and compassion, and the value of liberty does not" (Halleck 1974).

The current legal situation is exemplified by some recent court decisions that have a bearing on the confusing issues that arise.

The most important of these decisions comes from the U.S. Supreme Court (*O'Connor* v. *Donaldson* 1975). Kenneth Donaldson was civilly committed in a court proceeding to confinement as a mental patient, suffering from "paranoid schizophrenia," in the Florida State Hospital in January of 1957. He was kept there against his will for nearly fifteen years. Dr. J. B. O'Connor was the hospital's superintendent during most of that time. Donaldson repeatedly demanded his release, claiming that he was not mentally ill, that he was dangerous to no one, and that the hospital was not providing treatment for his supposed illness. Donaldson filed a lawsuit under the Civil Rights Act alleging that O'Connor and other members of the hospital staff had intentionally and maliciously deprived him of his constitutional right to liberty. The jury returned a verdict assessing both compensatory and punitive damages against O'Connor and a codefendant. The Court of Appeals affirmed the judgment and the U.S. Supreme Court agreed to hear the case because of the important constitutional questions presented.

At the trial in the District Court, the evidence showed (1) that the hospital had the power to release a patient, not dangerous to himself or others, even if he remained mentally ill and had been lawfully committed; (2) that the patient Donaldson posed no danger to others during his long confinement or at any point in his life; (3) that there was no evidence that Donaldson had even been suicidal; (4) that Donaldson could have earned his own living outside the hospital; (5) that Donaldson's confinement was a simple regime of enforced custodial care, not a program designed to alleviate or cure his supposed illness; and (6) that Donaldson's requests for ground privileges, occupational training, and an opportunity to discuss his case with staff members were repeatedly denied.

O'Connor's principal defense was that he had acted in good faith and was therefore immune from any liability for monetary damages, and that state law, which he believed valid, had authorized indefinite custodial confinement even if no treatment was given and the patient's release could harm no one.

The jury returned a verdict for Donaldson against Dr. O'Connor (and a codefendant) and awarded damages of $38,500, including $10,000 in punitive damages. The Court of Appeals affirmed the judgment in an opinion that held that the Fourteenth Amendment guarantees a right to treatment to persons involuntarily civilly committed to state mental hospitals.

However, the Supreme Court took the position that the constitutional issues dealt with by the Court of Appeals were not presented by the case, and "that there is no reason now to decide whether mentally ill persons dangerous to themselves or to others have a right to treatment upon compulsory confinement by the State, or whether the State may compulsorily confine a nondangerous, mentally ill individual for the purpose of treatment."

The Court did rule that the "State cannot constitutionally confine . . . a non-dangerous individual who is capable of surviving safely in freedom by himself or with the help of [others]." Since the jury found that O'Connor, as an agent of the State, did knowingly so confine Donaldson, it properly concluded that O'Connor violated Donaldson's constitutional right to freedom.

In disposing of the case the Supreme Court did two things. First, it referred back to the Court of Appeals the issue of O'Connor's immunity from liability for monetary damages, and second, the Court stated that the Appeals Court opinion, declaring a constitutional right to treatment to persons involuntarily civilly committed to State mental hospitals, had no precedential effect. In other words, the constitutional right to treatment of persons so committed as declared by the Court of Appeals remains open to debate and speculation.

On the question of the doctor's liability for monetary damages, it appears that the relevant question for the jury is whether O'Connor knew or reasonably should have known that the action he took within the sphere of official responsibility would violate the constitutional rights of Donaldson or if he took the action with the malicious intention to cause a deprivation of constitutional rights or other injury to Donaldson. Thus, the question of the doctor's qualified immunity or defense to monetary damages remains a matter to be determined by the jury in each case.

Another example of proscribed psychiatric conduct is illustrated in the case of *Semler* v. *Psychiatric Institute of Washington, D.C.* (1976). A state court suspended sentence on a criminal defendant and placed him on probation on condition that he receive treatment and remain confined in a psychiatric institute. The psychiatric institute, however, placed defendant on outpatient status without a court order. During the time he was an outpatient, he killed a person. This decision holds that the psychiatric institute and the treating physician breached their duty to protect the public by placing defendant on outpatient status without court approval and, in doing so, their action was proximately related to the murder. A judgment against the psychiatric institute and the doctor in favor of the mother of the victim was affirmed.

In the *Semler* case, the institute offered as a defense the fact that the probation officer in charge of the defendant had approved the change to outpatient status. This defense was rejected by the court because the probation officer had no authority from the court to change the defendant's status. Also, the probation officer was not immune from liability and was ordered to pay one-half of the judgment.

Further legal restrictions have been placed on psychotherapists by a recent decision of the Supreme Court of California (*Tarasoff* v. *Regents of the University of California* 1976). The facts were: A student at the University of California sought psychiatric help as an outpatient at the student health facility. After examination by a psychiatrist, he was referred to a psychologist for psychotherapy. The psychologist determined that the student was dangerous, based in part on his pathological attachment to a young woman who had rejected his love and evidence that he intended to purchase a gun. The psychologist notified the campus police, both orally and in writing, that the student was dangerous and should be taken by the campus police to a facility authorized by the state civil commitment statute to commit him.

The police, after interviewing the student, concluded he was not dangerous and released him with his promise to stay away from the young woman who had rejected him. Neither the woman nor members of her family were warned about the student's possible dangerousness. Two months later, the student killed the woman.

The parents of the victim sued the regents of the University of California, the therapist, and the police. The California Supreme Court held that the relationship between a therapist and patient imposes on the therapist a duty to use reasonable care to protect third parties against danger posed by the patient by warning third parties, or by notifying police, or some other form, depending on the circumstances. The court placed no similar duty to warn on the police.

Consider the dilemma of the therapist under this decision. He has a duty to protect the public and a duty to protect the confidentiality of his patient. He must also predict dangerousness with sufficient accuracy to arrive at a reasonable conclusion about his now new duty to protect others from the possible results of prognosticated dangerous conduct. As Judge Mosk stated in his separate opinion, the standard announced by the court "will take us from the world of reality into the wonderland of clairvoyance."

Not directly germane to our subject are the problems involved in predicting dangerousness. It may well be generally accepted that the natural experiment created by the release of 967 "patients" from Dannemora and Mattewan under a decision by the U.S. Supreme Court in *Baxstrom* v. *Herold* (1966) sufficiently demonstrated the over-prediction of dangerousness to justify discarding this concept in confining prisoners or patients involuntarily (Kozol, Boucher, and Garofalo 1972; Steadman and Halfon 1971; Steadman and Keveles 1972).

Finally, we note the most current impact of law on psychiatry. *Bartley* v. *Kremens* (1975) was first decided by a three-judge U.S. District Court in 1975.

The named plaintiffs in this class action are all persons under nineteen years of age who have been or are committed or admitted to mental health facilities in Pennsylvania under that state's Mental Health and Retardation Act. They contend that they are denied due process of law and equal protection of law because Pennsylvania allows children under nineteen years of age to be detailed—denied their liberty—in mental institutions without substantial procedural safeguards.

Kremens, a defendant and director of Haverford State Hospital, contended that due process does not apply since the purpose of the law is to meet the child's needs through treatment and rehabilitation, rather than to punish by incarceration for what he has done. A further defense was that since under the law the parents, guardians ad litem, or persons standing in loco parentis must set in motion the commitment machinery, these persons effectively waive any due-process rights of plaintiffs (children).

The court questioned whether or not a child's interest in not being institutionalized under the Pennsylvania law is safeguarded by the Fourteenth Amendment. After considering a number of decisions, including *O'Connor* v. *Donaldson*, the court concluded that children have the right to due process.

It then had to determine whether or not the child's parent may effectively waive the child's right to due process and what due process is applicable. On the question of waiver, the court concluded that in deciding to institutionalize their children, parents may at times be acting against the interest of their children, and in the absence of any evidence that the child's interests have been fully considered, parents may not effectively waive the personal constitutional rights of their children.

On the kind of due process applicable to children under the Pennsylvania law, the court ruled that before children under nineteen may be institutionalized, they are entitled to: (1) a probable-cause hearing within seventy-two hours from the date of their initial detention; (2) a postcommitment hearing within two weeks from the date of their initial detention; (3) written notice, including the date, time, and place of the hearing, and a statement of the grounds for the proposed commitment; (4) counsel at all significant stages of the commitment process, and if indigent the right to appointment of free counsel; (5) be present at all hearings concerning their proposed commitment; (6) a finding by clear and convincing proof that they are in need of institutionalization; (7) the right to confront and to cross-examine witnesses against them, to offer evidence in their own behalf, and to offer testimony of witnesses; but (8) no jury trial is required.

The court expressed the hope, in a footnote, that all of the above procedures would not be required in every case, that all of the rights, except notice and counsel, may be waived by the child and his lawyer if approved by the court and upon a finding that the child understands his rights and is competent to waive them.

Two of the judges agreed with the above decision. A third judge dissented. He felt that the procedures outlined by the Pennsylvania legislature, when balanced against the traditional rights of parents to control the rearing of their children, afford sufficient protection to the child. He noted that the law required agreement from two psychiatrists, after an examination, that the child is in need of institutionalization. He also mentioned that in voluntary commitments a periodic review must be had by the director every thirty days and children thirteen years of age and older are entitled to a hearing with counsel if he objects to institutionalization.

The dissent noted the concern of the majority about the warehousing of children which might result from the voluntary commitment procedure. His answer to this fear was the holding in the *O'Connor* v. *Donaldson* case by the U.S. Supreme Court that a state cannot constitutionally confine a "nondangerous" individual who is capable of surviving safely in freedom by himself or with the help of willing and responsible family members or friends.

The Supreme Court opinion notes that Bartley and four other "mentally ill" persons between fifteen and eighteen years of age initiated this action challenging the constitutionality of a 1966 Pennsylvania statute which established the voluntary admission and voluntary commitment to state mental health institutions procedures of persons aged eighteen or younger. The statute provided that a juvenile might be admitted upon a parent's application, and that unlike an adult, the admitted juvenile could withdraw only with the consent of the parent admitting him.

After the District Court held those provisions unconstitutional as violative of due process, and after the Supreme Court determined it would probably consider the case, Pennsylvania, in 1976, enacted a new law which repealed the provisions declared unconstitutional by the District Court except as they relate to mentally retarded persons.

Under the new 1976 law any person fourteen years of age or over may voluntarily admit himself, but his parents may not do so, and may withdraw from voluntary treatment at any time by giving written notice. Those fourteen to eighteen who were committed by their parents under the former (1966) law are treated as adults under the new (1976) law.

However, under the new law, children thirteen years of age and younger may still be admitted for treatment by a parent, guardian, or person standing in loco parentis, and may be released by the parent.

The Supreme Court ruled that since at the time the suit was filed in the District Court each of the five named plaintiffs was older than fourteen and "mentally ill," that the 1976 Pennsylvania law treats mentally ill juveniles fourteen and older as adults in that their parents may not voluntarily commit them, and those receiving voluntary treatment may withdraw at any time by giving notice, they, the five named plaintiffs, no longer have any complaint because of mootness. Accordingly, the judgment of the District Court was vacated as to the five named plaintiffs.

In the original action the five named plaintiffs sought also to vindicate the constitutional rights of all persons under eighteen years of age admitted or committed to Pennsylvania state mental health facilities. The decision relating to the five named plaintiffs (who were over thirteen years of age and "mentally ill") did not dispose of the claims of those "mentally ill" and under fourteen years of age and those eighteen years of age or younger who were mentally retarded. This issue was sent back to the District Court for further proceedings.

The Supreme Court carefully avoids ruling on the real issues. It does conclude that since the five named plaintiffs now have the same rights as adults they no longer have any complaint. Does this mean that minors must have the same rights as adults for due process, or can these rights be diluted by transferring some to the parent? And what of the rights of the mentally retarded eighteen and under, and the mentally ill under fourteen?

Two members of the Supreme Court (Brennan and Marshall) were critical of the majority opinion. They felt that the court failed in its duty to properly serve "the constituencies who are dependent on our guidance, by issuing meaningless" orders returning cases to the lower courts.

The majority took the position that its order refusing to adjudicate the issues was consistent with its policy that it will not "formulate a rule of constitutional law broader that is required by the precise facts to which it is to be applied."

Using Judge Brennan's words in his dissent we can sum up this discussion: "As written, today's opinion can only further stir up the jurisdictional stew and frustrate the efforts of litigants who legitimately seek access to the courts for guidance on the content of fundamental constitutional rights."

REFERENCES

Alexander, F., and Staub, H. 1929. *The Criminal, the Judge, and the Public*. Glencoe, Ill.: Free Press, 1956.

Bartley v. Kremens. 1975. U.S. 402 F. Supp. 1039.

Baxstrom v. Herold. 1966. 383 U.S. 107.

Durham v. United States. 1954. 94 U.S. App. D.C. 228, 214.

Halleck, S. 1974. *The Politics of Therapy*. New York: Science House.

Kozol, H.; Boucher, R.; and Garofalo, R. 1972. The diagnosis and treatment of dangerousness. *Crime and Delinquency* 18:371–392.

O'Connor v. Donaldson. 1975. 422 U.S. 563, 45 L. Ed. 2d 396.

Semler v. Psychiatric Institute of Washington, D.C. 1976. 538 F. 2d 121, Court of Appeals, 4th Circuit.

Steadman, H., and Halfon, A. 1971. The Baxstrom patients: backgrounds and outcomes. *Seminars in Psychiatry* 3:376–385.

Steadman, H., and Keveles, G. 1972. The community adjustment and criminal activity of the Baxstrom patients: 1966–1970. *American Journal of Psychiatry* 129:304–310.

Tarasoff v. Regents of the University of California. 1976. 551 P. 2d 334.

United States v. Brawner. 1969. U.S. 471 F. 2d.

31 JUVENILES IN ADULT COURTS: UNRESOLVED AMBIVALENCE

CARL P. MALMQUIST

With the increasing amount of publicity and discussion about juveniles who commit crimes of violence, there is a need to appraise the current mode of handling these juveniles after apprehension. Any clinician who deals with them is concerned about the fate of these adolescents when they are charged with a serious offense and brought before a court. There is always the potential that any adolescent may find himself in such a predicament, and therefore a need for those who work with them to understand the possibilities which can be brought into play. The consequences can be quite serious.

The ultimate issue is whether the juvenile will remain within the juvenile court system, or whether he will be arraigned and tried in adult criminal court. The various terms used in this context—"transferred," "remanded," "waived," and "certified"—are not all synonymous. Waiver hearings refer to the shift of a juvenile up to an adult criminal court from a juvenile court. Certification hearings are the bridge from an adult criminal court down to a juvenile court. In every American jurisdiction, except New York, both the juvenile and criminal courts hold concurrent jurisdiction over minors charged with certain crimes. A hearing can be held to determine which court has jurisdictional priority in all but three states. In Delaware, Louisiana, and Nebraska the prosecutor can choose the court at which the juvenile will appear for certain offenses. In forty-four states and the District of Columbia the juvenile court has the power to waive its jurisdiction in certain circumstances. In seven states (Alabama, Arkansas, Maryland, Pennsylvania, Vermont, Virginia, and Wyoming), criminal courts have authority to certify cases to juvenile courts under certain circumstances (Whitehead and Batey 1975). In some states there has also been a shift toward requiring mandatory institutionalization for certain categories of juvenile offenses after adjudication, but this remains within the juvenile system (Recent reaction to juvenile crime, 1977–1978).

Since referral processes raise questions at the heart of a system of juvenile justice, they present the opportunity to examine the issues raised from a combined legal and clinical perspective. Questions are raised with respect to the purposes served by maintaining a separate system of juvenile courts and the variability in application of these purposes to individual cases which can result in trial in adult criminal courts.

Increasing rates of juvenile crime, as well as publicity about the violent end of the spectrum, put juvenile courts under greater pressure not to permit such youths to be handled under traditional juvenile procedures. While on the one hand these figures raise serious questions about the effectiveness of whatever is being carried out under the banner of juvenile rehabilitation processes, they simultaneously make the system more vulnerable to community pressures to increase sanctions against juveniles who are allegedly not being dealt with adequately.

When the rates of violent crime committed by those in juvenile age categories are considered, one can see the source of concern. Those under eighteen years of age account for about 25 percent of all arrests. Fifty percent of property crimes and 25 percent of violent crimes against people are committed by juveniles. More juveniles under eighteen years are arrested than adults for burglary, larceny, arson, auto theft, and vandalism (FBI 1976). Further, juvenile recidivists commit more serious offenses than one-time juvenile delinquents (National Advisory Commission 1973).

Statutory Variation

All states and the District of Columbia provide some mechanism for certain juveniles to be handled outside the system of juvenile courts. Variations in procedures do exist. There are five conditions, which vary from state to state, under which a juvenile can be sent to an adult criminal court: (1) Some states provide for a judge to waive a juvenile to an adult criminal court before the facts alleged in a given petition are adjudicated. (2) Others allow a waiver during the process of determining what the facts are. (3) A waiver may occur after the facts have been established, the youth adjudicated, and a disposition required. (4) Yet other states may allow waiver after a minor has actually been committed to an institution for juvenile delinquents. (5) There is also a process in some states of retaining original jurisdiction in adult courts and not certifying down to juvenile courts. Without entering into a detailed legal analysis, there is potential for wide variation. Constitutional problems may arise involving double jeopardy (Note, 1972). Under the Fifth Amendment of the United States Constitution, applied to the states through the Fourteenth, a person cannot be "put in jeopardy" twice for the same offense. Questions have centered around what jeopardy entails. At present, the Supreme Court has decided that if a juvenile is adjudicated delinquent in a juvenile court, he cannot subsequently be waived and prosecuted in a criminal court. Transfers must take place before evidence is taken and an adjudication made (*Breed* v. *Jones* 1975).

There are limitations on the power of a juvenile-court judge to waive. In some jurisdictions statutes require certain offenses to have a mandatory waiver. Indiana has made the commission of an act of first degree murder by a youth, otherwise subject to juvenile-court jurisdiction, into a required waiver. In Nebraska, the prosecutor now has complete discretion as to whether a petition shall be filed in adult or juvenile court (Neb. Rev. Stat. 1974). In Virginia, the attorney for the commonwealth can present a juvenile's case to the Grand Jury on his own motion if the alleged offense could result in a sentence of death, life imprisonment, or over twenty years sentence if convicted as an adult, or if the juvenile commits a second offense which is a felony (Va. Code Ann. 1977). For murder, rape, or armed robbery, criteria of amenability to treatment can be required by the court (Va. Code Ann. 1977).

A different limitation on the power of the juvenile-court judge is in the opposite direction of minimum-age groupings. Again, there is state-to-state variation, and the range is from thirteen to eighteen years of age. Illinois and Mississippi hold that a minor under thirteen cannot be waived, while Hawaii and Idaho make the age limit eighteen, although, if the act in question is a felony, the age for possible waiver is lowered to sixteen (see Statutes). Some jurisdictions allow minors to be waived no matter what their age (see New Hamp. Rev. Stat. Ann.

1973). It is also a matter which differs among states, but the trend seems to be toward greater ease in waiving juveniles who are charged with a felonious act. The paradox is that publicity often attends juveniles who are handled leniently, while those that are handled in a severe manner often do not receive any.

Rationales for Certification

Appraisal of the reasons for waiving minors is inextricably bound to the rationales for the juvenile court system itself. Historically, why was such a system devised? Since political and social forces gave rise to the concept of the juvenile court, similar forces must now be operating to shift its manner of functioning. Historical antecedents are not seen as the prime governing criteria, but such a perspective allows us to gain insight into the justifications given which need clarification.

Innumerable articles and treatises have dealt with the juvenile-court movement in the United States. Only a few points germane to the issue of waiver will be noted. The first juvenile court, established in Illinois in 1899, and those which followed, were in part responsive to the harshness of the adult criminal system. Some have taken a critical view of the "do-gooder" influence behind the movement (Platt 1969). However, there was objective evidence of the adverse impact on children and adolescents of a system of criminal justice which was not performing adequately with its adult clientele. To accomplish the removal of a population of juvenile delinquents from the jurisdiction of adult criminal courts meant that a separate system of justice had to be devised. Never resolved was the conflict between two separate goals: separation of minors from adult offenders and their institutions was seen as desirable in itself, yet a rehabilitative ideology also permeated the procedures of the juvenile court. These two goals need not coexist, and in recent years they have tended to be seen as not always feasible.

It is possible to process juveniles separately and still employ rationales other than rehabilitation for an individual delinquent. For example, a juvenile might be adjudicated and committed to a juvenile correctional facility for purposes of deterring him from such behavior in the future. Or, a goal of general deterrence may be operating in hopes that other juveniles will not indulge in such behavior. It is also possible to argue in terms of a juvenile simply being punished for his behavior because of its unacceptability to society. While the degree and type of punishment might vary from the adult system, it would still be a punishment. Finally, a retributive rationale could be used whereby a society and some of its members who have been offended against exact some type of penance for the misconduct to balance the scales of justice. Over time, confusion arose in the juvenile system from mixing these various notions with the idea of treatment. In retrospect, a rehabilitative model (even as an ideal) was never fully subscribed to by the juvenile system. While the utilitarian model was often thought of as the guiding principle, it was never consistently applied, and there were always individual juveniles for whom it was never considered.

Legal Standards

The emphasis on the state as benevolent parent under the doctrine of *parens patriae* has been stressed by many, and yet even at the zenith of its advocacy as a means to curb delinquency and reform its clients, it was never the only rationale operating. In contrast was the prosecutorial adversary role, in which the main goal was to secure community protection. Other goals of the criminal law were noted as possibilities as well, such as punishment or restraint. At least one major justification for a separate system of juvenile justice was that the child would not have to face the same penal consequences for his antisocial behavior as would an adult, who is subject to a criminal conviction with its corollary sanctions. Therefore, certain disqualifications associated with being a convicted criminal would not accrue. Records were to remain confidential and evidence was not to be admissible in other courts. A type of justice was sought that would be based on the individualized needs of a particular delinquent and would involve approaches such as counseling and the rehabilitative processes of probation or correction. The price was the sacrifice of crucial due-process safeguards. A conflict remains, therefore, between a welfare emphasis and the extent to which constitutional standards should be sacrificed.

Not until the Gault case (1967) were specific protections given to juveniles, and then only if commitment to an institution could occur. These were right to counsel, notification of charges, right to confront and cross-examine witnesses, and protection against self-incrimination. Similarly, when a finding of delinquency could result in commitment to a state institution, the proof for guilt by an evidentiary standard of reasonable doubt was not established until 1970 (In re Winship 1970). Even now, the evidentiary standard used for waiver is independent from a finding of delinquency per se, since it is based on civil standards of preponderance of the evidence.

One way of viewing these changes is that rights are being restored to juveniles because their de facto handling approximates the adult model of criminal justice. Juveniles have still not been granted the right to a jury trial, and continued ambivalence toward the issue is seen in the statement of one court, which referred to a jury trial as a right ". . . which would most likely be disruptive of the unique character of the juvenile process" (*McKeiver* v. *Pennsylvania* 1971). Rights to receive a transcript of the legal proceedings, to bail, and to appeal remain unclarified. After analyzing which rights have been restored to juveniles and which have not, we realize that the idea that juvenile proceedings are noncriminal is progressively being challenged.

Since the Kent case (*Kent* v. *U.S.* 1966), decided before Gault, waiver of juveniles without a hearing has been interpreted as unconstitutional. Although the case legally involved an interpretation of statutory language, wherein a judge was required to conduct a full investigation before effecting a waiver, the Supreme Court applied constitutional principles relating to due process and the assistance of counsel. The Court was finally acknowledging the inconsistency of giving minors the right to a separate system of juvenile justice and then, without proper safeguard, allowing it to be undone. The Court stated, "There is no place in our system of law for reading the result of such tremendous consequences without ceremonies—that is, without hearing, without effective assistance of counsel, without a statement of reasons." What is often ignored is a follow-up of the original Kent case after it was remanded to the juvenile court and a hearing was finally given. The original waiver was sustained as entirely "appropriate and proper" (*Kent* v. *U.S.* 1968). The reason given for the waiver is most revealing, since it shows how psychiatry enters into the picture. The juvenile court held that Kent should be waived since long-term facilities which could provide the type of psychiatric treatment the boy required did not exist. Therefore, the decision was to waive him to the adult court to stand trial as a criminal. There is something about this type of reasoning that needs careful dissection. It logically amounts to accepting a conclusion that a certain treatment approach is necessary. However, if it is not then available, a totally contrary approach is offered which ignores the treatment needs of the juvenile. This type of double-talk of course infuriates those involved in these dilemmas. The basic sense of injustice attaches when the absence of facilities or adequate treaters can lead to adult criminal handling. It is the either/or approach that is striking in such decisions. For juvenile cases, some type of treatment interventions may have limited usefulness, but they are perhaps superior in many ways to a prison (and the great majority of juveniles who are certified get convicted in adult criminal courts).

Further ambivalence was seen in the new hearing of the Kent case, in which acceptance of a civil commitment of Kent as mentally ill was rejected "because of the defendant's potential danger to himself or others"—one of the major grounds on which civil commitment can take place. On a review of cases, it is the thread of protection for the community which is preeminent over rehabilitative efforts in most cases as determining waiver.

The rehabilitative model does not appear to gain primacy over what could be construed as a potential threat to a community by a juvenile. Part of the problem is connected with what courts at the time of a waiver hearing interpret and accept as adequate and relevant behavioral data to help them in reaching a decision. A skeptic may say that such data are not useful, and some courts do operate in such a vacuum. Decisions are based more along correctional data with a heavy emphasis on past records and contact with correctional facilities. Hence, data from police departments, sheriffs offices, and FBI arrest records are compiled as a basis for determining amenability to juvenile handling. The quality of probation reports varies widely, depending on the experience and quality of the probation officer. These types of reports can either aid or hinder the direction of waiver, depending on the data. They are admitted, even though they are perhaps hearsay, since the hearing is viewed as a transfer hearing and not an adjudicatory one which can lead directly to confinement or punishment. This again ignores data indicating that, once waived, the majority of juveniles are convicted.

Most waiver hearings lack any psychiatric evaluations, and those that have them often have inadequate data and take conclusionary forms. This may be no worse than what occurs in the remainder of the criminal justice system, but due to the greater lack of those with adequate training and expertise with adolescents, it is probably worse in its consequences. The result is either inadequate clinical data or a complete lack of it. Many games are played in this regard which give lip service to utilization of clinical material in its absence. In common practice, people who work in correctional facilities are given credence as overall experts, and their opinions regarding treatment are taken as expert with respect to clinical assessment and prediction. Personnel testifying for a waiver may be employed at the same institution where the juvenile will be sent if waiver is denied. Therefore, the people working at an institution decide whether the juvenile is someone who they wish to have at their institution or not. Of course, their opinion and testimony are not binding on the court, but a close working relationship often develops among people in the system. A variation is for a particular person who works at an institution, or who is used for testimony by a particular juvenile court, to become his own arbiter of standards to receive a juvenile or not.

As in many other areas of court work, testimony by experts is often conclusionary and unelaborated. At juvenile hearings, despite the serious consequences which may ensue, great latitude exists regarding those who may be permitted to give opinions. As indicated, the absence of treatment facilities often means that treatment is ignored. The next step is the conclusion that waiver is indicated.

It seems ironic that while more procedural protections, such as the right to a hearing before waiver, as in the Kent case (along with the assistance of legal counsel), have occurred, there is at the same time a laxity of standards as to experts who testify on key behavioral questions. Unless the standards simply resolve to waiver being contingent upon a certain type of charge pending, such as a serious felony charge automatically requiring a waiver statutorily, there would appear to be great need for clinical expertise at these hearings. Nor should legal counsel's failure to demand a high level of psychiatric expertise in their witnesses at these hearings be ignored. In part, this reflects the lack of knowledge of many of the parties as to what constitutes an adequate clinical evaluation of an adolescent. Much testimony of the type now often used might be better omitted altogether, since it does not do justice to the complex legal, psychiatric, and personal significance of waiver. It is the last and only time that a minor can assert his status as a minor relating to the act before trial and that he can show that he is in effect a fit and proper subject to be handled by the processes of a juvenile system of justice without bringing adult penal sanctions into play.

451

Specific Criteria

While the criteria used in transferring a juvenile to an adult criminal court are fairly uniform in their phraseology, the judge has great power to decide in this matter. In practice, the criteria utilized for waiver may include the following: (1) the recidivism of the juvenile; (2) a judgment that the juvenile is not amenable to the treatment processes of the juvenile court (which includes the lack of availability of juvenile treatment facilities as a basis to waive); (3) or a determination that the juvenile is a threat to public safety, in which case the community requires that he or she be handled in the adult criminal courts (if the offense involves force or violence or demonstrates what is viewed as vicious behavior). Indeed, so broad is the discretion of the judge that almost any type of offense against the person can be seen as posing a threat to the community so that public safety demands certification. Here, then, is further evidence for the unresolved ambivalence of the juvenile court in its handling of minors: When the criteria are phrased in terms of allowing waiver on the basis of community safety or the welfare of society, it becomes possible to certify almost any juvenile involved in a serious offense.

A typical statute may specify that a child be certified if he or she is either not suitable for treatment, or the public safety will not be secured (see Minn. Stat. 1974). In one case, a juvenile argued that it had not been shown that he was incapable of benefiting from the rehabilitative processes of the juvenile court (*State* v. *Hogan* 1973). The courts, noting the disjunctive nature of the criteria for certifiability, specified the factors that could threaten safety: (1) the seriousness of the offense in terms of community protection; (2) the circumstances surrounding the offense; (3) whether the offense was committed in an aggressive, violent, premeditated, or willful manner; (4) the reasonable foreseeable consequences of the act; and (5) the absence of adequate protective and security facilities available in the juvenile treatment system.

It would be difficult to conceptualize a case of any magnitude that could not meet one of these criteria of dangerousness and hence be certifiable. These are similar to the criteria in the appendix to the Kent case (1966), which made an attempt at establishing criteria in terms of the seriousness of the offense. Greater weight was given to such factors as offenses against the person, whether a Grand Jury would indict, the desirability of trying a juvenile with his adult codefendants, the sophistication of the minor, prior record, public safety, and the chances of rehabilitation. Similar problems are present in almost every state. The problems will persist as long as the unresolved duality with respect to juvenile courts persists—whether they are primarily to protect the public, or to rehabilitate juveniles. The vagaries and unreliability of predicting future dangerousness, despite a clinician or judge's certainty that they can do so, are well known (Livermore, Malmquist, and Meehl 1968). If we accept a completed act as dangerous, which it would assuredly be if it is something like a homicide, no independent appraisal is needed if this is taken as tantamount to requiring waiver. What is missing is any appraisal of the individual personality and the possible psychopathology present. Nor does a reference to pursue an insanity defense in the adult criminal courts meet the issue of why we have a system to deal with juveniles who need rehabilitation unless the juvenile court is actually seen as one existing solely for minor offenses.

In practice, various types of unclarified criteria continue to govern waiver. It may be that a long and contentious hearing is foreseen, which then influences a court to grant waiver. In some cases, the adverse publicity in a community dealing with the heinousness of a crime leads prosecutors as well as juvenile-court judges to press for prosecution as a criminal rather than face the political consequences of a public which feels that juveniles are being coddled. Yet special handling is precisely the justification given for the juvenile court. In one study, 17 percent of the judges in a survey admitted that public feelings influenced their decisions (Note, 1969).

In many cases, the court and all parties concerned become pessimistic about continuing to deal with young people in the juvenile system when their behavior raises threats to personal integrity and community safety. This occurs particularly when recidivism has also been present in particular adolescents. The failure of rehabilitative approaches has been cited as the justification to eliminate them from the juvenile system. This seemingly rational decision can be seen as beside the point when what has been customarily administered as treatment is closely examined. This is not the place, however, to consider the possible deficiencies of various approaches used in institutions dealing with delinquent or criminal populations. Lipton, Martinson, and Wilks (1975) have shown most of these approaches to be devoid of significant results on a review of the literature.

This gives rise to a different type of question. Should treatability of a juvenile, or the presence or absence of adequate treatment facilities with proper staff, be a major factor given reconsideration? Should such an assessment be made part of the dispositive question at all? It means that if past failures in rehabilitative programs exist, they may lack substantive credibility in determining whether a juvenile should be handled as a juvenile or as an adult.

The lack of quality or validity in many programs dealing with juvenile delinquents, and the lack of clinical sophistication noted in much treatment and research, make a treatment approach for juvenile delinquents appear to be more in the category of experimentation. Considering the different types of clinical and social pathology in the backgrounds of individual youths, programs in institutions for juvenile delinquents often do not attain sufficient validity from which to draw conclusions about the rehabilitative consequences for a given juvenile. This raises the issue of whether juveniles should be handled separately because of their age, or because they may be salvaged, rather than simply being transferred into the adult criminal justice system. Such a question is different from a lack of resources or inadequate treatment facilities. Inadequate resources do not determine the possible treatability of any given juvenile. Hence, basing waiver on what any particular institution is not equipped to carry out raises fundamental questions about whether what is called treatment is really in the nature of experimentation at best, or custodial maintenance at worst.

Conclusions

Four decades ago it was held that the juvenile court was not justified in transferring a case, no matter how serious, unless the child's own good and the best interests of the state could not be obtained by retention of jurisdiction (In re Heist 1938). We continue to be plagued by the same problems at present, since lists of criteria do not help to resolve the issues; they simply provide a means to justify a decision. The deficiency is in the arbitrariness of the process of waiver when individual cases are examined. This chapter has repeatedly emphasized that the criteria used allow almost any juvenile with a serious offense pending to be waived when it is wished. We continue to do this not only from a lack of clarity concerning why we have a juvenile-court system at all, but because it allows us to maintain the illusion that helping juveniles comes first, while simultaneously permitting such broad basic criteria that certification can be increased simply by changing attitudes or in response to community pressures. No changes in statutes are even needed.

Occasionally, a constitutional question about vagueness will arise, such as when a Michigan statute providing for transfer was struck down (*People* v. *Fields* 1972). However, it is amazing how rarely this occurs. Vagueness is desirable if the goal is one of accommodating to political goals by allowing an increased adaptability to diverse circumstances and community pressure. Decisions reached on that basis ignore human motives, defenses, and conflicts within the individual delinquent. In such a system both individuals and society remain prone to a feeling of ambiguity and arbitrariness.

The solution would seem to be toward either eliminating juvenile jurisdiction entirely for serious offenses, which at least serves clarity, or accepting the juvenile system of justice as having a mission for juveniles, even when their conduct involves serious offenses. At least these contrary alternatives have the merit of avoiding the myth that randomized discretion serves justice. That any coherent clinical end is met is then bypassed, but that would be tantamount to abandonment of the juvenile system for juveniles charged with serious delinquencies.

REFERENCES

Breed v. Jones. 1975. 421 *U.S.* 519.

Federal Bureau of Investigation. 1976. *Crime in the United States: Uniform Crime Reports*. Washington, D.C.: Government Printing Office.

Gault. 1967. 387 *U.S.* 1.

Heist. 1938. 11 *Ohio Op*. 537.

Kent v. U.S. 1966. 383 *U.S.* 541.

Kent v. U.S. 1968. D.C. Cir. 401 *F 2d* 408.

Lipton, D.; Martinson, R.; and Wilks, J. 1975. *The Effectiveness of Correctional Treatment*. Springfield, Mass.: Praeger.

Livermore, J. M.; Malmquist, C. P.; and Meehl, P. E. 1968. On the justification for civil commitment. *Pennsylvania Law Revue* 117:75–96.

McKeiver v. Pennsylvania. 1971. 403 *U.S.* 528.

National Advisory Commission on Criminal Justice Standards and Goals. 1973. *Corrections*. Washington, D.C.: Government Printing Office.

Note. 1969. Waiver of jurisdiction in the juvenile courts. *Ohio State Law Journal* 30:132–160.

Note. 1972. Double jeopardy and the waiver of jurisdiction in California's juvenile courts. *Stanford Law Revue* 24:874–902.

People v. Fields. 1972. 388 *Mich.* 66.

Platt, A. M. 1969. *The Child Savers: The Invention of Delinquency*. Chicago: University of Chicago Press.

Recent reaction to juvenile crime: are state legislatures "getting tough" with teenager delinquents. 1977–1978. *Children's Rights Report* 2:1–7.

State v. Hogan. 1973. 297 *Minn.* 430.

Statutes. Hawaii Rev. Stat., § 571-11 (Supp. 1973); Idaho Code Ann., § 16-1806 (Supp. 1974); Ill. Ann. Stat., Chap. 37, § 702-7 (Smith Hurd Supp. 1974); Minn. Stat., Ann., § 260.125 (1974); Miss. Code Ann., § 43-21-31 (1972); Neb. Rev. Stat., § 43-205 (Supp. 1974); New Hamp. Rev. Stat. Ann., § 169.21 (Supp. 1973); Va. Code Ann., § 16.1-176 (1977).

Whitehead, C. H., and Batey, R. 1975. Juvenile double jeopardy. *Georgetown Law Journal* 63:857–885.

Winship. 1970. 397 *U.S.* 358.

32 THE COMMITMENT OF MINORS: PROBLEMS OF CIVIL LIBERTIES

JONAS ROBITSCHER

W. H. Auden called the period before World War II the "age of anxiety." Our current period might be called the "age of antiauthority." We can contrast the structureless and fluid society of today, which makes few demands on the individual and promises him many supports, with a much crueler society which existed at least until World War I. That social period, which had manifestations that were felt for many years, consigned people to certain places and positions, allowed them no chance for protest, and penalized them severely for deviation. Wives obeyed husbands and did not have the right to challenge them. Employees obeyed their employers—the penalty for questioning authority could be unemployment and possible destitution. Soldiers obeyed officers—minor shows of independence and disrespect could lead to the stockade. Above all, children obeyed parents.

We now have a different societal situation. There is a questioning of authority, a rise of consumerism, an emphasis on the consumer as a participant, and an insistence on safeguards and checks so that the individual can keep the largest measure of his autonomy. In this context we have developed a much less authoritarian kind of practice of medicine. This has caused particular problems in psychiatry since some patients by their regressive behavior require that they be dealt with authoritatively. There is also an insistence on the rights of oppressed minorities, the handicapped, the sexually nonconforming, women, the mentally disabled, and children.

We are not just upgrading the rights of children—we are upgrading everyone's rights. We get into a great many legal and ethical problems when we upgrade the rights of adult psychiatric patients. We are put in a position where we are directed in many cases to deal with mental patients as if they were ordinary medical patients. When we apply the same kind of upgrading procedure to the rights of children, we find ourselves in even more confusing territory. The old concept of the therapist as the wise, parental figure is disappearing, but the newer concept of the therapist and patient as coadventurers in a voyage of mutual exploration—the concept proposed by Laing, Szasz, and others—does not always seem very practicable. As Wrightsman (1976) has said, "Children's rights is an issue whose time is now. At the same time 'children's rights' remains a slogan in search of a definition."

When we try to deal therapeutically with children and, in particular, with adolescents, we find they present many special problems. Most of them lack many of the major qualities that we ascribe to the good, adult psychiatric patient. When we work with adolescents we realize that they are not aware of intrapsychic conflict: They see their battle as one with their external environment, and their concept of successful psychotherapy would be to achieve a change in their parents' expectations of them. They find it extraordinarily difficult to develop a trusting relationship with an adult therapist. They are only comfortable with their peers; adults are seen as potential enemies.

Adolescents are aware that the therapist is playing a difficult role. He has to appease parents, who pay for the therapy, sometimes even sharing information or appearing to share information with them. Adolescents become aware of the tensions they can create in the relationship between therapist and parents, and they often manage to maximize this tension.

Freud, Piaget, Erikson, Klein, Winnicott, and others have emphasized the sensitivities of young children, their susceptibility to hurts, their need for self-assertion and rebellion, their need to establish their own identities, and the respect that must be accorded to their feelings. Our therapy is designed to accentuate the importance of understanding children's feelings and helping them with them. At variance with this, however, are the authoritarian and paternalistic procedures which accompany our treatments—breaches of confidentiality, imposed treatment, cooperation with third parties, and emphasis on the elevated stature of the therapist as compared with the patient. These go against our desire to respect children, but perhaps these cannot be completely dispensed with if we wish to give structure to children and control them.

Every legal problem in adult psychiatry is present in child psychiatry in a form more complicated and more difficult to solve (Robitscher 1973). Confidentiality is more of a problem in child than in adult psychiatry because parents and teachers are omnipresent third parties who demand information and need to be informed. Informed consent is especially difficult in child psychiatry where various kinds of incompetency are piled one on another—the kind attributable to age on top of the kind attributable to mental condition. Since it involves the major disruption of the life of the committed person and is a deprivation of liberty, commitment is a particularly sensitive topic. Informed consent and commitment are interrelated topics. The problem is that, although it is easy to support the idea of children's rights, it is much harder to implement it since in the process of implementation parents and therapists must relinquish some of their control of children.

Informed Consent

Today informed consent is a prerequisite for medical treatment. Without such consent medical treatment would constitute a battery and be the basis for a tort action. This is an exceedingly old legal doctrine and, until its recent revival, had been generally ignored. Theoretically, if a doctor did more than the patient expected him to do, he might be liable in damages to the patient. Juries, however, respected doctors, and were ready to impute good intentions to them; thus few patients could win a legal battle based on the argument that their physicians had not properly explained the possible consequences of the treatment.

All this changed with a line of law cases of the early 1960s in which courts found doctors negligent in not sharing enough information with the patient so that the patient could give a truly informed consent. Since then courts have refined the doctrine and tried to deal with the complex question of how remote the possibility of a bad effect—such as a drug reaction—must be before the doctor is obligated to mention it to the patient.

Our new emphasis on consumerism demands that we discuss treatment aims and consequences with patients. Doctors working with mental patients, however, do have some discretion to withhold such information—under the doctrine of the so-called therapeutic privilege—if in their clinical judgments the information would harm the patient.

At one time minors were presumed not to be able to give consent to medical treatment. We have had two developments which have led us to give older minors the chance to consent to their own treatment, without the knowledge of their parents. One was the necessity of providing treatment for venereal diseases, contraceptive information, abortion services, and drug counseling to minors. Many minors would not, of course, seek these services unless they could keep their need confidential from their parents.

The second factor has been the increasing independence of older minors, characterized by earlier sexual activity and other culture changes—although still dependent on parental financial help. Emancipated minors—those older minors, including college students, who are not dependent on their families or who live apart from their families—can give consent for their own treatment. Many legal authorities believe that children as young as fourteen years can give their own informed consent in some situations—such as for drug, obstetrical, or gynecological treatment—even without statutory authorization and must be asked to give joint consent with their parents for other kinds of treatment.

One problem here is that if the minor alone gives consent for treatment, either the minor or the state must pay for treatment. Obviously we cannot keep treatment a secret from parents and still submit the bills to them. Perr (1976) has noted that an anxious or unhappy adolescent of seventeen may be able to contract for psychotherapy—that is, he may have both the intellectual comprehension and the rational judgment necessary for contractual consent—but he will rarely be a private patient; instead, he will be a client at a clinic, mental health center, neighborhood drug unit, or student health service.

The problem of informed consent arises in the treatment of adolescents as to whether older adolescents should be allowed to come into hospitals as voluntary admissions. We are not always sure of the validity of the informed consent of some adolescents. We want to be sure that their parents' rights are not infringed upon and that the parents will be responsible for the expense of the hospitalization. In these cases we sometimes secure the consent of both child and parents, although we always secure the consent of the parents. If the adolescent refuses consent, we may not pay attention to his refusal since we were assuming that the wishes of the child were not material even when we asked for his consent.

Commitment of Minors

Patients need advocacy. However, too much attention to the legal rights of patients can lead to legalistic procedures which take up time and interfere with the autonomy of mental health professionals.

In 1972 an attorney brought a proposed case to my attention.[1] He was challenging the method by which minors were admitted to the hospital as voluntary patients on the substituted consent of their parents or guardians. He was challenging the "voluntariness" of the voluntary commitment when the minor patient resists entrance into the hospital but an adult has the power to force him into the hospital on the adult's signature. I was asked if I would be an expert witness to inform the court that most committed minors do not need the total care environment that a hospital provides, that there should be rigorous procedural safeguards that would help separate those few minors who need to be committed, and that the absence of an advocate created a lack of protection for that minor during the commitment process; above all I was asked to provide expert testimony that psychiatric hospitalization can stigmatize and otherwise harm minors.

Although genuinely sympathetic to these ideas and goals, I have had many questions and doubts about the attempt to make adult commitment more protected and more difficult to obtain. I have written (Robitscher 1976) about how our overemphasis on legalism is complicating the life of the psychiatrist and, in many cases, the patient. The overlegalistic approach to commitment makes it difficult to get a patient into a treatment situation quickly. Expensive and time consuming, it does not seem to me to be necessary if patients have easy recourse to court review.

Minors, however, are another matter: They are not able to assert their rights to a court review because their decisions are being made not by themselves but by their parent or guardian. In order to feel reassured that the minor is receiving justice, one must be convinced that the interests of the minor and the adults moving to commit him are identical. Often the move to commit comes when there are family differences: The minor who is being committed is not always the most pathological member of the family and there may be scapegoating, misuse of the mental hospital by parents who want to control the

461

behavior of their children, abandonment or dumping of a child by parents, and misidentification of honest attempts at change and growth as pathology. I decided I could not be an expert witness in spite of a good deal of sympathy for the cause because I felt that as a member of the psychiatric establishment I was being threatened by an excess concern with civil rights and was not familiar enough with the conditions under which minors were committed to be able to say with assurance that their rights were being violated.

The attorney proceeded with the case, *Bartley* v. *Haverford State Hospital*, later named *Bartley* v. *Kremens*.[2] The United States District Court for the Eastern District of Pennsylvania declared in this case that minors were being hospitalized too easily and that they needed elaborate legal protections. The case has the distinction of being one of only a very few cases dealing with the civil rights of the mentally disabled which the Supreme Court has been willing to review. The Supreme Court has availed itself of the privilege of refusing to hear most issues regarding mental patients.

The argument in *Bartley* v. *Kremens* was that patients up to the age of nineteen (eighteen or younger) were placed in a facility as "voluntary" patients under the Pennsylvania Commitment Act—which was not different in this respect from the commitment acts of many other states—upon the application of a parent, guardian, or individual standing in place of the parent without notice or hearing, without counsel or independent guardian ad litem (a guardian to act in his or her best interest), and without the procedural safeguards provided for adult patients under the stringent Pennsylvania commitment law.

Later, in a similar case brought by Georgia Legal Services and the Southern Poverty Law Center, *J. L. and J. R.* v. *Parham*,[3] a similar holding was issued by the Federal District Court for the Middle District of Georgia that the commitment of minors was unconstitutional because the minors were not given procedural protections and the services of a lawyer.

The American Bar Association and the American Psychiatric Association wrote friend-of-the-court briefs which were diametrically opposed to each other in the appeal of the *Bartley* case to the Supreme Court. The lawyers argued that commitment to a mental hospital was such a constitutionally significant deprivation of liberty that parental authority must give way to a proper safeguarding of the rights of the child. The psychiatrists argued that the Supreme Court had repeatedly emphasized the basic constitutional right of parents to control the upbringing of their children and that this right should be maintained. Dynamic psychiatrists did not make any concession in their general attitude toward legal interference, but then they did concede that in certain situations—and this eventually became a large concession—a due process hearing should be accorded the minor when the person initiating the commitment was an agency or a state department rather than a parent, when the child had reached adolescence, when the commitment was to an unaccredited institution, or when the detention was for more than forty-five days.

Although psychiatrists and lawyers were far apart ideologically, psychiatrists had conceded that in most of the situations in which children and adults are committed, procedural safeguards are needed. Many psychiatrists wished that less could have been conceded. One of the great problems with giving children the right to refuse hospitalization is that we have not fully conceptualized the situation at home when the child wins the right to remain out of the institution. Are the losing parents obligated to take their child, who they feel should not be home, back into the family? Should the court find an alternative domicile? Who would pay for this alternative domicile? Should the parents be forced to pay for the legal expenses their child incurred in fighting them?

The Supreme Court decided *Bartley* by declining to decide it; it remanded it to the district court for reconsideration in light of new Pennsylvania legislation. However, it later agreed to hear the Georgia case, which presented the same issues. Again the American Bar Association and the American Psychiatric Association submitted their friends-of-the-court briefs, which opposed each other ideologically but were not so far apart after the psychiatrists' concession that in the four circumstances described there should be a due process hearing.

The Court heard argument on the case in December 1977. From the justices' line of questioning, observers felt that the concept of parental rights was of great concern. In October 1978 the Supreme Court heard reargument on the case and on the same day it also heard argument on the *Bartley* case—returned under a new name, *Secretary of Public Welfare* v. *Institutionalized Juveniles*.[4] The two cases present the same issues except that the Pennsylvania case deals with private as well as public institutions, while the Georgia case includes the concept of "less restrictive alternative" placements.[5]

Conclusions

The Supreme Court has a difficult decision—individual rights of children versus parental rights and family rights. Eventually, either in this case or some other case, the Court will have to deal with the issue. This is the kind of problem that, once it has been presented to us—in spite of the fact that we were happily able to ignore it for years—will not go away.

Eventually psychiatrists will have to cede to children some greater say over the question of their commitments. We have had the influence of the consumerism and patient-participation movement, we do have the beginnings of a doctrine of the right to refuse treatment, and we have an increased recognition in the law of the autonomy of older minors—all legal arguments for giving minors more legal protection. We also have increased psychiatric recognition that parents often use hospitalization of minor children as retribution or as pressure in a power struggle. They do not always act in ways that unbiased observers would see as in the best interest of the child.

Increased procedural safeguards will certainly have to be worked out at least for (1) adolescents and (2) children whose commitment is initiated not by a close relative but by an impersonal state agency. Because children have special vulnerabilities, special protection for children in the commitment process will have to be accorded. An example is a twelve-year-old, hyperkinetic child who had been in a state hospital for the previous seven years. Hospital authorities had told his parents that he did not require hospital care, but he did require specialized foster care. He was not eligible for Aid to Families with Dependent Children and was subsequently released by the order of the three-judge federal court and returned to his home. Within a short period of time there were reports that his stepfather was mistreating him. Before authorities had a chance to intervene, the boy hanged himself. The stepfather was convicted of child abuse and sentenced to five years in jail. Thus, not committing children as well as committing children can have its adverse consequences.

NOTES

1. David Ferleger, a former student and organizer of the Mental Patient Civil Liberties Project in Pennsylvania.

2. Bartley v. Kremens, 402 F. Supp. 1039 (E.D. Pa. 1975), vacated and remanded to District Court, 431 U.S. 119 (1977); Secretary of Public Welfare v. Institutionalized Juveniles, prob. juris. noted, 98 S. Ct. 3087 (1978), argument heard October 10, 1978.

3. J. L. and J. R. v. Parham, 412 F. Supp. 112 (M.D. Ga. 1976), prob. juris. noted, 431 U.S. 936 (1977), reargued October 10, 1978.

4. 47 U.S.L.W. 3263 (1978).

5. Since the preparation of this chapter for publication, the Supreme Court has issued its opinions in the child hospitalization cases, J. L. and J. R. v. Parham and Secretary of Public Welfare of Pennsylvania v. Institutionalized Juveniles. The Supreme Court decision was handed down on June 20, 1979, too late for the article to be revised. The article predicted that we were entering an era of the greater protection of the rights of minors and assumed that the Supreme Court decisions would extend protection to children being committed on substituted voluntary consents (at least in the cases of older children), children being committed by state welfare departments, and when the commitment was to an unaccredited institution. Counter to this prediction, the Supreme Court decision, by a six-to-three vote, gives the child as his only protection the examining physician's medical judgment that the commitment is justified, vitiating the hope that the rights of children in commitment would receive greater recognition.

REFERENCES

Perr, I. N. 1976. Confidentiality and consent in psychiatric treatment of minors. *Journal of Legal Medicine* 4:12–16.

Robitscher, J. 1973. Child psychiatry and the law. In S. L. Copel, ed. *Behavior Pathology of Childhood and Adolescence.* New York: Basic.

Robitscher, J. 1976. Moving patients out of hospitals—in whose interest? In P. I. Ahmed and S. C. Plog, eds. *State Mental Hospitals: What Happens When They Close?* New York: Plenum.

Wrightsman, L. S. 1976. *Children's Rights and the Mental Health Professions.* New York: Wiley.

RICHARD C. MAROHN, DANIEL OFFER, ERIC OSTROV, AND JAIME TRUJILLO

Following upon Freud's (1950) finding that certain character disorders and perversions were the reverse of the psychoneuroses, a number of investigators have attempted to formulate juvenile delinquency and adolescent behavior disorders from a psychodynamic point of view. Aichhorn (1925) utilized the classical transference situation in an attempt to reach and modify the delinquent's neurotic conflict, but with a certain kind of delinquent he had to establish a relationship first and then work with the narcissistic transference. Alexander and Staub (1931) observed that certain criminals acted out of a sense of guilt which they hoped to expiate by being caught and punished. In this tradition Friedlander (1960) postulated that it was important to convert delinquent character disorders to neuroses by blocking the avenues for acting out discharge and creating an internalized conflict which could then be worked with psychotherapeutically.

In a similar vein, Anna Freud (1958, 1965) viewed delinquency as a failure of the socialization process but also noted that some delinquency develops because of the chance availability of delinquent peer groups onto whom the adolescent, separating from his parents, displaces his investments. The focus here is on delinquent value systems, which are also emphasized in the work of Johnson and Szurek (1952) who described a number of children responding to the unconsciously transmitted delinquent urges of their seemingly upright parents.

Glover (1950) distinguished two kinds of delinquents: the structural who gives evidence before and after adolescence of significant psychopathology, and the functional whose delinquent behavior is a result of the temporary psychic imbalances of the adolescent maturation process. Blos (1966, 1967, 1971) has offered a variety of psychodynamic explanations, including separation struggles, precocious ego development, the propensity for action language, and delinquency as a symbolic communication. Redl's emphasis (1966) has been on the vicissitudes of ego development and ego functioning and has underlined the importance of a psychodynamic understanding of the delinquency in an attempt to engage the child therapeutically. Finally, Winnicott (1958, 1973) focused on the early and primitive object hunger for the mother, once possessed but later lost, whom the delinquent hopes to recapture through his behavior.

In our work with hospitalized juvenile delinquents, we have attempted to proceed along two parallel lines: a clinical treatment program and an investigative research project (Marohn, Dalle-Molle, Offer, and Ostrov 1973; Offer, Marohn, and Ostrov 1975; Ostrov, Offer, Marohn, and Rosenwein 1972). Adolescents who performed delinquent acts were referred to us primarily by the juvenile court, but also by schools, private psychotherapists, social agencies, parents, and themselves. We excluded those who did not require institutionalization and those who gave evidence of psychosis, serious mental retardation, or brain damage. As a result, we excluded the very healthy and the very disturbed delinquent. Patients were hospitalized on the delinquency unit at the Illinois State Psychiatric Institute and engaged in a comprehensive hospital program which includes individual, family, group, and milieu therapy, with extensive emphasis on activities, school, and limit setting. Data were collected about the subjects and their families through interviews, inventories, self-report questionnaires, observations and impressions of others, and regularly monitored quantified measures of antisocial behavior on the unit, as well as the usual psychological testing and psychiatric interviewing. Those adolescents who did not stay on the unit for a minimum of thirteen weeks had to be excluded from our project because we felt a certain baseline was necessary in order to eliminate the effects of the initial phases of hospitalization. As a result, fifty-five subjects described in table 1 were studied intensively from 1969 to 1974, and subsequently in follow-up interviews, and form the foundation for two monographs.[1]

Methodology

To reduce these data to a smaller number of underlying dimensions, factor analysis was performed on forty-three of the original variables.

TABLE 1

DEMOGRAPHIC CELL BREAKDOWN OF SUBJECTS IN A STUDY OF PSYCHODYNAMIC
TYPES OF JUVENILE DELINQUENTS ($N = 55$)

	Males			Females		
	Higher SES	Lower SES	Blacks	Higher SES	Lower SES	Blacks
Younger	4	6	7	2	3	5
Older	5	4	4	8	6	1

NOTE.—In the study were 30 males, 25 females, 18 blacks, and 38 whites. Their mean age was 15 years, 6 months; range, 13 years to 18 years, 2 months; SD = 14 months. The mean Socioeconomic Status (SES) was 41.38; range 11–77; SD = 19.44. For the SES Hollingshead (1965) uses a two-factor scale; 11 is the minimum possible, 77 the maximum. SES and race were treated along one dimension to prevent the occurrence of empty cells and because, in this sample, almost all the black subjects were below the sample mean for SES; whites were divided into higher and lower SES categories according to the median score for whites only; subjects were divided into younger and older categories along the total sample median for age.

To reduce the influence of demographic effects of intercorrelations among these variables, subjects were grouped into cells based on their age, sex, race, and social class. Cell means were subtracted from subject's scores on each variable. The resultant scores were then intercorrelated and factored using the principal axes method, and varimax rotations were performed yielding a series of multiple-factor solutions. The five-factor solution[2] was chosen for exposition since it was the most stable solution and made the most sense clinically. Subsequently, variables making up each factor were standard scored using demographic-cell means and standard deviations as reference points. Each subject's standard scores on the variables making up the various factors were added, yielding five-factor scores per subject.

These data were treated in two ways. First, within each demographic cell, subjects highest and lowest on each factor scores were listed. Second, note was made of the number of factor scores each subject had which were more than one standard deviation above the mean for the total sample. The first approach yielded demographically matched groups of subjects who were high and low, respectively, on each factor score. Using these groups, two lists of names for each factor score were given in random order and with no further information to clinical staff who knew and worked with all the subjects in the total sample.

That is, raters were given, without identifying information, a list of names of subjects who were high on each factor score along with another list which presented the names of subjects who were low on the same factor score. Staff were then asked, individually and without consulting one another, to describe clinically and impressionistically how each group differed from its paired group. The resulting comments were used to enrich our understanding of the clinical meaning of each factor dimension. The second approach to the data enabled us to generate a list of subjects who scored high on one factor only or, alternatively, on a combination of factors.

Results

Four factors and the variables they comprise are presented in table 2. These four factors seem to correlate with types of delinquents with whom we have worked clinically and who can be understood in psychodynamic terms. These impressions are borne out by the fact that various blind ratings of delinquents grouped according to these factors were substantiated by a number of senior members of the treatment staff. We believe we have identified four psychodynamic types which can be described as an impulsive delinquent, a narcissistic delinquent, a depressed delinquent, and a borderline delinquent.

THE IMPULSIVE DELINQUENT

This delinquent was viewed by his therapist as the most disturbed psychiatrically, and in his behavior on the unit he showed significantly more antisocial behavior, both violent and nonviolent. He was seen by teachers as having little social sensitivity and gave the impression to staff members of being very impulsive, as well as not being particularly likable on first meeting. He seemed to have some awareness of wanting to change. These patients were described as quick to action with little forethought, maintaining high drive levels, having outbursts, aggressive, engaging, diffuse, anxious, and having poor impulse control. A good example of this group is Victor Q:

TABLE 2

Variables Composing Four Factors of a Five-Factor Solution
Generated by a Factor Analysis of 43 Variables in a Study
of Psychodynamic Types of Juvenile Delinquents (*N* = 55)

Factor, Variable Name, and Definition	Loading on Factor*	Communality
1. Impulsive:		
Therapist rating overall health—poor	.689	.503
BCL—violence toward others—high	.658	.577
Teacher rating of social sensitivity—poor	.639	.625
Staff rating of impulsivity—impulsive	.620	.619
BCL—nonviolent—high	.532	.528
Self-image from background Q-like to change	.529	.348
Early likability—not likable	.496	.379
2. Narcissistic:		
OSIQ—total score—well adjusted	.784	.656
OSIQ—impulse control—well adjusted	.733	.616
Delinquency checklist—total score—low	.730	.628
Video interview—interviewee depressed	.516	.325
3. Depressed:		
Staff rating of depression—depressed	.827	.702
Background Q: physical punishment? yes	.580	.508
Teacher rating—initiative—high	.455	.288
Power score, father vs. mother—father wins	.434	.339
Change in likability—become more likable	.418	.362
Use narcotics? Yes†	.403	.260
4. Borderline:		
Video interview—passive	.740	.591
Therapist rating—emotional expressiveness—low	.672	.476
Therapist rating—emotional experience—low	.609	.408
Parents' SIQ—total adjustment score—low	.591	.458
Video interview—what kind of person? negative†	.423	.534
Video interview—pessimistic	.408	.278

Note.—BCL = Behavior Check List, OSIQ = Offer Self-Image Questionnaire, both available from authors Marohn and Offer.

*Absolute values of loadings are given because direction of variables is arbitrary. Variables are listed only if their primary loading is on the factor in question and if they loaded .40 or more on that factor.

†These variables were not stably associated with this factor across factor solutions but were associated with this factor in the five-factor solution. They were not used to generate subjects' factor scores.

Victor, a sixteen-year-old, black male, was referred by his probation officer after spending time in a detention center for attacking his mother and sister. A year before admission, he had been shot in the chest and suffered spinal injury. He had been paralyzed two weeks before recovering some movement in his right toes. He worked out on parallel bars, started walking on crutches, and at time of admission walked with the help of the cane. During the previous year he was involved in many fights in school, hit his mother with his cane, and fought with his fourteen-year-old sister when she called him names.

As a child, Victor used to catch grasshoppers to break their legs. At eight years of age he set the house on fire by throwing a lit match into a clothes hamper. When he was nine, he was described as "nervous," easy to scare, and was in outpatient treatment. During that period he stole some fishing rods from a parked car. He also shot dogs with a BB gun and described this in a matter-of-fact way. At age thirteen he was in and out of different schools and was involved repeatedly in fights, riots, and truancy. Currently, his sixteen-year-old girl friend was expecting a baby whom he said he fathered. Their relationship had thus far lasted three years, and he was planning to live with her and take care of the baby.

Victor's mother suffered from hypertension and was described as a very irritable person who shouted a lot and then withdrew to her room to lie down. She had been married and divorced twice and had one common-law relationship. Victor was one of six children. Delivery was normal, and no problems were described before age eight. More recently he had become involved with gangs and his defiance and violence had escalated.

At the start of hospitalization, Victor was watchful and began playing the tough guy. In individual therapy he spent many sessions bragging about his sexual prowess and expressing his anger toward staff. On the unit, he tussled with male patients and befriended the female patients. He was furious with staff when limits were set after he acted aggressively and sexually toward his girl friend when she was visiting him. On one occasion, he tried to enter the nursing station to get a piece of equipment and ended up in restraints. After this, he threatened staff, pushed, spat at, and hit one male staff member, and was administratively discharged.

Victor, because of his impulsive behavior, both violent and nonviolent, was readily seen by all to be disturbed. He was quite insensitive to others' social needs, and his unpredictability, high anxiety level, and propensity for aggressive outbursts characterize him an an impulse-ridden delinquent. He was unable to delay or modulate urges, to tolerate frustration, or to conceptualize. He demonstrated a marked deficiency in fantasy life and a marked tendency to discharge through action.

NARCISSISTIC DELINQUENT

These delinquents saw themselves as well adjusted and described little delinquency prior to hospitalization. However, when parents and staff were interviewed about these adolescents they appeared depressed and pessimistic about the prognosis. These subjects were described as resistive, secretive, superficial, cunning, leaders; they appeared to develop a therapeutic alliance. Our impression is that this subgroup exhibits an exaggerated sense of self-worth and tends to deny problems. We anticipate, however, that they will continue to do well at follow-up principally because their pathology is more of a characterological nature. They function fairly well, may have problems in self-esteem regulation, and for the most part tend to use other people for their own needs, yet maintain a fairly stable integration and cohesion. A good example of a delinquent from this group is Kenneth E:

Kenneth was a good-looking fourteen-year-old who, after he was admitted to the hospital, talked sincerely about straightening up and not repeating his delinquent acts. He was referred to us after he became involved with the police for repeatedly forging checks and stealing a bicycle. At another time, neighbors called the police when they observed him beating a dog that he was paid to walk. Kenneth's mother said that she had found him uncontrollable and often found herself involved in angry outbursts with him. These arguments occasionally became violent on both sides.

Kenneth's mother related a normal delivery and early developmental tasks within normal limits. When he was ten months old Kenneth's parents were divorced after much conflict. A year and a half later a younger sister was born, fathered by a different man. This fact, however, was never told to Kenneth by his mother, who told him instead that the divorce occurred when he was three years old. Kenneth began to have behavior problems shortly after his sister was born. At first he hit other children; later, in kindergarten, he was disruptive in class. The teacher described him as willing to do anything to attract attention. Still later, he started stealing and was sent to live with his father, who had remarried when Kenneth was five years old. He was disappointed with his father's involvement with his new family and did not get along well with his stepmother. He returned to his natural mother, but lived with her only a few months before she sent him to his maternal grandmother. His grandmother could not control him and she returned him to his mother once more. When living with mother, he began bullying other children, lying, stealing, truanting, and, more lately, hitting and engaging in sex play with his sister. From his point of view, he felt that his mother always preferred his sister to him because she was a girl. He remembered many times when he experienced a sense of terror about the possibility of his mother's abandoning him. This usually happened to him when he was falling asleep. Often he felt like dying. On psychological tests, Kenneth revealed a focus on narcissistic issues, with thinly disguised fantasies of winning oedipal victories.

Kenneth was hospitalized for six months. During this time peer relationships were characterized by many verbal arguments and a few times by overt hitting. He was sarcastic, provocative, and at one time called another handicapped adolescent a monster. On one occasion, he schemed to declare himself the winner in a ping-pong competition. In individual therapy he became aware of how he externalized his conflicts and manipulated others. At the same time he expressed a great deal of rage toward his mother. He was discharged to his mother with the understanding that he would continue outpatient therapy, attend school, and work in a bike shop.

Kenneth demonstrates the narcissistic delinquent's resistance to psychotherapy; his defensiveness and tendency to deny problems cause many staff members to feel pessimistic about his prognosis. These adolescents are changed very little by the hospital program, primarily because they need to protect themselves constantly against experiences which might lead to lowered self-esteem; yet, they are not so disturbed that they fragment under either painful narcissistic injury or grandiose narcissistic exhilaration and elation. Kenneth, once able to establish a supporting environment with minimal involvement in intimate relationships, should function fairly well, though his narcissistic character disorder would continue to be evident to careful clinical scrutiny.

DEPRESSED DELINQUENT

This next type of delinquent was characterized as depressed by staff members. He described physical punishment as being important in his rearing. He showed a considerable amount of initiative and compliance in school, perhaps because of strongly internalized values and aspirations from an actively functioning superego. Father tended to dominate decisions. The adolescent, himself, became significantly more likable during the course of his hospitalization. There was frequently a history of narcotic abuse. These subjects were described as depressed, confused, having poor boundaries, likable, having labile affect, really involving staff, and often noticed modeling themselves after staff, asking for advice and trying to use it. Their depression may be based on superego functions, and as a result they tended to be neurotic achievers with high interpersonal awareness; the etiology of this configuration might be due to parents who used physical punishment as a training modality and the presence of a dominant father determining the family value system, leading to a child with a more clearly internalized value system and more distinct psychic structure. These patients tended to present more structuralized conflicts than the second group whose conflict was with the environment primarily and the first and fourth groups whose problems were primarily psychological deficits. A good example of someone from this group was Martha V:

Martha was seventeen years old when she was transferred from a detention home to our hospital for treatment because "I am doing too much to get along with the crowd, but I am not getting along with my parents."

Four years of turmoil preceded our contact with her. It began with her running away from home to go to movies with boyfriends. After stealing five dollars from her mother, to avoid confrontation she spent two days away from home with friends. On returning home, she continued to steal—money from her mother and cigarettes from her father. At high school, she was "guy crazy" and chased boys with "sharp cars." At fifteen her "real family" was her peer group; they engaged in drinking, smoking, and sexual intercourse at drive-in theaters. Once the police caught them, but Martha claimed she had been raped while drunk. She then ran off several times, using LSD and other drugs heavily and forging her father's checks. She spent time in detention and a psychiatric hospital, was involved in outpatient psychotherapy, but eventually was expelled from school for stealing and truancy.

Martha had become pregnant and took an overdose of barbiturates "to get rid of the baby." After hospitalization for an abortion, she ran from her suburb to the city and became more heavily involved in LSD, amphetamines, marijuana, and prostitution, which she found "fascinating" and "exciting." She was hospitalized for gonorrheal peritonitis and pneumonia, but left against medical advice. She continued prostituting herself, abusing barbiturates, and stealing checks. After another runaway to a distant state and continued use of hallucinogens, she was referred to our program.

Martha's early developmental years were described as uneventful. In grade school she was well behaved and an A student, talented in art. Her grades began to decline in the eighth grade when she had conflicts with teachers about poems she wrote in which she made repeated references to sexual intercourse.

Martha's mother was the domineering person at home. She had sudden mood swings, frequently felt martyred, had been depressed after the death of her own mother, and would slap her husband and children when angry. She would hit and insult Martha and would say to her: "Everyone in the family hates you, bitch." She demanded perfection from her children, but tried to discover faults. For instance, she intercepted Martha's mail and asked her about sexual involvement with boys well before Martha's sexual activity began. Martha remembers herself as compliant and eager to please until the age of twelve. She remembers thinking about killing herself after her mother slapped her. On a few of these occasions she put scarves around her neck and started pulling them until it began to hurt. Once, while in the eighth grade, after one of these incidents she drank drain cleaner in an attempt to kill herself.

Martha's physical appearance was disheveled. She was over-weight. She seemed very tense, anxious, and in spite of manifest depression was pleased to be in the hospital.

Soon after admission, and during her entire hospitalization of ten months, she tested and tried to bend the rules. Moreover, she could not believe the staff meant what they said about going to her room, wake-up routines, etc. She eloped from outside trips at least twice, but was found by staff members and returned to the unit. On at least three other occasions she was discovered planning elopements with other patients.

Only slowly could she begin to take responsibility for her own behavior. When she stole someone else's food, after many community meetings, she finally admitted that she stole. She then left the meeting, went to her room, and set a fire, almost trapping herself in the smoke-filled room. Most of her interactions with peers involved telling them of her anger with staff and her therapist. She was demanding and accusatory when she was not gratified and instigating destructive activities. She was eventually discharged administratively after several incidents of physical abuse of staff.

Martha demonstrated not only overt clinical depression, but also the kind of neurotic character structure with stongly internalized values and a need to achieve academically and artistically, typical of so many adolescents in this category. Her involvement with her family and her acting-out behavior were also quite characteristic. Her utilization of physical punishment, even to the point of brutality, had resulted in the internalization of a severely punitive superego. Her delinquent behavior, including heavy drug usage, was an attempt to relieve herself of a severe depression which at other times manifested itself in suicidal and self-destructive behavior.

THE BORDERLINE DELINQUENT

This type of delinquent was viewed as a passive person who tends not to be well liked and whose future was viewed pessimistically. He experienced little affect, was not emotionally expressive, and was seen by his parents as having adjusted poorly. Clinically these subjects were described as passive, depleted, not future oriented, not as aware of having internal problems, empty, disorganized, nonverbal, withdrawn, affect flat, less engaging, especially unattractive and unappealing, outcasts or keeping to themselves, more openly needy, more withdrawn, with more idiosyncratic thinking. A typical delinquent from this group is Lorraine G:

Lorraine was seventeen when admitted to the unit for check forging. A white girl, from an upper-middle-class home, it was difficult to obtain a clear history from her because she was vague and seemed to be blocking. However, one fact that did emerge was that five months prior to admission she received permission from her mother to live with a boyfriend.

Lorraine's mother was an attractive woman in her early forties, college educated, and described by a social worker as very neurotic, self-centered, and full of negative feelings for Lorraine. Lorraine's parents were divorced when she was six because Lorraine's mother had been having affairs. Four years later, Lorraine's mother married another man and stayed married to him for three years. A year later, she married another man ten years her junior. They separated after a year. After her second divorce, Lorraine's mother was hospitalized for three weeks for depression.

Lorraine was described as a difficult delivery and a colicky baby, a fact which made her mother very angry. At two, Lorraine was hospitalized for asthma and at five underwent a bilateral, inguinal herniorrhaphy. She was described as well behaved and good in school until eighth grade. At that time Lorraine was sent to live with her natural father after her mother's divorce and hospitalization. While with her father she dated boys he disapproved of, started using a variety of drugs, and was frequently truant from school. When she returned to live with her mother she was uncooperative at home, sarcastic, associated with drug users, and argued frequently. At that time, too, she began running away for short periods of time and fought physically with her mother over her drug taking. Lorraine described her mother as unloving, hateful, and promiscuous, but added that she was just like her mother.

Lorraine was hospitalized for over one year. In a psychological test report she was described as having little sense of self-worth and at the same time continuously looking for affirmation of her own worth. She was also depicted as depressed and ready to handle bad feelings with anything available: sex, drugs, or running away. On the unit, staff discovered she had been ten weeks pregnant upon admission. She appeared homesick, anxious, and uncertain, and saw staff as intrusive. She argued with other female patients, was very upset during visits with her mother, and cried when visited by her boyfriend. She decided to have an abortion and was tearful after she returned from the hospital in which the abortion was performed. At one point she tried to bring drugs on the unit by means of her boyfriend's visits. When confronted about this by staff, she became angry and made plans to elope. Later on in the course of hospitalization she became quarrelsome, swore a lot, and sent a list of things she could not tolerate to her mother. With time she became more pleasant and willing to follow the rules of the unit. After five months she appeared more sophisticated and able to get along with other patients. However, at times she still was haughty, sarcastic, and prodded other girls to rebel against staff. Before discharge she became depressed and irritable and began refusing to go to school, saying she was under a lot of pressure from staff and her mother.

In individual therapy, she manifested a growing alliance with her therapist, moving from vague anger to denial of feelings about the abortion to talking about feelings of abandonment when her therapist announced a vacation. Gradually, she related more and more unhappy incidents between her and her mother. Eventually, she expressed feelings of worthlessness, emptiness, and confusion. However, after ten months, she accused her therapist of violating confidentiality and betraying her. She said she felt worthless and unable to control her destiny. While preparing to leave the hospital, she confused her therapist with her mother during psychotherapy sessions. Somatic complaints reappeared as well as complaints that her mother did not care for her.

Lorraine demonstrates the typical emptiness and need for merger union, or reunion, with a maternal self-object so characteristic of the borderline. Because of her emotional depletion, her future tends to be seen in somewhat pessimistic terms. She, herself, was for the most part incapable of planning or orienting herself to the future and would vacillate between a schizoid withdrawal or an open clinging neediness, frequently engaging in delinquent behavior designed to fill her up or to support her shaky boundaries.

Discussion

Using factor analysis and clinical experience, we have described four types of juvenile delinquents. These factors resonate with good clinical sense and fit our experiences in working with these patients both in individual psychotherapy and in the hospital milieu. In our hospital work, we expect that various members of the treatment team provide data collected from different vantage points: the intrapsychic, the interpersonal, the family, the peer group, the classroom, and the group or social milieu. In our team meetings we take the position that if our theories are valid data from these various perspectives must be able to be integrated with each other and explained in a unified manner which embraces all the systems involved. This approach to behavioral science research is in the tradition of Grinker (1956, 1968), Offer (1969), and Offer and Offer (1975) because we have attempted not only to utilize in our analysis data from a number of perspectives but also to integrate statistically valid data with our own clinical experiences.

However, one sees mixtures of these factors with various degrees of intensity. Often, for example, a delinquent who best typifies a particular subgroup or factor may not demonstrate that particular form of psychopathology as obviously as another delinquent who may also be beset by other motivating forces. The case examples described here are relatively pure types and typify the specific factor involved without much contamination, if any, by other factors.

We also attempted to consider what different combinations of these factors would produce clinically. For example, we predicted that a patient who was both seriously impulsive and narcissistically inclined would turn out to be dangerous. We expected that a subject who gave significant evidence of both impulsivity and depression would tend to act out in order to relieve himself of depression. We guessed that someone who was both depressed and gave evidence of narcissistic pathology might be a chronic depressive character. And we thought that someone who was depressed and also exhibited significant border-

479

line features would show tendencies to cling and to merge. All of these features were borne out by the clinical material, with some surprises in the last clustering. The patients in this group tended also to be somewhat exhibitionistic, but more in a passive way, revelling in their being noticed rather than actively seeking and provoking it.

Because our sample was small, though studied in depth, we have not been able to assess fully the effects of socioeconomic status, race, age, and sex differences, although we have attempted to control statistically their contribution to interrelationships among the variables studied. We do not deny the impact of demographic factors on the causation of juvenile delinquency, but we wish to highlight the psychological factors associated with delinquent behavior.

These factors and their clinical correlations not only add another dimension to our overall understanding of delinquents but also have implications for treatment. Staff should help patients identify affects, teach patients that behavior has meaning and flows from internal psychological states, identify psychological deficits in patients, provide for those deficiencies externally through psychological interventions, work in a psychotherapeutic atmosphere to help the patients begin performing those psychological functions for themselves, teach patients to introspect, and help patients convert motor behavior into verbal behavior. Our therapeutic interventions organize themselves around our understanding of the delinquent's use of space, time, objects, and personal relationships. Yet each clinical type of delinquent may require particular modifications and shifts in emphasis. The borderline's tendency to merge with his objects, his inability to distinguish himself from another person, his inability to identify an internal psychological life, and his poorly integrated concepts of space and time all point more toward attempting to help him structure his experiences on the hospital unit. To set limits in an attempt to help the delinquent develop internal controls may be more useful with the impulsive delinquent where one is attempting to develop certain kinds of psychological functions and shift the pathology inward. Separating delinquents statistically into subtypes that have clinical meaning helps develop specific preventive and therapeutic interventions.

Conclusions

Four empirically derived and clinically meaningful psychodynamic subgroups of delinquent adolescents are presented. The data were obtained from an ongoing hospital treatment program and investigative research project, some aspects of which are described. Psychodynamic thinking about delinquency, its causes, and its treatment has contributed to the exposition of the four subgroups: the impulsive, the narcissistic, the depressed, and the borderline.

The impulsive delinquent shows more violent and nonviolent antisocial behavior. He is considered quite disturbed by his therapist, socially insensitive by his teachers, and unlikable and quick to action by most staff members. Yet, he seems to have some awareness of a need for help. His delinquency derives from a propensity for action and immediate discharge.

The narcissistic delinquent sees himself as well adjusted and not delinquent. However, parents and staff recognize his difficulties in adapting and characterize him as resistant, cunning, manipulative, and superfical. He denies problems, only appears to engage in therapy, exaggerates his own self-worth, and in his delinquency tends to use others for his own needs, especially to help regulate his self-esteem.

The depressed delinquent shows school initiative, is liked by staff, and tries to engage with staff therapeutically. Relationships with parents lead to strongly internalized value systems, and these delinquents tend to show structuralized or neurotic conflicts, from which delinquent behavior serves as a relief.

The borderline delinquent is a passive, emotionally empty and depleted person, who is not well liked, is an outcast sometimes, needy and clinging at other times, and whose future seems pessimistic. These adolescents behave delinquently to prevent psychotic disintegration or fusion and to relieve themselves of internal desolation.

The variables which make up the four factors and appropriate case reports are discussed. The psychological subgroups contribute to our understanding of adolescent delinquent behavior, regardless of age, sex, socioeconomic status, or race. The resulting psychodynamic formulations enrich psychotherapeutic interventions. Further research is needed to refine subgroups and to verify their presence in each of the demographic groupings.

NOTES

1. Offer, Marohn, and Ostrov (1979) and Marohn, Dalle-Molle, McCarter, and Linn, in preparation.

2. One of the five factors, a factor made up almost entirely of Rorschach variables, will not be described in this paper.

REFERENCES

Aichhorn, A. 1925. *Wayward Youth.* New York: Viking, 1935.

Alexander, F., and Staub, H. 1931. *The Criminal, the Judge and the Public.* Reprint ed. New York: Collier, 1956.

Blos, P. 1966. *A Developmental Approach to Problems of Acting Out.* New York: International Universities Press.

Blos, P. 1967. The second individuation process of adolescence. *Psychoanalytic Study of the Child* 22:162–185.

Blos, P. 1971. Adolescent concretization: a contribution to the theory of delinquency. In I. M. Marcus, ed. *Currents in Psychoanalysis.* New York: International Universities Press.

Freud, A. 1958. Adolescence. *Psychoanalytic Study of the Child* 8:255–278.

Freud, A. 1965. *Normality and Pathology in Childhood: Assessments of Development.* New York: International Universities Press.

Freud, S. 1905. Three essays on sexuality. *Standard Edition* 7:123–243. London: Hogarth, 1953.

Friedlander, K. 1960. *The Psychoanalytic Approach to Juvenile Delinquency.* New York: International Universities Press.

Glover, E. 1950. On the desirability of isolating a "functional" (psychosomatic) group delinquent disorder. *British Journal of Delinquency* 1:104–112.

Grinker, R. R., Sr. 1956. *Toward a Unified Theory of Human Behavior.* New York: Basic.

Grinker, R. R., Sr.; Werble, B.; and Drye, R. C. 1968. *The Borderline Syndrome.* New York: Basic.

Hollingshead, A. B. 1965. Two factor index of social position. Mimeographed. New Haven, Conn.: Yale Station.

Johnson, A., and Szurek, S. A. 1952. The genesis of antisocial acting out in children and adolescents. *Psychoanalytic Quarterly* 21:323–343.

Marohn, R. C.; Dalle-Molle, D.; McCarter, E.; and Linn, D. In preparation. *Adolescent Behavior: A Psychodynamic Perspective.*

Marohn, R. C.; Dalle-Molle, D.; Offer, D.; and Ostrov, E. 1973. A hospital riot: its determinants and implications for treatment. *American Journal of Psychiatry* 130:631–636.

Offer, D. 1969. *The Psychological World of the Teenager*. New York: Basic.

Offer, D.; Marohn, R. C.; and Ostrov, E. 1975. Violence among hospitalized delinquents. *Archives of General Psychiatry* 32:1180–1186.

Offer, D.; Marohn, R. C.; and Ostrov, E. 1979. *The Psychological World of the Juvenile Delinquent*. New York: Basic.

Offer, D., and Offer, J. B. 1975. *From Teenage to Young Manhood*. New York: Basic.

Ostrov, E.; Offer, D.; Marohn, R. C.; and Rosenwein, R. 1972. The impulsivity index: its application to delinquency. *Journal of Youth and Adolescence* 1:179–196.

Redl, F. 1966. Ego disturbances and ego support and the phenomena of contagion and "shock effect." In *When We Deal with Children*. New York: Free Press.

Winnicott, D. W. 1958. The antisocial tendency. In *Collected Papers*. New York: Basic.

Winnicott, D. W. 1973. Delinquency as a sign of hope. *Adolescent Psychiatry* 2:363–371.

MEYER SONIS

In searching for a structure within which to present my comments on the acting-out behavior of adolescents, I could find no more fitting framework than to quote old friends who have walked this path before.

In 1909, in a letter to Julia Lothrop, William Healy stated:

The need is for work, extensive, solid work, to be done in determining as much as possible the causation of delinquency and other mental unfitness, in deciphering for diagnoses the proper values of the various physical and mental stigmata which we know exist in most of these cases, in developing a classification of the individuals according to their needs, and estimating results obtained in the various private and public schools for defectives which are now on the various experimental bases. I have been over the field fairly thoroughly and I am convinced of the need for a work that may be as classical as that of Lombroso, that may be much more scientifically founded and a thousand times more practically beneficial. But it can only be accomplished by long labor in competent hands. [Healy 1971]

In 1934, Sheldon and Eleanor Glueck (1934), in their review of 1,000 juvenile delinquents and their records between 1917 and 1922, gave this composite picture of the boys who passed in and out of the Boston Juvenile Court and the Judge Baker Foundation:

To a larger extent than the general population, they are native born sons of foreign born parents, a situation likely to make for cultural friction. Their parents have had a very meager education. The boys are members of unusually large families, which even in happier economic times would continually be on the ragged edge of poverty. These families have disintegrated early; often the parents have become separated or divorced, or are unduly quarrelsome, and the home life has been distorted by inadequate care and discipline of the children. The standards of the parents, as interpreted through evidence of thrift, temperance and moral decency, are very low, and criminality on the part of the parents, brothers and sisters of our young delinquents is an all too frequent phenomenon. . . . These findings lead to the conclusions that the working relationship between clinic and court might be considerably improved; that the success of both institutions is greatly dependent upon the adequate collaboration of other social agencies; that the work of all organizations concerned with various aspects of the prevention and treatment of delinquency needs to be effectively integrated; that additional specialized community facilities for coping with delinquency are necessary; that the court needs to have greater power over the families of delinquents; and the major conclusion which is inescapable, that the treatment carried out by the clinic, court and associated community facilities had very little effect in preventing recidivism.

In a dedication to August Aichhorn on the occasion of his seventieth birthday, Archibald (1949) summarized a major presentation she had made by stating:

To sum up, numerically, this may not seem to constitute a very serious problem, since the number of London children of school age charged with indictable offenses is only 1.2 percent of the school population; nor are the vast majority of offenses of a serious nature. The gravity of the situation lies in three facts: first, that in spite of all the progress that has been made in the treatment of delinquent children and despite the outstanding improvement in social conditions that have taken place in the last few years, there is no sign of a real decline in total numbers; second, the fact that

485

recidivism appears to be on the increase, and all of this may be a temporary phenomenon, our ignorance of its causation leaves it a mystery; third, while all pre-war statistics show the early adolescent years as the peak for delinquency, the established trend has changed, and for the first time since records existed, the youngest boys equal the adolescents.

With this as a framework, the purpose of this chapter will be twofold: first, to present a brief report on a study, yet in process, of juvenile acting-out behavior; and second, to ask several questions: Of whom are we speaking in our reference to the acting-out adolescent? Is the acting-out behavior of the adolescent a role for which he had been preparing and prepared all of his previous life? Is the acting-out behavior of some adolescents the price they must pay for insufficient intervention in the past and overdue intervention in the present? And finally, are those of us who serve adolescents in a position to do anything more today than we have been able to do in the past?

In many ways we are in a much better position to answer such questions today. Our current state of knowledge in the information sciences can define questions for us in almost any set of parameters, whether by number, color, income, families, households, population, rural or urban residence, sex, education, and many other terms and characteristics. In the United States are we talking about the 15–18 percent of our population which is now in its adolescent years, or are we also talking about the almost 25 percent of the population yet to become adolescents? Of the adolescent population in the United States, is the target population of our concern that portion of the population of adolescents who act out by becoming mothers before they have successfully been teenagers, who may be mentally ill or emotionally disturbed, who run away, or who flow in and out of our juvenile courts? If our target of concern is the acting-out adolescent population, are we also talking about the children of the 10 percent of white families or the 32 percent of black families below the poverty level, the 17 percent of children of families below the poverty level, the 17 percent of children who do not live with their parents, or the 9 percent of white teenagers and the 15 percent of black teenagers who are not in school (Sonis and Sonis 1975)?

I suspect that our answer to the question would theoretically encompass that population of adolescents whose range of behavior can include acting out against others, against themselves, against their independence, against their dependence, and against values established by others as a way of finding one's own values. We have elected to focus our attention on a target population of adolescents whose total number is small in comparison with all other adolescents but whose total cost to themselves, their families, and society is enormous. Our population also includes those whose acting-out behavior has brought them to the attention of a juvenile court and its judicial process of deciding whether the behavior of the juvenile requires treatment, remediation, correction, containment, or a combination of these.

During the past two years this author has been engaged in a study of the juvenile population which flows into and out of the Allegheny County Juvenile Court because of alleged or adjudicated delinquent behavior (Sonis 1976). This study has focused on the nature of the juvenile population which is brought to the attention of a juvenile court and the nature of human services this population receives and requires. Though this study involves one county in the United States and the population of juveniles from this county who are brought to the attention of a juvenile court, it can be said that the information and data specific to this county and population would be generally applicable to other counties and their juvenile populations.

Allegheny County has a population of approximately 1.65 million people, of whom approximately one-third are under the age of eighteen. In the course of a year about 9,000 different juveniles flow into and out of the court approximately 12,000 different times. Though the incidence of juvenile delinquent behavior for the county is 3 out of every 100 juveniles between the ages of five and seventeen, the range of this incidence varies from 7 per 100 juveniles in some geographic areas to .6 per 100 juveniles in other areas. It is interesting to note the comparison of some characteristics of the geographic areas of highest and lowest incidence. For example, the median income in the former is $5,500, compared with $8,000 in the latter; 12 percent of the population is in poverty in the former, 5 percent in the latter; 39 percent of the black population is in poverty in the former, 27 percent in the latter; 12 percent of the households with children are headed by females in the former, 5 percent in the latter; 81 percent of children are living with both parents in the former, 92 percent in the latter; 13 percent of children are living at the poverty level in the former, 4 percent in the latter; and 45 percent of the female-headed households with children are black in the former, 20 percent in the latter.

Of the 9,000 juveniles flowing through the court during the course of the year, 78 percent are male and 22 percent are female, compared with their distribution in the general population of 51 percent male to 49 percent female. Seventy percent are white and 30 percent are black in comparison with the distribution in the general population of 90 percent white and 10 percent black. The age range for this population of juveniles flowing into the court is five to eighteen years, with 90 percent of these juveniles ranging in age from thirteen to eighteen and 10 percent below the age of thirteen. Approximately 70 percent are brought to the attention of the juvenile court for the first time, while 30 percent have had previous contact. Of these approximately 3,000 juveniles who have had previous contact with the court, 73 percent have had two contacts, 13 percent three contacts, 4 percent four contacts, and 10 percent between five and nine contacts. Of these 9,000 juveniles, 13 percent have been brought to the attention of the court because of aggressive acts against persons, such as murder, voluntary manslaughter, involuntary manslaughter, aggravated assault, rape, robbery, arson, or simple assault; 45 percent for aggressive acts against objects, such as burglary, auto theft, theft, or purse snatching; 16 percent for offenses in the form of minor status offenses such as running away or incorrigibility; 3 percent for offenses relating to traffic, such as hit and run, driving without a license, or other traffic offenses; and 23 percent for offenses such as possession and sale of marijuana and alcohol or possession, use, and sale of drugs, criminal mischief, and other offenses.

It is interesting to note the various characteristics of offenses or acting-out behaviors which distinguish the juvenile population. For example, no female was found acting out in the form of the serious offenses of murder or manslaughter; of all juveniles whose acting out behavior was in the form of the serious offense of aggravated assault against another, 38 percent of them were white males, 51 percent were black males, 1 percent were white female, and 10 percent were black females. Of all the juveniles manifesting acting-out behavior in the form of the serious offense of robbery, 34 percent were white males, 59 percent were black males, 2 percent were white females, and 5 percent were black females. While burglary was perpetrated by 74 percent of white males and 22 percent of black males, purse snatching was committed by 15 percent of white males and 82 percent of black males. While females make up 12 percent of those juveniles acting out in the form of aggression against persons, females constitute almost 42 percent of the minor-status offenses. Of the juveniles acting out in the form of possession and sale of marijuana and alcohol, 73 percent were white males, 12 percent were black males, 12 percent were white females, and 3 percent were black females. Of the juveniles brought to the attention of the court for the minor-status offense of running away, 37 percent were white males, 14 percent were black males, 33 percent were white females, and 16 percent were black females. Of those juveniles brought to the attention of the court because of incorrigibility, 39 percent were white males, 20 percent were black males, 21 percent were white females, and 20 percent were black females.

Of the 9,000 juveniles who were brought to the attention of a juvenile court during the course of a year, the bulk of them, estimated at 70–80 percent, can be characterized as: (*a*) juveniles who are predominantly first offenders, though not exclusively so, and for offenses which can be classified predominantly as aggression against objects, antisocial behavior as a nonspecific result of abusive nature, or behavior of a minor-status nature; (*b*) juveniles whose behavior may be explained as primarily symptomatic of a crisis in the course of their normal growth and development and juveniles who may require the intervention of those human services ordinarily available within a community; (*c*) juveniles whose behavior may be explained as primarily symptomatic of deviation in their emotional, cognitive, and/or central nervous system development and juveniles who require the direct intervention of the public or private mental health or mental retardation services; (*d*) juveniles whose behavior may be explained as primarily symptomatic of deviation in their characterological and social development and whose development now reflects a later sequela of earlier social, emotional, and intellectual deprivation; and (*e*) juveniles who require the intervention of human services such as group homes, social and welfare agencies, and vocational training programs.

Of concern and pertinence to this chapter are the 20–30 percent of this juvenile population of 9,000. It is this population which can be categorized as: (*a*) juveniles who predominantly, but not exclusively, are more than first offenders; (*b*) juveniles who have been brought to the attention of the court predominantly for offenses of a very serious nature in the form of aggression against persons and objects; (*c*) juveniles who are brought to the attention of the court repetitively for minor-status acting-out behavior and whose serious behavior may be explained as symptomatic of deviation in their characterological and social development but whose intensity, extensiveness, and duration of developmental deviation offer a poor prognosis for correction or remediation; (*d*) juveniles whose offense is of a serious nature and whose records now reflect previous and repetitive contacts with the court, including repetitive contacts in detention; inability of the juvenile to effectively utilize human services provided in the past; previous contacts with a variety of human services; suggested earlier signs and symptoms of developmental deviation in any one of several areas of development, that is, social, emotional, cognitive, physical, etc.; incomplete past studies and inadequate follow-up of earlier studies; fragmented human services provided to them in the past, that is, the "turnstile child"; an extensive history suggesting problems in differential diagnosis between psychopathology, social pathology, neuropathology, environmental pathology, earlier deprivations; serious problems in disposition; and (*e*) juveniles whose behavior is of an intense nature and whose deviation in development is multiple, extensive, and of long duration and whose behavior following serious and comprehensive diagnosis cannot be explained on the basis of a primary psychiatric disorder but on the basis of multiple etiological factors suggesting a poor or guarded prognosis.

It is in a study of 500 records of this latter group of juveniles that the following information emerges: 80 percent of them are male and 20 percent female; 57 percent are white and 43 percent black; 38 percent of them have been residents in nonpsychiatric public institutions in the past; 5 percent have previously had a psychiatric hospitalization history; 68 percent come from families that are not intact; 23 percent have a recorded psychological test rendering a full-scale IQ above 100, 50 percent with a registered IQ of 82–100, and 27 percent with a recorded IQ of below 100; 70 percent come from families with five or more siblings; prior to this contact, 38 percent of them had lived with both parents, 38 percent with one parent, 12 percent with relatives, and the remainder had been in institutions; about 15 percent have been identified as having some form of chronic health problem, such as epilepsy, diabetes, orthopedic problems, hearing loss, etc.; 60 percent were identified as having difficulties in learning; 85 percent were identified as coming from backgrounds of social pathology, such as family dysfunction, parental family instability, or neglect; 68 percent had recorded information of sibling dysfunction in the form of siblings who were school dropouts or who had court records, mental illness, or mental retardation; and 70 percent had over three previous recorded contacts with human service agencies.

In a study of these juveniles during the time of their residence in the detention center, it was found on ophthalmological and audiological referral that 38 percent of this population has refractive problems and 17 percent has problems in hearing, in comparison with nationally reported data on this age population of 3 percent for visual problems and 4 percent for hearing problems. Furthermore, it is of interest to note that the grade placement of this population on the Stanford Primary Achievement Test indicates that 19 percent are at or above their grade placement, 12 percent one grade below their grade placement, 31 percent three grades below their grade placement, and 38 percent five grades below their grade placement.

Of these 9,000 juveniles, for how many has their acting-out behavior been a role for which they have been preparing and prepared during their earlier period of growth and development? For most of the adolescents in our population who do not come to the attention of the juvenile court, it can be said that their acting-out behavior may be an age-appropriate version of mastering the developmental tasks of adolescence, tasks for which the adolescent has been prepared by successful past mastery. For most adolescents who come to the attention of the court for offenses such as possession of alcohol or drugs, traffic violations, and minor-status offenses, it can be said that this acting-out behavior may be a phase of the developmental process in which the adolescent attempts to achieve independence from the environment while forcing the environment to increase control and surveillance. This suggests deviations in development which arise in the process of growing up but does not suggest a quality of child rearing and caretaking which has been destructive. For some of these juveniles, whose number is small, acting-out behavior is such as to unequivocally reflect signs, symptoms, and histories which lead to diagnoses of mental illness, mental retardation, or chronic brain syndrome, with all of their implications for earlier failures at developmental tasks.

And finally, for some of our juvenile population, acting-out behavior is a role for which they have been prepared as the final payment for a whole succession of failures in development. This is the juvenile population which comprises the bulk of those who have repeated contacts with the court for aggressions against persons and objects and for minor-status offenses. This is the population of juveniles whose acting-out behavior reflects deviations in physical, cognitive, social, and behavioral development. The pathology is produced by a combination of etiological factors, such as psychopathology, social pathology, and neuronal pathology. Such pathology reflects the presence of a child-rearing and child-caretaking environment which has not been and is not supportive of constructive development, a documented chronic history of developmental failures manifesting themselves sequentially in every one of the juvenile's earlier human service contacts, and a potential diagnosis reflecting characterological and/or personality defect or inadequacies and a prognosis which is guarded to grave.

The following vignettes are presented to illustrate this latter group of juveniles.

1. Case example A: A fourteen-year-old white male's repeated fire setting brought him into contact with the court. He was from an intact family with a mother forty-six years of age and father forty-nine. His mother had been suffering from arthritis and phlebitis for approximately twenty years, and father was reported to be a severe asthmatic and alcoholic. At the time of his birth his parents had been married for nine years. He was a premature baby and spent the first two months of his life in an incubator. He is reported as "soft-boned," with a history of frequent fractures of his limbs. When he was six, the school psychological report revealed an IQ, on the WISC, of 69. When he was nine, the school psychological study reported that he had a full-scale IQ of 77, that he repeated kindergarten, and that overall he tested toward the top of the educable, mildly retarded range of ability. When he was ten the school reported that the quality of his afternoon work differed so drastically from that of the morning that the teacher wondered if he had suffered a mild brain injury. The Bender Gestalt, however, appeared to be within expected ranges of performance for mildly retarded children of his age. When he was twelve the school reported that he tended to be quiet. The record reveals that, when he was thirteen, his older brother was involved with the correctional system in an armed robbery attempt, and an older sister returned home to live with her illegitimate child. His contact with the court began when he was fourteen because of repeated fire setting in various public facilities. In the next two years he spent eight months in a youth development center, two months in a general psychiatric hospital, and five months in a state psychiatric hospital where he was diagnosed as manifesting a social aggressive reaction. At age seventeen he was committed to a state correctional institution.

2. Case example B: At the time of his birth the parents of this sixteen-year-old black male had been married two years and were

twenty-one and thirty-two years of age, respectively. He had one older sibling and four younger ones. When he was ten years of age his father died of an unknown cause. Mother, a high school graduate, reported that he was a problem as a youngster in that he was nervous, hyperactive, and clumsy. School reports indicated that he failed two grades in elementary school and had been placed in six different schools. In the eighth grade he was reading at the fourth-grade level and failing many subjects.

During a three-year period, prior to his initial contact with the court, three of his siblings had been brought to the attention of the court for various offenses, including indecent exposure, disorderly conduct, and armed robbery. At the age of sixteen he was brought to court and charged with rape, sodomy, and robbery—all of these occurring within a period of three months. He was charged with robbery, indecent exposure, and forcible rape of an older woman, all with a knife. Psychiatric examination indicated that he was not psychotic. He was diagnosed as having a personality disorder and was reported to have an average IQ. He was committed to a state correctional institution.

3. Case example C: A fourteen-year-old black male's parents, married for fourteen years, were separated when he was six years of age. He had four older and two younger siblings. There is a social service exchange listing of twenty-four different contacts with agencies over a fifteen-year period. Prior to his birth his four older siblings had been placed with Child Welfare Service because of dependency and neglect. When he was five years of age his mother was admitted to a state hospital and diagnosed as an antisocial, aggressive person with primary syphilis. When he was seven years of age his mother brought him to juvenile court because he was uncontrollable, and she reported that he frequently ran away. At eight years of age he was placed by his mother. When he was nine years of age his mother disappeared and did not return for two years. When he was twelve years of age he was placed in a group home and was discharged one year later because of chronic running away. A psychological evaluation indicated that he had a full-scale IQ of 92 but was developmentally at the level of a nine-year-old youngster. At thirteen he was brought to the court because of vandalism. At the age of fourteen he was brought to the attention of the court because he burglarized two houses and was referred for treatment to a group home. Three months later he was brought to the attention of the court because of repetitive running away from the home.

Summary

There is an ever-increasing number of juveniles who time and again flow into and out of our juvenile justice system and who demonstrate the evolutionary history of our collective scientific and clinical attempts to understand and remedy their acting-out behavior (Hendelang 1973).

It is this group of juveniles who at one time fostered the belief that such severe behavior could be produced only by poor constitutional endowment and required punishment and incarceration as means of control. Later it was thought that such behavior could be produced only by psychopathology and required psychological treatment to effect its change. Still later it was believed that such behavior could be produced only by the detrimental and deprived effects of social pathology, and therefore these juveniles required separation from their environmental pathology in order to manage and rehabilitate their behavior.

It is this group of juveniles who now present us with a market basket of pathologies to explain their behavior, a shopping list of developmental problems they have developed under the eyes and ears of the human services provided them, and the dilemma of furnishing them with the scope of human services best equipped to match their market basket of pathologies and their shopping list of developmental problems.

Conclusions

As a result of this revisit of old freinds, are there conclusions we can draw beyond the conclusion that their past comments and concerns are still valid today? For myself, there are several additional conclusions which can be drawn.

To begin with, there is so little we know about the violence and aggression of our juvenile population. For this reason our human services, ordinarily designated responsibility for the diagnoses of pathologies and the identification of developmental disorders, must assume responsibility not only for recommending plans for programs to match the identified needs of this juvenile population but also for monitoring the ongoing validity of diagnoses and developmental assessments.

Second, as responsible professionals, we must, painfully and sadly, acknowledge to ourselves and to others the limits of our current knowledge for explaining the violent and aggressive acting-out behavior of some of our juvenile population, and the limits of our current human resources for effecting major change, through acceptable and safe procedures, in this behavior of some of our juvenile population. We must also acknowledge that for the immediate future such juveniles will continue to be identified within the human service network. For this reason the scope of human services available to this juvenile population must include services which can provide the security for containment of this behavior while they remedy the identified developmental problems.

And finally, we do know that behavior which is multiply determined and developmental problems which are manifested in multiple developmental areas require multiple solutions. For this reason the spectrum of human services required to match the needs of this juvenile population must be such as to allow for the crossover relationship between the separate streams through which human services are delivered (Stone 1975).

REFERENCES

Archibald, D. 1949. Some services for London's difficult boys. In K. Eissler, ed. *Searchlights on Delinquency.* New York: International Universities Press.

Glueck, S., and Glueck, E. 1934. *One Thousand Juvenile Delinquents.* Cambridge, Mass.: Harvard University Press.

Healy, W. 1971. Letter to Julia Lothrop. In R. H. Bremner, ed. *Children and Youth in America.* Vol. 2. Cambridge, Mass.: Harvard University Press.

Hendelang, M. 1973. *Sourcebook of Criminal Justice Statistics.* Washington, D.C.: Government Printing Office.

Sonis, M. 1976. "Report of Task Force of Allegheny County Juvenile

Court and Regional Office of Mental Health for Western Pennsylvania." Unpublished manuscript.

Sonis, M., and Sonis, A. 1975. Children, youth and their gatekeepers. *Journal of the American Academy of Child Psychiatry* 14(1):95–113.

Stone, A. 1975. *Mental Health and Law: A System in Transition.* Washington, D.C.: Government Printing Office.

DEVELOPMENTAL ISSUES AND THEIR
RELATION TO DUE PROCESS IN THE
FAMILY COURT

MICHAEL G. KALOGERAKIS

The movement to give children rights which society has long granted only to adults is most welcome and manifestly overdue. Children may indeed be the last disadvantaged group. Justine Wise Polier was for years a lone clarion reminding us that America's greatest hypocrisy may well be its pretended child-centeredness. The reality is that we have ignored our children, who undeniably, are our greatest resource—ignored them often to the point of renunciation. Of course, in the rarified atmosphere of the psychiatric profession there are no renouncers. We are all believers and we are keeping the faith, each in his fashion. Nor would most of us question very seriously the need for continuous protection of children by the state. How sadly this lags in some states is evidenced by some statutory rape laws. In Maine, Georgia, and Puerto Rico a girl can consent to sexual intercourse at fourteen years of age; in Louisiana and Tennessee the age of consent is twelve; and in the state of Delaware, it is only seven. An attempt to change the Delaware statute by raising the age from seven to twelve as recently as 1972 was defeated.

Many of the rights for children being discussed would today be considered inalienable, though the battles fought over them have been long: the consent to medical treatment for the emancipated youngster; the right to confidentiality; and the right to legal representation in the court. Hofmann and Pilpel (1973) have stated that the deprivation of rights has been nowhere more evident than in juvenile courts and

© 1979 by Federal Legal Publications, Inc., 157 Chambers St., New York, N.Y. 10007, *Journal of Psychiatry & Law* 3, no. 4 (Winter 1975):75. Reprinted by permission of the publisher.

schools. In my remarks, I shall deal with particular regard to the efforts to introduce due process into the handling of children who come before the court. Unanticipated consequences of the legal moves have been less than felicitous in some cases and need to be examined carefully by both the law and psychiatry.

The landmark Gault (1967) decision spurred the movement for due process in the juvenile court. The result of a suit launched by the Arizona Civil Liberties Union, it established that children before the court on a charge of delinquency had to be given timely notice of charges, notification of the right to counsel and appointment of counsel by the court if necessary, the right to confront and cross-examine a witness, adequate warning of the privilege against self-incrimination, and the right to remain silent. This served to curb flagrant abuses of due process that had been routine in many courts for years.

As with all good laws, however, the implementation of *Gault* has not been without problems. As an example, it is not rare in our experience that an adolescent remanded by the Family Court for examination is felt to require, as a primary need, the provision of external controls to compensate for his serious lack of internal controls. The recommendation in such cases is likely to be for a well-supervised secure setting, which in New York State usually means a training school. Now, the law guardian appointed by the court to represent the youth is occasionally caught in a bind which forces him to take a position that, to the mental health professional, has often seemed inimical to the best interests of the child. The function of the lawyer as an adversary in the court is clear: "If we agree that the adversary system is the most reliable and just method of fact-finding, then children are entitled to its benefits. If a juvenile does not desire incarceration in a reform school, he has a right to a lawyer who will defend him vigorously and to the best of his ability. One who will consider it his obligation to prevent that result if possible. A lawyer who would fail to do that because he feels that his client might benefit from a court imposed treatment program is behaving unethically" (Wizner 1971).

However justifiable this stance may be from the standpoint of the law, one can see how it can bring the lawyer and the psychiatrist into open conflict in certain cases. My quarrel with this view, and my major thesis here, is that it involves an unjustifiable application of adversary procedure used with adults to the child whose dependent status and developmental immaturity distinguish him in many ways from the adult. To be specific:

498

1. In contrast to the adult, the child or adolescent is not an independent human being having all the rights that accrue to one who has reached the age of majority. He is dependent on his parents for support and guidance and their wishes for him are important considerations in any decisions that materially affect his life. For example, he cannot, in opposition to his parents' wishes, choose to live with another family or, before he is sixteen (in New York), withdraw from school.

2. Cognitive development is not yet completed in most younger adolescents, who may not achieve abstract reasoning until the age of fifteen or older (Inhelder and Piaget 1958). The relevance of this fact to the capacity to exercise judgment in determining what is in one's best interest is self-evident.

3. Biologically, EEG patterns have been shown not to change definitively until the age of eighteen, and the brain increases in size and continues to undergo myelinization until that time. The implications of these findings for adolescent behavior are by no means clear, but they serve to highlight the fact that developmental differences with adults exist and must be kept in mind.

4. Emotionally, the normal adolescent is struggling with problems of individuation in which breaking the bonds of dependency which have tied him to his parents is a paramount concern. In this vital quest for autonomy, the teenager commonly sets up situations of conflict with his parents, in which he differs, opposes, and often rebels. It is essential to be able to interpret such behavior correctly and not ascribe to it significance it does not have. This would lead him, for example, to deny any need that betrays infantile strivings and to resist any plan that might satisfy the wish to be cared for, whether by his parents or by the child care system. It is obviously hazardous to side with the adolescent when his protestations about being sent away may belie an unconscious (or preconscious) wish for that very thing.

5. His struggle with his parents and his turning away from them frequently leave him with a profound sense of guilt, particularly if his behavior has taken a hostile turn. This may then lead to an inordinate need for punishment, and many maneuvers designed to bring that about. In more pathological situations this dynamic plays a major role in delinquent activity. Typically, when society fails to respond by restraining or punishing such a youth, he escalates the antisocial character of his delinquency until he forces the desired response.

6. Closely related is the need for limit setting which all children have, but which becomes particularly acute during adolescence when sexual

and aggressive impulses are spilling over. The consequences of a lack of such limits are particularly noticeable in fatherless families, overwhelmingly the majority of family court cases. Depression, acting out, and manipulation of the adult world are common direct outgrowths of this particular form of deprivation. The fact that a particular adult (e.g., the law guardian) is visibly committed to helping the youth in no way precludes his being the victim of such manipulations.

7. Deriving from much of the above, and abetted by the adolescent's typical concern for saving face, is the commonly observed clinical fact that adolescents frequently do not say what they mean or mean what they say. How then are we to take their verbal expressions as representative of their true wishes? Their nonverbal communications are far more reliable, as any student of adolescence will readily attest.

For the lawyer, society's appointed guardian of our legal rights, a difficult dilemma arises. His ethical code is binding, every bit as much as the Hippocratic Oath is on physicians. But it was drawn up with the adult client in mind at a time when the complexities of children's rights had not yet exploded on the scene. Even with adults, it was clear that the commitment to do precisely what the client wished was based on the assumption of reason: severe psychopathology interfering grossly with judgment would lead to either substitution of the lawyer's judgment on behalf of his client or withdrawal from the case. No professional code of ethics would consciously support a position that risked being regularly detrimental to the client. There was an implied concern for best interests, but it was felt that in the overwhelming majority of cases, this would be best represented by the client's stated wishes. Besides, what was the alternative? A totally unacceptable substitution of one man's concerns for another's—an unconscionable abrogation of individual liberty.

We have seen that in the child an alternative must be found. When he is before the court, we no more have a choice about determining independently what is in his best interests than do his parents in the home. The age at which this changes is one of the great unsolved problems of the day. Until we have clearer definition, I would suggest that we take mid-adolescence, say fifteen, as the age when parental and societal prerogatives must begin to yield to the individuating wishes of the youth. This would effectively cover almost all who come before the Family Court in New York State, where the cut-off point is sixteen. This transition point should logically be kept fairly loose—frustrating though this be to the legal mind—since precocious maturity in a healthy individual can move it down a few years and significant disturbance will delay it. We come to the knotty problem of who makes the determination.

It should be clear that such a determination does not fall within the expertise of the lawyer. The determination of stage of development, cognitive functioning, personality organization, and presence or absence of psychopathology and the implications of same are the province of the child or adolescent psychiatrist. If these issues are critical to the establishment of what is in the best interests of the child at any given point, how can we reasonably expect that a lawyer can serve alone as the advocate for a child, particularly if his code clearly precludes such a role? In a word, if not the lawyer, who is to advocate for a child's best interests?

I propose the establishment of a clinician-advocate position to serve children who come before the court. Such an individual would be equipped to assess the true meaning of a child's assertions, evaluate conflicting wishes, deal with ambivalence toward parents, and weigh the implications of personality disturbance. A psychiatrist, psychologist, or social worker not part of any delivery system and assigned to the child as is the law guardian, one specially trained to understand fully the workings of juvenile court procedure, could fill such a role. Unless he were to be an accredited attorney as well, which would be highly desirable, he would of course be unable to argue the case, so the continued presence of a defense lawyer is essential. However, the latter's functions could then be confined to assuring due process, the task of arguing for the child's best interests falling on the clinician-advocate.

Conclusions

This is not a proposal for extending the use of the psychiatrist currently used as a consultant in cases in which conflict over evaluation done by other psychiatrists exists. Rather, its aim is to provide clinical, legal, and psychological expertise in each and every case that comes before the court, while in no way implying that psychopathology is present each time. Short of such a solution, true advocacy for children before the court will continue to elude us.

REFERENCES

Hofmann, A. D., and Pilpel, H. F. 1973. The legal rights of minors. *Pediatric Clinics of North America* 2:989–1004.

Inhelder, B., and Piaget, J. 1958. *The Growth of Logical Thinking from Childhood to Adolescence*. New York: Basic.

In re Gault, 387 U.S. 1, 1967.

Wizner, S. 1971. The defense counsel: neither father, judge, probation officer or social worker. *Trial* 7(5):1–15.

36 DELINQUENCY IN ADOLESCENT GIRLS: DEVELOPMENTAL ASPECTS

PERIHAN A. ROSENTHAL

In the last two decades, new images of womanhood, rapid changes in social mores, and greater options for females have increasingly led adolescent girls to express their conflicts with earlier attachments through delinquency, suicide, depression, running away from home, and identity confusion (Adler 1975).

Adolescence is a period of transition with a resurgence of instinctual processes accompanied by reactivation of unwelcome preoedipal ties to the parents. Previously unresolved conflicts combined with instinctual impulses, both aggressive and sexual in nature (oedipal), express themselves during mid-adolescence (Galenson 1976). With some adolescents, the available defenses do not work and regression takes place. The adolescent then introjects the negative side of the ambivalence toward the parents, which has a most destructive effect (Jacobson 1961; Kestenberg 1972).

Our study group of fifteen delinquent girls, ages thirteen to seventeen with a median age of fourteen, are middle or lower-middle class and of mixed ethnic and religious backgrounds. Eighty percent are from intact families. This group of girls had long-standing feelings of deprivation because their mothers were not available to them due to work, depression, rejection, or other causes. The girls had developed severe conflicts and were truant from school. Most of them were involved with the courts for shoplifting, gang fights, drug abuse, aggression toward parental figures, suicidal attempts, promiscuity, running away, and pregnancy.

The mothers of these girls had been distant or unavailable. Some, because of employment, left their children with multiple caretakers;

others were depressed, had been away physically, were rejecting, or had severe problems of separation from their daughters. Rochlin (1961) has stated that "psychoanalytic work with young children who have experienced loss in fact or fantasy, through separation, deprivation, or in whom adequate object relationship has failed to develop has shown that the clinical picture is ruled by the infantile vicissitudes of aggression." Because these mothers were themselves needy and narcissistic, they were not able to see their children's needs. They projected onto their children their own demands for love, help, and comfort, thus pushing the children into premature maturity. These children learned quickly to take the mothering role and to become self-reliant.

The fathers of these girls were, in some cases, extremely rejecting. In other cases they were seductive, which is a threat to an adolescent girl who feels strongly pushed toward her father. These girls felt increased incestuous guilt and frequently resolved the guilt by running away, because their mothers were not available to help them solve the problem in another fashion.

Particularly disturbing to the adolescent girl are preoedipal ties to the mother. The intensity of these feelings depend on the mother's conflicted feelings concerning her own femininity (Benedek 1973). This also affects the adolescent girl's negotiation and integration of these feelings with her new identifications as she strives to become autonomous and independent of her mother. Traditionally, transition from latency to adolescence has been easier for girls than for boys because the female-dominated childhood provided a role model. However, environmental changes, the loss of objective standards of conduct for women, and the opening of many different life choices have accounted for increasing identity confusion, depression, and delinquency among girls (Adler 1975). The internal and external conflict, generated by the usual disruption of puberty, plus the ambiguity of new roles, creates complex identity problems for girls, perhaps more intense than for boys at present.

If the adolescent girl is strongly conflicted about her feminine role, she may rebel against it or exaggerate and distort it. Often her feelings devalue her mother, make her feel guilty, and give rise to rebelliousness and antagonism toward women, often with destructive hostility and unconscious violence. These responses seem to stem from a lack of warmth, protection, and/or the setting of a positive role identity and strict demands on sexuality by the mother (Ginandes 1964). Such girls

504

may develop hypochondriacal feelings and fears of being unattractive. Their relationships with their mothers are full of guilt and rage, which the girls usually turn against themselves. They have problems with peer relationships, low self-esteem, and unsupportive parents, all of which throw them into loneliness, despair, and sometimes suicide. They may find themselves competing freely with men, identifying with them, or following male modes of action in a more archaic form by forming gangs.

A girl in early adolescence feels empty and depressed if her preoedipal love object was ambivalent about her and if her dependency needs were unmet. These girls have a very negative view of themselves and struggle with identity problems (Erikson 1950). At this age, peers give intense support to members of the same sex. Conformity becomes very important. This support by members of the same sex in early adolescence is an attempt to supply the mothering each is lacking. Since they are all needy but cannot really meet each other's dependency needs and be sufficiently supportive, they indulge themselves with heavy drug use, alcohol, and promiscuity (Hartmann 1969; Wieder and Kaplan 1969).

When instinctual-incestuous impulses threaten to emerge, the adolescent girl deals with them by seeking new relationships and using a new object to displace the preoedipal parents. At times in this new relationship, the intensity of the attachment becomes so important that the adolescent girl tries to keep it at the expense of everything else. Otherwise, the fear of merging with the earlier love object (the mother) causes severe regression. The new relationship is like the transitional object of the young child and offers the adolescent illusory bridges to the earliest period in her life (Winnicott 1963). It is a cushion against the distress of frustration (instinctual-aggressive-sexual) before reality testing is secure (Bush, Nagera, McKnight, and Pessarossi 1973; Greenacre 1969).

This intense and destructive new object attachment is usually with an older delinquent or an assaultive boy who has a long court record. The adolescent girl recreates the earlier sadomasochistic relationship with the transitional object and retains her devalued self-image. These girls feel both hatred and guilt toward their mothers and, as a result, turn against them (Wolfenstein 1969). They are unable to compete with females or males, because they either lack or feel too strong an affectionate attitude toward their fathers.

Therapeutic Approaches

In approaching these delinquent girls therapeutically, I found two pathological types that required different techniques. One type has severe problems with separation-individuation and defensively used transitional objects, whether animate, such as older boys who had criminal records, or inanimate, such as drugs or alcohol. If the adolescent girl, struggling with issues of separation and individuation, displaces her earlier parental feeling onto the transitional object, she must be treated individually on the issues of the psychodynamics of the transitional object representation, with separate counseling for her parents. Therapy for these adolescent girls must explore the feelings toward and the relationship with the new object (in most instances a boyfriend) without making judgments or interfering with the pathological relationship. Like the transitional object of a young child, the attachment figure of the adolescent prevents a regression to the oral stage (a merging with the mother) and becomes an auxiliary ego for the adolescent.

If the parents, in their own therapy, are helped to become aware of the meaning of their daughter's new relationship, they can become supportive and empathize with her. The adolescent girl slowly develops a sense of reality and establishes her own identity with separation-individuation from her transitional object (boyfriend).

In the second pathological type, the delinquent adolescent is still struggling with separation-individuation and continuation of the symbiotic relationship with the original love object. The therapist needs first to work together with the adolescent and her mother, separating them, before starting individual work with the adolescent.

Case Examples

CASE EXAMPLE 1

The patient was a fifteen-year-old delinquent adolescent girl who used a transitional object to prevent intense regression. Referred because of her bouts of depression, academic failures, marijuana use, and intense sexual involvement with her boyfriend, she and her mother have been in conflict for the past three years. While she does get along well with her father and they have good communication, both parents were very concerned about her behavior and heavy drug use during the last year.

The patient was a precocious and friendly child. The mother reportedly had no difficulty with her until she was twelve years old, when she developed a gastric ulcer and a mild form of anorexia, losing a considerable amount of weight. At that time, she developed friendships with a different group of girls, most of whom were heavily involved with drugs, alcohol, and promiscuity.

The oldest of four siblings, she has three younger brothers, all active in sports. Both father and mother, who have taken a great deal of pleasure in their involvement with these activities, are in their late thirties and from upper-middle-class families. The patient's mother had a very conflictive relationship with her own mother, while the patient's father had a somewhat deprived childhood because his mother was ill with hemiparesis since he was four years old. He remembers always having multiple housekeepers and being very lonely and sad.

The patient is a tall, attractive girl with a short, afro haircut. Her affect was depressed, and she spoke with a low voice. She complained that she has been unhappy with life in the last three or four years and that her depression was getting worse. She felt that her mother is temperamental like her, but that her father is quiet and even-tempered. Her mother becomes angry easily, yells, and throws things. The patient also found herself losing her temper easily and becoming violent with her friends.

When she was a little girl, she was treated like one of the boys by her father and she felt close to him. The family did things together, like fishing, baseball, and skiing. Now, she would like to be a boy, since she has felt alienated and lonely for the last four years. Her mother told her the facts of life when she was twelve years old, after which she lost her appetite, suffered stomach pains, and became anorectic. When she was sick, her parents took a lot of interest in her and took her to Florida for a week.

For the past six months, the patient had a boyfriend of her own age who was everything to her. They were always together, and she talked to him about her problems. She had no other close friends, since she had grown to dislike her junior high school friends because they were athletes who looked down on everybody else. She reported that in the last year she was so "wild" that she did not know "if it was day or night." When she was in the eighth grade, she began to take drugs and found herself staring into space and becoming very withdrawn. Her marks were poor; she skipped classes sometimes and became friendly with lower-class kids. She spent most of her time with her boyfriend Bob.

The patient made the connection in therapy that Bob and her father were both kind people who made her feel safe and comfortable. She felt it was her obligation to let her parents know that she had a sexual relationship with him. When she suggested that her boyfriend come to see me also, I told her that I would like to get to know her first and then I might see him with her. She went on from there to say that it was difficult to talk to her mother, who often became violent and whose reactions were unpredictable. She felt that her mother asked too many questions and did not trust her because of her delinquency and involvement with drugs over the last two years. She could not understand why her mother was so "bitchy" and ungiving to her, while she was very close to the boys and gave them a great deal of freedom and love. The girl felt that her parents expected too much from her and that she disappointed them frequently.

At one point during therapy, the patient found herself fighting a great deal with her boyfriend and smoking too much pot. Her alienation from the "super athletes" started to bother her.

From the beginning of the diagnostic evaluation, she was intensely involved in the therapeutic relationship. The patient saw herself as devalued and rejected by her original peers and her family. Because of her ambivalent and conflictual relationship with her own mother, whom she felt rejected her, she tried to get close to her father, but the sexual aspect frightened her and led to depression, which expressed itself with anorexia nervosa and a gastric ulcer.

The patient spoke of her early years, remembering how she was sad at seven when their housekeeper was fired; she missed her close relationship with this woman. During her childhood, she rarely saw her mother, who spent her time traveling, playing cards, or taking her brothers out. She had had a sheepdog whom she loved, but her mother gave him away because he had fleas. She was very sad and cried a lot at this loss and still thinks sadly about him. Also when she was seven, her mother sent her to camp for the whole summer, where she was lonely and cried a lot. She was now able to make friends only with boys and had very little to do with girls.

When her brothers were not around, the patient and her mother were able to sit down and talk to each other without yelling. As therapy progressed, she still spent a lot of her free time after school with her boyfriend, but things began to get very tense between them because he wanted to know her every thought. He yelled at her, showed his violent temper, and beat her up a few times. Once he threw a knife at her because he was jealous. At times she encouraged his violence, and at other times it upset her. She saw him as inferior because he had and still has severe dyslexia. Because they were seeing each other too much, they began to irritate each other. She got very mad at him and also yelled and threw things at him.

The patient reported that her boyfriend worried that she would become crazy and that he would lose her. Slowly, the girl was able to see that her interaction with him was a replication of her relationship with her mother and father. After this insight, she started to go out with another boy and liked being with him. At the same time, however, she worried about her boyfriend's reaction if he were to find out. While struggling with these ambivalent feelings, her mother caught her smoking pot, grounded her, and prohibited her from seeing her boyfriend for a week. Before, she would have gotten very upset about this type of intervention; this time, however, she was somewhat relieved.

Gradually, she tried to break her ties with her boyfriend. She felt that he was acting like her parents and that one set of parents was enough. She became very concerned about his violence toward her and told him that if he hit her again, she would stop seeing him. She then found herself happier, no longer staring into space or depressed. The patient now felt that, although she and her mother were still temperamental, her mother did not scare her anymore. Her school grades improved, and she began to mingle with other boys and feel more comfortable in general.

The goal of therapy with symbiotic, delinquent girls is the ultimate separation and individuation of the girl and the mother. This is best accomplished when the two are seen together. In individual sessions, they cannot distinguish their own thoughts and actions and distort and project on both sides, each sabotaging improvement of the other. These adolescent girls and their mothers never finalized their separation-individuation. Both seem fixated at the level of rapprochement, where the toddler sees the maternal, caretaking figure as unavailable, unpredictable, insensitive, or intrusive. The toddler then deals with this through restlessness, increased motor activity, and anxiety about separations from the maternal figure due to unresolved conflict over separation (Mahler, Pine, and Bergman 1975).

CASE EXAMPLE 2

The patient was a fourteen-year-old girl, an only child, living with her single mother. The mother, now in her thirties, conceived when she was a teenager and refused to marry the father. In the patient's early years, while her mother was acting out her own adolescent conflict—going out with different boys, drinking, and being promiscuous—she was taken care of by her maternal grandmother. When the girl was of school age, she and her mother moved away from her grandmother's home. Although the mother never thought she was ready to nurture her on her own, she felt guilty about leaving the child with her grandmother. The patient's mother had been trying to finish college, had lived with different men (changing her partner every two or three years), was very aggressive, and felt that her life came first. Superficially, she presented herself as a capable, independent woman who was happy at what she was doing.

At puberty, the patient became uncontrollable; was violent toward her mother, peers, and teachers; continually ran away; drank heavily; and took drugs. She felt that her mother's interest in men and school was a rejection of her and saw her mother as a vulnerable little girl who was not capable of mothering. When the patient tried to follow in her mother's footsteps, creating a pseudo-independence with her behavior and boyfriends, she was ostracized by school authorities (Harley 1970). She tried to involve herself with an older boy in an attempt to displace her mother and to fulfill her unmet dependency needs. Unfortunately, this relationship was discontinued abruptly by her mother, and when she made an attempt to establish a relationship with another male, this time a teacher at school, her behavior was taken by the school and her mother as a sexual threat.

The patient's only choice seemed to be regression. This was very threatening because, although she did wish to be closer to her mother, she feared intimacy with women. Her anxiety was especially intense because it was difficult for her to control her aggressive, as well as sexual, impulses any time there was emotional or physical closeness with her mother, due to her mother's own conflict in the same area. They were merged in their conflict of tenderness, sexuality, and aggression. She and her mother, to keep from merging (regressing to the oral stage) and to maintain distance, used physical aggression (sadism) defensively. When her preoedipal dependency needs were frustrated, she acted silly and childish and developed a school phobia to help her deal with her instinctual aggressive and destructive feelings. It was quite obvious, in this case example, that the mother was interrupting her daughter's growth and development by preventing heterosexual relationships.

Ambiguity concerning her feminine role created complex identity problems for the patient. When she challenged many different social restrictions, including those which limit female activities to an established female role, she was thrown into chaos. Her unhealthy identification with her mother made her feel emotionally deprived and led to acting-out behavior, such as stealing, shoplifting, drinking, running away, and rage attacks against other females.

I saw her mother as consciously identifying herself with an idealized female role, while unconsciously holding onto a depreciated and devalued image of herself as a female (Greenacre 1969). She had difficulty from the beginning in accepting her daughter because of her ambivalent feelings and confusion about her own role as a woman and mother, a confusion the patient was quite aware of.

During the diagnostic evaluation, it was obvious that the patient and her mother were locked into preoedipal issues. The mother was pushing the patient into premature maturity and projected her own conflict onto her child. From the time the patient was six years old, her mother demanded that she be self-reliant and left her alone when she was away.

The problem was intensified when the patient turned thirteen because of unresolved, frustrated instinctual processes. Precocious physical maturation was an added burden because of her conflict about her sexuality and her pathological identification with her mother. The patient became sexually active, involved with drinking, and abusive toward her mother and female teachers. The lack of controls pushed her into the street, where she became involved with a male gang.

When the mother and daughter failed to gain any insight from individual therapy, I decided to see them together. Unfortunately, whatever they learned in therapy, they were not able to apply to their daily life. The patient saw her violence toward her mother and her delin-

quency, running away, and shoplifting as expressions of earlier deprivation. Finally, we recommended separating the child and her mother
by placing the patient in a therapeutic boarding school.

CASE EXAMPLE 3

The following is an example of a symbiotic relationship which was
amenable to conjoint treatment of the mother and the daughter. The
patient was a sixteen-year-old high school girl, the youngest of four
girls. She was truant from school and heavily involved with drugs.
She shoplifted and was aggressive toward female teachers. Her father was
a paranoid schizophrenic with a violent temper. Her mother was chronically depressed, had a low self-esteem, and was abused by her husband. For two years, the patient was involved with a notorious motor-
cycle gang. Her boyfriend, who had a long court record of assault and
battery, badly beat up the patient, breaking her arm and smashing her
face. She could not leave this boy, however, because she was not able
to see what he represented. During individual therapy with the patient
and her mother, the father refused to be involved. In individual therapy, we saw projection on both sides, and neither the patient nor her
mother were able to look into themselves. When they were seen
together, it was obvious that the mother was encouraging the patient's
delinquent behavior somewhat under the auspices of protecting her
from her violent father. The mother drove the patient anywhere she
wanted to go, helped her shoplift, and covered up information about
her bad companions. However, when the mother was given insight into
her role in her daughter's behavior problem, she was able to take a
competent, supportive mother role. She stopped being intrusive and
separated her thoughts and unconscious fantasies from her daughter,
thereby helping the patient become a more autonomous, separate individual and a responsible adolescent.

Conclusions

During adolescence, transitional phenomena with unique adaptive
and defensive purposes serve the same functions as those of a teddy

bear or a blanket for the younger child, namely, a self-applied soother in the face of separation anxiety, depressive affect, and feelings of loneliness. Like an auxiliary ego, they help the adolescent to keep from regressing to a psychotic oral stage (Erikson 1950). With this defense mechanism, the adolescent can remain in contact with reality in the face of primitive conflicts involving separation from transitional objects. Losing this capacity may bring on psychosis (Fox 1977). In symbiotic relationships, the adolescent girls were not psychotic but were fixated at the rapprochement subphase and, as Mahler et al. (1975) wrote, their conflicts were characterized by ambivalence. When the mother is unavailable, unpredictable, intrusive, or insensitive to the child's needs, the child becomes restless and motor activity and separation anxiety increase. On the one hand the child wants to hold onto the good side of the mother, but on the other hand he wants to push away the bad side.

The internal and external conflict generated by the usual disruption of puberty, plus the role change ambiguity of her new role, creates complex identity problems for the adolescent girl, more intense in nature and scope than those faced by boys (Adler 1975; Galenson 1976). The increasing antipathy which adolescent girls feel to the traditional female role can easily lead to increased acting-out behavior.

There are two aspects of the formation of the ego ideal during adolescence. The first is biological, derived from identification with the mother from the earlier experiences of nurturing, mothering, and comforting. There are very few changes in this over time if the object relationship is good and harmonious. The second is the sociocultural aspect of the ego ideal, which is likely to be influenced by cultural changes, women's liberation, and an increasingly wider variety of options. Adolescents must integrate these biological and social ego ideals (Gaddini 1975). If there are conflicts between the two, we see the conflict expressed in extreme behavioral changes, aggression, depression, delinquency, and suicide.

Erickson (1950) describes adolescence as follows: "The integration now taking place in the form of ego identity is more than the sum of the childhood identifications. It is the accrued experience of the ego's ability to integrate these identifications with the vicissitudes of the libido, with the aptitudes developed out of endowment, and with the opportunities offered in social roles" (p. 228).

REFERENCES

Adler, F. 1975. *Sisters in Crime*. New York: McGraw-Hill.

Benedek, T. 1973. Parenthood as a developmental phase. *Psychoanalytical Investigation*. New York: Quadrangle.

Bush, F.; Nagera, H.; McKnight, J.; and Pessarossi, G. 1973. Primary transitional objects. *Journal of the American Academy of Child Psychiatry* 12:193–214.

Erikson, E. 1950. *Childhood and Society*. New York: Norton.

Fox, R. P. 1977. Transitional phenomena in the treatment of psychotic adolescents. *International Journal of Psychoanalytic Psychotherapy* 6:147–165.

Gaddini, R. 1975. Brief communication: the concept of transitional object. *Journal of the American Academy of Child Psychiatry* 14:731–736.

Galenson, E. 1976. Psychology of women: late adolescence and early childhood. *Journal of the American Psychoanalytic Association* 24(3): 631–647.

Ginandes, S. C. 1964. Children who are sent away. *Journal of the American Academy of Child Psychiatry* 3(1): 68–69.

Greenacre, P. 1969. The fetish and the transitional object. *Psychoanalytic Study of the Child* 24:144–164.

Harley, M. 1970. On some problems of technique in the analysis of early adolescents. *Psychoanalytic Study of the Child* 25:99–121.

Hartmann, D. A. 1969. A study of drug-taking adolescents. *Psychoanalytic Study of the Child* 24:384–398.

Jacobson, E. 1961. Adolescent moods and remodeling of psychic structures in adolescence. *Psychoanalytic Study of the Child* 16:164–183.

Kestenberg, J. 1972. Phases of adolescence. *The Adolescent: Physical Development, Sexuality and Pregnancy*. New York: Mss Information Corp.

Mahler, M. S.; Pine, F.; and Bergman, A. 1975. *The Psychological Birth of the Human Infant*. New York: Basic.

Rochlin, G. 1961. The dread of abandonment. *Psychoanalytic Study of the Child* 15:451–469.

Wieder, H., and Kaplan, E. G. 1969. Drug use in adolescence:

psychodynamic meaning and pharmacogenic effect. *Psychoanalytic Study of the Child* 24:399–431.

Winnicott, D. W. 1963. Transitional objects and transitional phenomena. *International Journal of Psycho-Analysis* 34:89–97.

Wolfenstein, M. 1969. Loss, rage and repetition. *Psychoanalytic Study of the Child* 24:432–460.

37   SEVERE FEMALE DELINQUENCY: WHEN TO INVOLVE THE FAMILY IN TREATMENT

BRET BURQUEST

Most therapists working with delinquents agree that delinquency is a family problem and that usually the family should be involved in the treatment process. In this chapter we discuss a method by which the therapist can decide when and how to involve the family in treatment of the nonpsychotic, seriously delinquent, adolescent girl who has failed repeatedly in treatment and is detained in a residential setting. The issues here are of timing and flexibility. If the parents and other family members are involved appropriately at the most propitious time, their involvement will generally be helpful. Frequently it will be crucial. This may be so even if they are unwilling to regard the delinquency as a family problem, since their major contributions may be to clarify how little they are able or willing to do for the adolescent and to allow the adolescent to interact with them openly and constructively in a therapeutic setting.

There are excellent discussions in the literature of the indications and contraindications for family therapy (Offer and Vanderstoep 1974; Wynne 1965). Generally, much less is written about deciding when rather than if to involve the family. When a delinquent girl is sent by the court to a closed treatment facility, the therapist seeks a way to maintain the cooperation of the family while deciding whether the girl should be returned to live with that family. The fragility of some of these families is so great that special consideration must be given to the possibility of premature separation of the delinquent from the family because of therapeutic involvement. Some families will tolerate no stress in therapy. Other families will appear to agree with almost anything the therapist suggests in order to have the delinquent returned home. In modifying our approach to a wide range of family types, we utilize a flexible mixture of individual and family treatment as advocated by Ackerman (1958), Brown (1970), and Williams (1968, 1973).

Herein are guidelines to help the average family therapist avoid involving the family too soon or too routinely, common errors in our observation. Very skilled and experienced family therapists need no such guidelines, but we believe that these guidelines can be helpful to others. This is a simple and practical method derived from the experience of working with 150 delinquent girls over the past seven years in a Los Angeles County Probation Department School called the Dorothy Kirby Center.

These guidelines were developed with a certain kind of very difficult delinquent, namely, girls from age thirteen to seventeen, who before being sent by court order to the school, have had at least one trial in most if not all of the following treatment modalities: individual therapy, group therapy, family therapy, group-home and/or foster-home placement, and two months of intensive treatment in another closed facility run by the probation department. Some have also been in psychiatric hospitals. All are screened before admission to the school, and those diagnosed as mentally ill or mentally retarded are not admitted. Because of their long histories of delinquent activities and repeated failures in rehabilitation with every modality of therapy in the community, they have been confined to this school for a period of at least six months. This program is an effort to interrupt the destructive behavior patterns before the girls qualify for incarceration by the State of California or become eighteen, when their delinquent activities are viewed as criminal by the adult court.

These adolescents have established solidly delinquent behavior patterns. In addition to the usual truancy, curfew violation, and running away from home, they have used virtually all street drugs. Most have abused at least one drug and/or alcohol extensively. Most also admit to shoplifting, burglary, or auto theft. Many admit to crimes of violence and/or to prostitution. This behavior often has some support from the parents as has been reported by Johnson and Szurek (1952) and Reiser and Kaufman (1959). Their parents are mostly unsophisticated, lower-middle-class working people and are not fully aware how they support the girl's delinquent behavior. Others are not aware that they have choices of how to raise children, and they raise their children as they were raised. Some know they are encouraging delinquent behavior, and they do so because they enjoy their daughter's escapades.

In our experience with these families who have had so many failures at therapeutic interruption of the daughter's chronic delinquency, it is the unusual family that is again ready for immediate, constructive, therapeutic involvement of the whole family. Some therapists advocate "jumping in" with the whole family in an interview at the start of the girl's detention. We have not held such immediate family interviews here in recent years. We have noticed that in programs which involve immediate family therapy, daily group-therapy meetings of the girls are louder, there is generally more upset in the lives of the institutionalized girls, and there are more episodes of behavior requiring restriction by the institution. We believe that girls in such programs experience more chaos and less constructive working together than our girls. We work to avoid recreating the family chaos so familiar to many of our girls. We believe that they can learn best in a quiet, nurturing, close group.

We do not permit the adolescents to see their families until they have established a cooperative relationship with both the personnel in the school and with the girls with whom they live. We interview the parents or family early in the girl's incarceration, but we do not see the girl with her parents until all have established therapeutic relationships with the treatment staff. We allow no unsupervised visiting until all have begun to work together, clarifying their relationships and probing the difficulties within the family. Hence the progressive involvement of the family in the closed treatment of the severely delinquent adolescent girl can be conveniently divided into six phases: (1) separate interviews for the delinquent and family, (2) the establishment of therapeutic relationships between the therapist and each family member, (3) family interviews and elective family therapy with the delinquent, (4) unsupervised visiting between the family and the delinquent at the school, (5) a home visit by the therapist with the family and the delinquent, and (6) home visits by the delinquent without a therapist.

If the family interviews clarify that the best plan will be not to return the girl to her family, then family therapy will not be undertaken. In those cases there will be little direct contact between them during the balance of the detention. If during the unsupervised visiting the family undermines the therapy or encourages delinquency, the unsupervised visiting is stopped and the family is confronted with this behavior in therapy. The home visit is particularly important diagnostically and can tell the therapist a great deal about heretofore concealed problems at home and the readiness of the family to live together without delinquency.

The parents of chronically delinquent girls may be conveniently divided into three groups according to how they handle the delinquent behavior: (1) those who collude in the girl's delinquency, (2) those who oppose the delinquent behavior but cannot tolerate emotional demands from the daughter and/or any further challenge to their authority, and (3) those who do not try to restrict their daughter's behavior because they are symbiotically bound to her or have given up struggling to control her delinquency. These groups are not completely exclusive, and parents of type 1 (collusive) commonly appear as type 2 (intolerant) or more commonly as type 3 (permissive).

Daughters of the first type tend to continue living with their parents. Case example 1:

Suzi was a seventeen-year-old daughter of a fifty-five-year old movie producer, who described himself as an "overaged hippie." She was in intense competition with her sister for their father's approval. The parents had separated, and father had as a frequent weekend guest his girlfriend, whom he asked his daughter to keep secret from her mother. When Suzi was allowed home visits with father, he permitted her to spend her visits unsupervised in her bedroom where she became intoxicated and had sex with her boyfriend, while her father was in another part of the house. They had a tacit agreement that each could do whatever they wanted without fear of being reported to someone who might disapprove. Of course it was necessary to interrupt the home visits and work intensely, both individually and in family therapy, to stop the covert encouragement of her delinquency.

This case illustrates how a flexible approach is necessary to handle forcefully the behavior that was acted out during the treatment. It also illustrates that where there is collusion between the parents and the delinquent, family therapy should begin earlier than with the two other types of families. It is sometimes necessary to permit early, carefully controlled home visiting by the delinquent in order to clarify the covert parental encouragement of her delinquency.

The daughters in the second type of family (intolerant) have usually run away or been abandoned by the parents. There is a surprisingly high number of parents who have had little personal and comfortable contact with their daughters for months and who have virtually given up the idea of ever being able to live with their daughter again. Some refuse any kind of therapeutic involvement with the school or their child. In these cases it is important not to involve the family during the initial period of the adolescent's therapy until she has done some basic work with the treatment staff, establishes a strong relationship with them, feels less deprived, and is less selfish and hostile toward her parents. This is because when the parents and daughter are brought together for treatment, this type of parent generally does not trust her, and the daughter has to tolerate a great deal of verbal abuse before any work can be accomplished. Some adolescents work with the treatment staff for many weeks before they can feel secure enough to tolerate this parental attack. The opposite danger, of course, is that the child will express so much hostility toward the parent that she will totally alienate the parent. In such cases, the daughter forces a continued separation because the parent refuses to have anything to do with the daughter's treatment. This premature separation is usually not accompanied by significant individuation and, in fact, frequently brings about regression, which results in depression or acting out. Case example 2:

Molli was a fourteen-year-old whose mother took good care of her until she was three years of age. At that point mother went away for a month to have an affair. During the next ten years, the daughter was raised by her mother and her second husband, but both parents admitted to not taking care of Molli's emotional needs. In fact, her serious delinquent behavior began when her mother impulsively sent her to live with Molli's father at age twelve. She ran away to return to her mother's home. However, not long afterward, mother traveled to South America with her boyfriend for a few months and left Molli with a friend of hers. By the time mother returned from South America, Molli had been in enough trouble to be confined to juvenile hall where it was recommended that she be sent to the Dorothy Kirby Center. The girl desperately wanted to live with her mother, but knew she could not make any demands on her emotionally. A long period of intensive work with the girl alone was necessary to meet some of her dependency needs and to permit expression of a great deal of anger so that mother would not abandon her totally when faced with her daughter's anger. Mother was willing to take Molli home only on the condition that the girl obey. Although it seemed questionable whether mother would be able to provide the kind of home Molli needed, it was clear that Molli would run away from any placement to be with her mother. Despite mother's intensive individual and weekly family therapy, she did not become much warmer. However, she did develop the capacity to tolerate some disobedience from her daughter so that Molli would not have to behave in a delinquent manner to get her attention.

Daughters from the third type of family (permissive) are generally living with the parents, but frequently spend a few days at a time away from home without their parents' permission. Case example 3:

Keri was a seventeen-year-old with a history of drug abuse. She was addicted to heroin and maintained her habit by stealing, particularly burglarizing homes. She was a bright and verbal girl, but lacked inner controls and seemed to need to test limits. Her parents, however, were completely unable to control her. Mother, feeling extremely guilty about being a "bad parent," was easily manipulated by her daughter. Her father was also ineffective as a disciplinarian since he was symbiotically bound to her and was willing to have her at home under any conditions. Although we worked first with the parents and the daughter separately, and then with them together in family treatment, it became apparent that the parents were never going to develop the capacity to set limits for her. Ultimately she was placed with the Job Corps.

Perhaps the most difficult cases are those of the third type (permissive) in which the daughter has been adopted by a gang, relates to the gang as her family, but has continued to live at home. In such cases, after being arrested, the adolescent knows the parents will put up with almost any behavior and are unable or unwilling to assume the parental role. Consequently, if family therapy is to be tried immediately, the parents require a period of time and support to regain the ability to set reasonable limits.

By forcing separation of the daughter from her parents, we gain much more control in the treatment. However, recent changes in the law have diminished this control by allowing girls and parents to correspond confidentially. Some parents now continue their antitherapeutic permissiveness through the mails, while they present a therapeutic facade in interviews. Case example 4:

Jodi is a fifteen-year-old who was adopted by a childless couple at age nine months because her adoptive father became alarmed at the neglectful conditions under which she was living. The adoptive parents were fifty and sixty years of age. They viewed her as a sweet girl and denied her gang involvement. They blamed the police and the probation department for her troubles even though she was a gang leader. When during a family interview she confirmed that she was a gang member, they said she had to leave the gang in order to continue living with them. But immediately following this session, they wrote that they did not agree with the therapists and they would never make her leave home no matter what she did.

With these families, the most important therapeutic task is to confront the parents with their unwillingness to set limits and their ability to undermine the therapeutic efforts.

In the treatment of almost all of these acting-out delinquents, it is more effective to begin with separate interviews. We have seen a few families, however, who have appeared to continue struggling with daughters who have not run away for long periods. The parents behave as though their daughters are totally out of their control and ignore the daughters' willingness to work together despite all the difficulties. Families of this type are more amenable to immediate family interviewing and therapy. When families do not collude with the girl in continuing her delinquency, there is a healthier family structure, the girl is usually less disturbed, and the whole family responds more quickly in treatment.

Conclusions

Our experience in working with delinquent girls has clarified how to approach families that have experienced massive delinquent behavior and have been unsuccessful in many treatment attempts. After proper classification and treatment, both parents and the adolescent girl are able to continue visits together. Thus, for families in which delinquent behavior has been truly severe, enforced separation, followed by controlled reuniting of the families, has resulted in more effective treatment.

REFERENCES

Ackerman, N. W. 1958. *The Psychodynamics of Family Life.* New York: Basic.

Brown, S. L. 1970. Family therapy for adolescents. *Psychiatric Opinion* 7:1–13.

Johnson, A., and Szurek, S. 1952. The genesis of anti-social acting-out in children and adults. *Psychoanalytic Quarterly* 21:322–343.

Offer, D., and Vanderstoep, E. 1974. Indications and contraindications for family therapy. *Adolescent Psychiatry* 3:249–262.

Reiser, D. and Kaufman, I. 1959. *Character Disorders in Parents of Delinquents.* New York: Family Service Association of America.

Williams, F. S. 1968. Family therapy. In J. Marmor, ed. *Modern Psychoanalysis.* New York: Basic.

Williams, F. S. 1973. Family therapy: its role in adolescent psychiatry. *Adolescent Psychiatry* 2:324–339.

Wynne, L. C. 1965. Some indications and contraindications for exploratory family therapy. In I. Boszormenyi-Nagy and J. S. Framo, eds. *Intensive Family Therapy: Theoretical and Practical Aspects.* New York: Harper & Row.

ELISSA BENEDEK

The girl (myself) is walking through Branden's, that excellent store in a suburb of a large, famous city that is a symbol for large famous American cities. The event sneaks up on the girl who believes she is herding it along with a small, fixed smile, a girl of 15, innocently experienced. She dawdles in a certain style by a counter of costume jewelry. Rings, earrings, necklaces. Prices from $5.00–$50.00, all within reach, all ugly. She eases over to the glove counter where everything is ugly, too. In her close fitted coat, with its black fur collar, she contemplates the luxury of Branden's which she has known for many years. Many mild, pale lights, easy on the eye and the soul, its elaborate tinkly decorations, its women shoppers with their excellent shoes and coats and hairdos, all dawdling gracefully, in no hurry.

The girl's heart is pounding! In her pocket is a pair of gloves! In a plastic bag! Airproof, breathproof, plastic bag, gloves, selling for $25.00 on Branden's counter! In her pocket! Shoplifted . . . In her purse is a blue comb, not very clean. In her purse is a leather billfold (a birthday present from her grandmother in Philadelphia,) with snapshots of her family in clean, plastic windows, in the billfold are bills, she doesn't know how many bills. In her purse is a lot of dirty yellow kleenex. Her mother's heart would break to see such very dirty kleenex, and at the bottom of her purse are brown hairpins and safety pins, and a broken pencil and a ballpoint pen, stolen from somewhere forgotten and a purse size compact of *Cover Girl* makeup, Ivory Rose. Her lipstick is Broken Heart, a corrupt pink; her fingers are trembling like crazy; her teeth are beginning to chatter; her insides are alive; her eyes glow in her head; she is saying to her mother's astonished face: "I want to steal, but not buy." [Oates 1970][1]

Delinquent behavior is a norm-violating behavior of a juvenile which, if detected by an appropriate authority, would expose the author to legally prescribed sanctions. The charge "official delinquency" is the identification of and response to delinquent behavior by the courts (Williams and Gold 1972). Those acts performed by juveniles which are considered delinquent fall into three basic categories: (1) those which are considered delinquent regardless of whether they are committed by a juvenile or an adult, because they violate criminal laws—for example, stealing, assault on human life; (2) those which violate societal mores as agreed upon generally by our particular society, regardless of whether the person is a juvenile or an adult—for example, forms of sexual behavior; and (3) those which are violations only because the person is a minor—for example, truancy from school, teenage drinking, runaway behavior. Adolescent girls are judged delinquent and committed to training schools most frequently for the "big 5 offenses" (Veder and Somerville 1970): runaway behavior, ungovernability, sex offenses, truancy, and curfew violations. In contrast, boys are referred to juvenile courts, in order of frequency, for larcency, burglary, and auto theft. Just as there are a variety of definitions for juvenile delinquency and for the juvenile delinquent, each of the offenses has a different legal definition, depending on city, county, or state. Juvenile delinquency discussed in this chapter excludes acts of terrorism or political crimes.

Demography and Epidemiology

Commenting on the art of criminal statistics, Doleschal (1972) cautions that anyone who tries to uncover facts and figures about crime and criminals learns quickly that there are many figures but few facts. Whether data exist that are adequate for any particular purpose depends on the exact nature of that purpose. If little more is required than an impression of a condition in criminal justice, some available information, if used with extreme care, can be of limited use. Doleschal cites the following important information that should be provided by the criminal justice system: (1) information about the types of crime committed; (2) information about circumstances surrounding crime; (3) information about the kinds of persons involved; (4) information about disposal decided upon by the courts or other authorities; (5) information about first offenders, including sex, age, and other social and psychological data; and (6) cost of maintaining services connected with detection and prevention of crime. Each of these categories might be examined if one wanted to discover statistical data about the juvenile female offender, but the searcher would quickly discover little or no data in most categories.

The official criminal justice system provides little or no relevant statistical information about the incidence and types of female crime which might help the researcher to describe its nature and to determine if it is increasing. Four sources of data illustrate problems in data collection: (1) self-report data, (2) FBI statistics (which are supposed to be a reflection of police apprehension), (3) HEW statistics (which are supposed to reflect cases handled by the juvenile court; and (4) Washtenaw County (an urban county in Michigan) statistics (1967–1972). An exact statistical portrayal of the female juvenile delinquent, however, is impossible to obtain. Although the mass media, via newspapers and television, indicate that female juvenile delinquency is on the rise, official statistics offer no conclusive evidence. Statistics might be broadly interpreted to show the following trends: (1) the lesser incidence of female juvenile delinquency, compared with male juvenile delinquency, in all reported statistics, and (2) the different type of crimes committed by females. I caution the reader, however, that professionals in the field almost unanimously agree that major statistics cannot be used for comparison between one locality and another, or between one time period and another.

One of the first sources of data about the female in the criminal justice system is self-report data. Williams and Gold (1972) have emphasized the importance of collecting self-report data on female delinquents. They observe that if one considers official delinquency—that is, delinquency recorded in police records and on court dockets to be representative of all delinquent behavior—the notion that delinquency is a black, male, lower-socioeconomic-class phenomenon is supported, since officials treat young, white, female first offenders differently and certainly do not record their delinquent behavior as often in court records or on court dockets. Using data drawn from interviews and records of the 847 thirteen- to sixteen-year-old boys and girls comprising the probability sample of a 1967 national survey of youth, Williams and Gold (1972) show that self-report data on delinquency and police-contact data differ greatly from those data found in police and court records. In general, they note: "It is clear that if authorities were omniscient and technically zealous, a large majority of American 13–16 year olds would be labelled juvenile delinquents but it is also clear that the number of adolescent delinquents decreases sharply as the measures indicate more frequent and serious delinquent behavior" (p. 210). It is especially important to note that 88 percent of the teenagers in their sample confessed to committing at least one chargeable offense in the three years prior to interview, but less than 3 percent of the offenses reported by the teenagers were detected by the police and less than 2 percent of the youngsters had ever been under judicial consideration. According to these authors, then, self-report data, police-contact data, and juvenile-court data all show an increased incidence of juvenile delinquency, if one simply looks at the statistics.

For our purposes, it is also important to note that Williams and Gold report that American girls describe themselves as exhibiting much less delinquent behavior than American boys. When girls are delinquent, they are delinquent less often and less seriously than boys. The self-report data also indicate that more boys are caught by police for delinquent acts; however, once caught, approximately the same percentages (19 percent of the boys and 17 percent of the girls) had been put on the police blotter and officially identified by the police. Williams and Gold subsequently searched court records but could come to no conclusion about court dispositions related to the sex of the offender. Incidentally, their self-report data conflict with Pollock's (1950) hypothesis that, once caught, female adult offenders are treated in a more chivalrous fashion by police and courts.

Turning from self-report data, let us look at the first official source of data about female crime. Local police reports are compiled nationally in the Uniform Crime Reports. Simon (1975) offers a word of special caution about interpreting FBI statistics in regard to women. She notes that FBI statistics describe arrests, not known or observed behavior at the scene of the crime. From arrests, we can infer participation in the crime, but, in discussing women in crime, this inference might be especially fanciful because of the discretion possible for police and the way in which they have in the past been presumed to exercise that discretion. Simon, however, has interpreted the 1972 FBI arrest data to

527

show an increase in female arrest rate owing almost entirely to women's greater participation in property offenses, especially larceny. Interpreting these statistics, she demonstrates that female arrest rates for violent crimes have hardly changed at all over the past two years. Arrest rates for homicide, for example, have been the most stable of all violent offenses. She does note that arrests for offenses showing the greatest increases are embezzlement and fraud, forgery, and counterfeiting. Simon does not feel that police are becoming less chivalrous to women suspects and that women are beginning to receive more equal treatment at their hands since there is a sharp increase in occupationally related crime—larceny, fraud, and embezzlement—but not in crimes of violence. Her explanation for this increase is that women's opportunities to commit crime are increasing as they enter the work force, and their criminal behavior is commensurate with their opportunity.

The next source of quasi-reliable data available to us as we attempt to interpret the most reliable statistics about female crime is data from the Department of Health, Education, and Welfare which is said to reflect the number of delinquency cases handled by juvenile courts, excluding traffic offenses. These data, then, exclude all delinquents who are apprehended by police, but were not officially charged. Stone (1975), in discussing the national increase in juvenile crime, cites statistics obtained from the department: "In 1971, 1,125,000 delinquency cases were handled by all juvenile courts." He observes that the actual number of cases handled by courts had increased every year since 1960, and the rate of increase has been greater in each succeeding year. He, too, interprets HEW statistics as showing that delinquency among girls is rising faster than among boys, and the ratio of girls to boys adjudicated by juvenile courts has dropped from four to one to three to one.

Finally, one last source of statistics is the Washtenaw County Juvenile Court (1967–1972), a sophisticated urban court whose officials, too, feel that female delinquency is on the rise and support their intuition with the following statistical information. The local court administrator notes that the ratio of boys to girls in traffic court, 85 percent to 15 percent, has remained constant between 1967 and 1972, but the percentage of girls among those referred on delinquency petitions is increasing. In 1971 adolescent girls represented 30.59 percent of the court population (we would assume this means cases adjudicated by the court), but that number rose to 37.28 percent in the last half of

1972, to give an average of 35.25 percent of court population being girls. The court also reports that 35 percent of all the allegations directed toward girls have to do with sexual misbehavior.

Even casual perusal of the material cited above makes it clear that the art of statistic keeping in regard to female delinquents is primitive. Self-report data, arrest data, and court data are not comparable. Each set of data is flawed. In self-report data, youngsters, fearful of detection, may not accurately declare the number of delinquent acts they have been involved in, whereas other youngsters, in a mood of bravado, may brag to investigators. The FBI data report only arrests, and there is no measure for those who may be guilty but are not arrested and those who may be innocent and are arrested. The HEW statistics simply show the number of cases handled by the juvenile court and give no information as to innocence or guilt and disposition, and, finally, when one looks at local court statistics, it is difficult to discover what, in fact, administrators are measuring. However, all who interpret statistics seem to agree that female delinquency is on the rise.

Etiology

The girl thinks as a stubborn and wayward child (one of several charges lodged against her) and the matron understands her crazy, white rimmed eyes that are seeking out some new violence that will keep her in jail, should someone threaten to let her out. Such children try to strangle the matrons, the attendants or one another . . . they want the locks locked forever, the doors nailed shut . . . and this girl is no different up until that night her mind is changed for her. [Oates 1970]

The etiology of female delinquency can best be categorized under three general classifications: psychological, sociological, and organic. Psychological theories of female delinquency find their origin in Freud's (1933) conception of the healthy female with passive, emotional, narcissistic, and deceitful tendencies. The healthy female is cursed with a weak superego because of a difficult resolution of the oedipal conflict. Later psychological theorists expanded the concept of the weak superego, adding the notion of parental superego lacunae which allow delinquent adolescents to act out vicariously parental fantasies and wishes (Johnson 1949). Blos (1963) comments on two types of female delinquents, adolescent females who have regressed to preoedipal stages and youngsters who desperately cling to a foothold in the oedipal stage.

Konopka (1966) presents a more encompassing psychological theory. She postulates a biological onset of puberty in the adolescent girl and a more complex psychological identification, that is, the adolescent girl must resolve her oedipal conflict by reidentifying with her mother or the person who nurtured her as a baby. "This creates special resistance and explains the frequent conflict with mothers in early adolescence." She suggests that the sexual promiscuity of these girls is not really for pleasure but, rather, is used by them to demonstrate that they are not afraid of men or intercourse when actually they are very much afraid and often express real guilt over their actions. However, Konopka begins to touch on some of the more sociological theories of delinquency, suggesting that prevalent culture and cultural changes affect all women and especially female delinquents. She cites the following sociological factors as impacting on a delinquent girl's behavior: only traditional vocational training for women, leading to stereotyped and low-paying employment, thwarted ambition, little legitimate outlet for aggressive drives with the ideal image of a girl still being sugar and spice, and increased awareness and resentment of the sexual double standard.

Maccoby and Jacklin (1974), in their volume reviewing the nature and extent of sexual differences, made the following psychological observations about commonly assumed myths that have application to female delinquency. Concerning unfounded beliefs about sexual differences, they dispute suggestions that girls are more socially oriented than boys, more suggestible, more auditory, less visual, and less analytic but better at rote learning and lower in self-esteem and achievement motivation. They do, however, comment that boys more often see themselves as strong, powerful, dominant, and potent than do girls. They find the following important sex difference well established: "The sex difference in aggression has been observed in all cultures in which relevant behavior has been observed. Boys are more aggressive, both physically and verbally. The sex difference is found as early as social play begins at age 2 or 2½ although the aggressiveness of both sexes declines with age, boys and men remain more aggressive through college years."

530

Klein (1973), in a critique of psychological theories, deplores the tendency to see persons moving in a sociological and political vacuum and believes prescriptions for individual or group therapy are useless if recommendations for environmental change dealing with racism and sexism are ignored. Felice and Offord (1971) support this position after an extensive review of psychological testing in female delinquents. They summarize data suggesting that, in general, studies on female delinquents utilizing personality tests are poorly controlled and inconclusive. These authors find no clear associations between female delinquent behavior and any specific personality characteristics. However, in describing the family of the female delinquent, they are able to distinguish between middle-class delinquency and lower-class delinquency. In children from unstable economic backgrounds, they note the following family patterns: an abusive or absent father, an overworked mother who may turn to alcoholism and prostitution, parental promiscuity, and high illegitimacy rates. Delinquents from middle and upper socioeconomic classes, in contrast, are described as suffering from some form of "parental exploitation." This may be comparable to the parental behavior described by Johnson (1949).

Sociologists, in contrast to psychologists, have concentrated on an investigation of such factors as the broken home, lack of discipline, bad companions, lack of organized leisure time, economic conditions, and anomie or normlessness. According to Reckless (1967), the behavioral scientists of the United States would not accept a solely biological or psychological causality of delinquency and tend to focus more on sociology. Shaw and McKay (1931) noted high delinquency rates in areas of declining population, physical deterioration, and high concentrations of foreign-born and black populations. These authors describe the high concentration of delinquent youngsters found in slum areas of a city inhabited by lower-socioeconomic classes.

Debate has centered, however, on whether sociological conditions, such as poverty, racism, and broken homes, have a causal factor in female delinquency or simply play a role in the official identification. Both Sarri and Gold (1975) note that "getting caught" is related to social class, race, and previous delinquency. Their data clearly indicate differences in regard to race when juvenile-court referrals are made. Halleck (1967), too, comments on the role of socioeconomic class in getting caught. He contrasts the college girl who flaunts rules and regulations and is seen as a healthy, rebelling adolescent involved in pranks with the lower-socioeconomic-status adolescent whose promiscuity and shoplifting are labeled "delinquency." He also describes the differential treatment of such behavior in the community. In his experience, upper- and middle-class girls are put on probation or sent to a mental hospital, whereas female adolescents who come from "nonrespectable or broken homes" end up in training schools.

Datesman, Scarpitti, and Stephenson (1975), looking at female delinquency from the perspective of self and opportunity theories, caution that most sociological research has been done by social scientists who oriented their research instruments toward the male role and its particular articulation within the economic and occupational structure. They raise questions about the validity of any sociological research where scales designed for males are applied to females, and they further elaborate that the study of female delinquency requires, first of all, an understanding of the female role as it is embedded in the social structure. Sutherland and Cressey (1960) attributed differential crime rates to the social positions of girls and women as compared with boys and men. They hypothesized that the differences in social position determine either the frequency or intensity of delinquency and antidelinquency patterns (whatever they may be) and determine the frequency of opportunities for crime which were available to them. These authors, too, looking at differential sex roles and the socialization of girls —that is, the tendency to teach girls to be nice and boys to be rough and tough—postulate that sex-role socialization contributes to the lesser incidence of delinquency in females. They observe that the female crime rate shows some tendency to approach closest to the male crime rate in countries where females have the greatest freedom and equality with males, such as Western Europe, Australia, and the United States, and vary most from the male rate in countries where females are still closely supervised, such as Japan and Algiers.

Simon (1975) and Adler (1975) focus on the role of opportunity in criminal acts by young women. These two authors have a different perspective from past authors who perceived lack of opportunity as a factor in juvenile crime. Simon and Adler hypothesize that women's liberation opens new opportunities to women to participate in the labor force. They suggest that increased opportunity will present new vistas of criminal activity to employed teenagers. They also postulate a large increase in white-collar crime, including embezzlement.

Generally, though, sociologists have attributed similar causality to male and female delinquency and have not separated out the relationship between sex-role and other social variables. Datesman, Scarpitti, and Stephenson (1975) caution researchers about the biasing factors inherent in using studies designed and tested on male adolescents with females and state, "The usefulness of interpreting a female response within a framework designed for males is limited." Parlee (1975), too, has questioned the effect of the sex of the researcher, generally male, on design of research study. Parlee notes that when aggression is studied the research subject is primarily male and when sexuality is studied the research subject is primarily female. The importance of sex-role socialization and its impact on adolescent delinquency has only recently come to the attention of researchers. Grosser (1958), in an early study, pointed out that stealing is a typical delinquency behavior. This articulates poorly with society's current definition of the female role, as stealing requires skill, courage, and prowess, none of which are acceptable female behavior patterns but all of which are accepted male behavior patterns. Grosser pointed out a twofold relationship between crime and sex roles: crime is a means of attaining some goals specified by the sex role, and crime can express through a deviant form behavior patterns which are valued because they are role appropriate.

Finally, although psychological and sociological theories for female delinquency are more prevalent, mention must be made of organic dysfunction, especially in three important areas: brain dysfunction, chromosomal abnormality, and hormonal relationships. Lombroso (1958), the putative father of the constitutional approach, stresses the thesis that criminals differ physically and physiologically from noncriminals, and, as one descends the developmental scale, the most poorly developed and physiologically deficient order of criminal behavior is the female offender. The relationship of brain dysfunction, including epilepsy and minimal brain dysfunction, to criminal behavior is controversial. Some authors describe clinical and EEG evidence (Monroe 1970) of brain dysfunction, especially in violent offenders (Mark and Irvin 1970). Other authors dispute this research, and the issue is unresolved at the present time (Rodin 1973). In males, a chromosomal abnormality XYY has been described, studied, and linked to institutionalized populations. In recent studies, however, other factors in the background of institutionalized patients are more correlative with their institutionalization than are their genes.

Questions about the effects of hormonal changes on young women's behavior have been posed for a long time but never answered definitively. Deutsch (1944) commented on primitive fantasies delinquent girls had about menstruation, including ideas of damage, castration, dirty feelings, and concerns about an inability to stop the menstrual flow (also see Dalton 1964). Some question whether, in a youngster with a delinquent character formation, ego and superego deal with universal fantasies differentially. Seiden (1977) notes that, surprisingly, after all these centuries of human menstruation, we do not have data about the subject. She suggests, as does Parlee (1975), that prolonged stressful situations culminating in attempted suicide, violent crimes, or poor examination performance prior to menstrual periods can sometimes represent tension-delayed menstruation instead of premenstrual tension. Others, such as Cowie, Cowie-Slater, and Somerville (1968) and Veder and Somerville (1970), have correlated both early and late maturation with delinquent behavior, but the research methodology has not been confirmed.

Treatment of the Female Delinquent

Princess Andali, a little white girl of maybe 15, hardy, however, is a sergeant in the House of Corrections for Armed Robbery. Corner her in the lavatory at the farthest sink and the other girls look away and file to bed, leaving her. God, she is beaten up. Why is she beaten up? Why do they pound her? Why such hatred? Princess vents all the hatred of a thousand silent Detroit winters on her body, this girl whose body belongs to me fiercely. She rides across the midwestern plains on this girl's tender, bruised body. [Oates 1970]

An extensive discussion of the treatment of the female offender in the juvenile justice system is beyond the scope and intent of this review. Needless to say, she is treated differently. Pollock (1950) reported his speculations that women are treated more leniently by the machinery of law enforcement, a sentiment which was echoed by others. He described patrolmen and male detectives who did not like to arrest women, prosecutors who had difficulties in achieving convictions, and judges and juries who were chivalrous and acquitted women despite extensive evidence of their guilt. In contrast, Chesney-Lind (1973) postulated a theory that the court sees female offenses in sexual terms and then severely sanctions them. She supports her position with data from the Honolulu Juvenile Court. She sees courts as a reflection of the morality of the community. In the community, female adolescents have traditionally had a narrower range of acceptable behavior. Even minor deviance is seen as a substantial challenge to the authority of the family. The double standard is incorporated into the courts and serves to maintain the system of sexual inequality. She comments: "It is the symbolic threat posed by female delinquents to these values that best explains: 1) why the juvenile court system selects aspects of female deviance which violate sexual expectations rather than those which violate legal norms and 2) why female delinquency is therefore, more severely sanctioned." Her conclusions are supported by evidence of differential administration of physical examinations, especially gynecological, and differential predetention and detention policies allowing for more females with minor offenses to be detained before trial and subsequently confined in correctional facilities.

Sarri and Gold (1975) observed that in their experience women once sentenced are more likely to be dealt with punitively by the criminal justice system. She notes that the placement of juvenile females in jails is increasing more rapidly than that of males in several states. For example, she cites Wisconsin, where there were 2,875 males and 768 females in adult jails in 1961. In 1972, there were 7,032 males and 2,892 females, a 277 percent increase for females versus 145 percent for males. She also cites the following areas of concern: (1) an overrepresentation of females in institutional populations as compared to day treatment centers or group homes—that is, females are more likely to be assigned to programs which involve removal from their homes; (2) a more limited range of dispositional alternatives for females; (3) females in correctional programs were disproportionately committed for status offenses (57 percent status, 16 percent drug, 12 percent property, and 12 percent personal offenses); (4) females were committed disproportionately for offenses which have little, if any, relationship to protection of the community, yet they were placed in institutions more frequently and held for longer periods of time; (5) younger, rather than older, youths were placed in institutions as compared to residential or day treatment programs, and thus the concept of lesser penetration has not been applied, since these younger females are more often status offenders. Analysis of prior correctional experience indicates that, despite the fact that juvenile females commit fewer felonies and misdemeanors than males, they have extensive contact with the justice system. Arrested females have a mean arrest rate of 4.6 times, an average of 3.8 times in detention, 2.0 times in jail, and 1.3 times in an institution. Foster care and probation are underutilized compared to these more stringent sanctions, with a mean of 1.5 and 1.4.

Sarri and Gold (1975), reviewing institutional programs for female delinquents, note that there are fewer internal education programs with less diversity and fewer external programs, fewer work release programs, and fewer alternatives to institutionalization. Felice and Offord (1971), reviewing institutional problems, note a high incidence of homosexuality and gynecological and obstetrical problems in female institutions. Previously, we have discussed the role of the social system in supporting a certain mythology in sex-role stereotyping. Institutions are notoriously slow in changing the internal education programs that exist for females. Training schools feature jobs in domestic service and an occasional enlightened program has a course in cosmetology. Alternative vocational programs which are more likely to interest these deviant girls are nonexistent and are not likely to be funded as they are considered luxurious by the general public and a form of pampering. The lack of treatment alternatives for the female juvenile delinquent is the most serious problem confronting our juvenile justice system. As right-to-treatment issues become more prevalent, it might be that litigation, such as class-action suits in which juveniles have claimed a deprivation of liberty for promise of treatment which is not forthcoming, will force legislators to examine their budgeting priorities and the public to probe its consciousness. Such litigation may act as a stimulus prodding community mental health centers to develop a range of treatment programs and options for female delinquents.

Conclusions

The female juvenile delinquent does exist. We do not know her numbers. She is defined by law, apprehended by police, sentenced by juvenile judges, and treated in juvenile institutions. Professionals do not understand the etiology of her actions, nor are they equipped to rehabilitate her. The dilemma of female juvenile delinquency is not a new one, but its solutions will have to be innovative and creative. I look to two areas, hopefully, for insight and resolution:

1. *Research by interested female and male professionals in this understudied area.*—A theory which can correlate sociology, biology, and psychology to a meaningful theory of delinquency is nonexistent. Most authors agree that we know little about female juvenile delinquency for two readily apparent reasons: (1) the low social status of female delinquency and (2) the low social status accorded researchers in that area. Seiden suggests, and I concur, that a new group of young women interested in women's problems may be productive of new hypotheses and formulations. "Research done on women by women will often ask different questions and examine different data than research conducted from male points of view" (Seiden 1977). She is optimistic that there will be a continued growth of research attention bearing on women's lives and that the influx of women researchers interested in women's areas will generate a scientific theory which will explain and help understand the behavior of the female.

2. *Right-to-treatment cases.*—As *Gault* (1967) and *Winship* (1970) have begun to legalize treatment of the juvenile offender, there have been unanticipated side effects. Constitutional rights of the female offender have been examined and extended. Right-to-treatment class-action suits have forced the close of some institutions for juveniles (*Morales* v. *Turman* [1973]) and the deinstitutionalization of others. Federal regulations dealing with treatment of status offenders have improved their lot, and I look to the courts for further improvement in the identification and treatment of these young women. I hope that research and legal activity will shed light on the identification and understanding and treatment of the youngest and the most neglected female in our society, the female juvenile offender.

NOTE

1. The quotations at the beginning of each section are from Joyce Carol Oates, *The Wheel of Love: How I Contemplated the World from the Detroit House of Correction and Began My Life over Again* (Fawcett Crest Press, 1970). Reprinted with permission.

REFERENCES

Adler, F. 1975. *Sisters in Crime*. New York: McGraw-Hill.
Blos, P. 1963. Female delinquency: three typical constellations. Paper

537

presented at the Annual Conference of the American Orthopsychiatric Association, Washington, D.C., March 1963.

Chesney-Lind, M. 1973. Judicial enforcement of the female sex role: the family court and the female delinquent. *Issues in Criminology* 8(2): 51–61.

Cowie, J. V.; Cowie-Slater, E.; and Somerville, D. B. 1968. *Delinquency in Girls*. London: Heinemann.

Dalton, K. 1964. *The Premenstrual Syndrome*. Springfield, Ill.: Thomas.

Datesman, S. K.; Scarpitti, F. R.; and Stephenson, R. M. 1975. Female delinquency: an application of self and opportunities theory. *Journal of Research in Crime and Delinquency* 7:107–123.

Deutsch, H. 1944. *The Psychology of Women*. Vol. 1. New York: Grune & Stratton.

Doleschal, E. 1972. *Criminal Statistics*. Publication No. (HSM) 729094.

Felice, M., and Offord, D. R. 1971. Girl delinquency: a review. *Corrective Psychiatry and Journal of Social Therapy* 17:1–26.

Freud, S. 1933. *Conception of the Healthy Female*. New York: Norton.

In re Gault. 1967. 387 U.S. at 1.

Grosser, G. H. 1958. Juvenile delinquency in contemporary American sex roles. Ph.D. dissertation, Harvard University.

Halleck, S. 1967. *Psychiatry and the Dilemmas of Crime*. New York: Harper & Row.

Johnson, A. M. 1949. Sanction for superego lacunae of adolescence. In K. R. Eissler, ed. *Searchlights on Delinquency*. New York: International Universities Press.

Klein, D. 1973. The etiology of female crime: a review of the literature. *Issues in Criminology* 8:3–29.

Konopka, G. 1966. *Adolescent Girl in Conflict*. Englewood Cliffs, N.J.: Prentice-Hall.

Lombroso, P. 1958. *The Female Offender*. New York: Wisdom Library.

Maccoby, E., and Jacklin, C. 1974. *The Psychology of Sex Differences*. Palo Alto, Calif.: Stanford University Press.

Mark, V. H., and Irvin, F. R. 1970. *Violence and the Brain*. New York: Harper & Row.

Monroe, R. 1970. *Episodic Behavior Disorders: A Psychodynamic and*

Neurophysiologic Analysis. Cambridge, Mass.: Harvard University Press.

Morales v. Turman. 1973. 364 F. Supp. 166.

Oates, J. C. 1970. *The Wheel of Love: How I Contemplated the World from the Detroit House of Correction and Began My Life over Again*. Greenwich, Conn.: Fawcett Crest.

Parlee, M. 1975. Psychological aspects of menstruation, childbirth and menopause: an overview of suggestions for further research. Paper presented at the Conference on New Directions for Research on Women, Madison, Wisconsin, May 31–June 2, 1975.

Pollock, O. 1950. *The Criminality of Women*. Philadelphia: University of Pennsylvania Press.

Reckless, W. 1967. *The Crime Problem*. New York: Appleton-Century-Crofts.

Rodin, E. A. 1973. Psychomotor epilepsy in aggressive behavior. *Archives of General Psychiatry* 28:210–213.

Sarri, R., and Gold, M. 1975. *The Female Offender: An Annotated Bibliography*. Ann Arbor: University of Michigan School of Social Work.

Seiden, A. M. 1977. Overview: research on the psychology of women. I. Gender differences, sexual and reproductive life. *American Journal of Psychiatry* 133(9): 995–1007.

Shaw, C. R., and McKay, H. D. 1931. *Social Factors in Juvenile Delinquency*. Washington, D.C.: National Commission of Law Observance and Enforcement.

Simon, R. 1975. *Women and Crime*. Lexington, Mass.: Heath.

Stone, A. 1975. *Mental Health and the Law: A System in Transition*. Rockville, Md.: National Institute of Mental Health Center for Studies of Crime and Delinquency.

Sutherland, E. H., and Cressey, D. R. 1960. *Principles of Criminology*. Chicago: Lippincott.

Veder, C. B., and Somerville, D. B. 1970. *The Delinquent Girl*. Springfield, Ill.: Thomas.

Washtenaw County Juvenile Court. 1967–1972. Six year report. Mimeographed. Washtenaw County, Michigan.

Williams, J. R., and Gold, M. 1972. From delinquent behavior to official delinquency. *Social Problems* 20:209–229.

In re Winship. 1970. 397 U.S. at 358.

THE AUTHORS

DAVID P. AGLE is Associate Professor of Psychiatry, Case Western Reserve University School of Medicine, Cleveland, Ohio.

ROBERT L. ARNSTEIN is Clinical Professor of Psychiatry, Yale University School of Medicine, and Chief Psychiatrist, Division of Mental Hygiene, Yale University Health Services.

ELISSA BENEDEK is Clinical Associate Professor of Psychiatry, University of Michigan Medical Center, and Director of Training and Education, Center for Forensic Psychiatry, Ann Arbor, Michigan.

SAMUEL BLACK is Assistant Clinical Professor of Psychiatry, University of California at Los Angeles.

PETER BLOS is Lecturer, New York Psychoanalytic Institute and Columbia Psychoanalytic Clinic for Training and Research. He received the 1969 William A. Schonfeld Distinguished Service Award of the American Society for Adolescent Psychiatry.

ELIZABETH BRETT is Assistant Clinical Professor of Psychology in Psychiatry, Yale University School of Medicine.

HILDE BRUCH is Emeritus Professor of Psychiatry, Baylor College of Medicine. She is the 1978 recipient of the William A. Schonfeld Distinguished Service Award of the American Society for Adolescent Psychiatry.

ALBERT BRYT is Clinical Assistant Professor of Psychiatry, New York University School of Medicine, and Training and Supervising Analyst, William Alanson White Institute, New York.

BRET BURQUEST is Assistant Clinical Professor of Psychiatry, University of California at Los Angeles Center for Health Sciences.

DENNIS P. CANTWELL is Associate Professor of Child Psychiatry, University of California at Los Angeles.

GABRIELLE A. CARLSON is Research Fellow in Child Psychiatry, University of California at Los Angeles.

ALEXANDER DEUTSCH is Clinical Assistant Professor of Psychiatry, New York University School of Medicine, and Chief, Psychiatric Outpatient Clinic, Cabrini Medical Center, New York.

SHERMAN C. FEINSTEIN is Clinical Professor, Pritzker School of Medicine, University of Chicago, and Director, Child Psychiatry Research, Psychosomatic and Psychiatric Institute, Michael Reese Medical Center. He is Past President, American Society for Adolescent Psychiatry and a Managing Editor of this volume.

PETER L. GIOVACCHINI is Clinical Professor of Psychiatry, Abraham Lincoln College of Medicine, University of Illinois, and a Managing Editor of this volume.

JAMES S. GORDON is Research Psychiatrist and Consultant on Alternative Forms of Service, Center for Studies of Child and Family Mental Health, National Institute of Mental Health.

RAPHAEL GREENBERG is Chief of Psychiatry, Blythedale Children's Hospital, Valhalla, New York, and Faculty Member, William Alanson White Institute for Psychoanalysis, New York.

MICHAEL G. KALOGERAKIS is Associate Commissioner, Bureau of Children and Youth Services, State of New York. He was President, American Society for Adolescent Psychiatry, 1978–1979.

HENRY O. KANDLER is Assistant Clinical Professor of Psychiatry, Albert Einstein College of Medicine, Co-Director of the Adolescent Psychiatry Services at Bronx Municipal Hospital Center, and Director of the School Consultation Service.

OTTO F. KERNBERG is Professor of Psychiatry, Cornell University Medical College, and Medical Director, New York Hospital–Cornell Medical Center, Westchester Division. He is also a Training and Supervising Analyst for Psychoanalytic Training and Research.

PAULINA F. KERNBERG is Associate Professor, Cornell University Medical College, and Director, Child and Adolescent Psychiatry, New York Hospital–Cornell Medical Center, Westchester Division.

CLARICE J. KESTENBAUM is Associate Clinical Professor of Psychiatry, Columbia University College of Physicians and Surgeons, and Director, Division of Child and Adolescent Psychiatry, St. Luke's Hospital, New York.

JONATHAN E. KOLB is Instructor in Psychiatry, Harvard Medical School, and Assistant Psychiatrist of Outpatient Services, McLean Hospital, Belmont, Massachusetts.

SAUL V. LEVINE is Professor of Psychiatry, University of Toronto, and Coordinator of Adolescent Psychiatric Services, Hospital for Sick Children.

JOHN G. LOONEY is Staff Child Psychiatrist, Timberlawn Psychiatric Hospital, Dallas.

CARL P. MALMQUIST is Professor of Law and Criminal Justice, University of Minnesota.

RICHARD C. MAROHN is Director, Adolescent and Forensic Services, Illinois State Psychiatric Institute, and Attending Psychiatrist, Michael Reese Hospital and Medical Center. Dr. Marohn is also Treasurer, American Society for Adolescent Psychiatry.

AKE MATTSSON is Professor of Child Psychiatry, New York University School of Medicine.

MICHAEL J. MILLER is Consultant Psychologist, Cabrini Medical Center, New York.

DANIEL OFFER is Professor of Psychiatry, Pritzker School of Medicine, University of Chicago, and Chairman of the Institute for Psychosomatic and Psychiatric Research and Training, Michael Reese Medical Center. He is Past President, American Society for Adolescent Psychiatry.

ERIC OSTROV is Research Director, Adolescent Program, Illinois State Psychiatric Institute, Chicago.

JONAS ROBITSCHER is Henry R. Luce Professor of Law and the Behavioral Sciences, Emory University, Atlanta, Georgia.

PERIHAN A. ROSENTHAL is Associate Clinical Professor of Psychiatry, Tufts Medical School, Boston, and Chief of Child Psychiatry, University of Massachusetts.

JOHN L. SCHIMEL is a Training and Supervising Analyst, William Alanson White Institute of Psychoanalysis, New York.

EDWARD R. SHAPIRO is Assistant Professor of Psychiatry, Harvard Medical School, and Director, Adolescent and Family Treatment and Study Center, McLean Hospital, Belmont, Massachusetts.

ROGER L. SHAPIRO is Clinical Professor of Psychiatry and Behavioral Science, George Washington University School of Medicine, and Chairman, Washington-Baltimore Center of the A. K. Rich Institute.

JON A. SHAW is Clinical Associate Professor, Georgetown University Medical School and the Uniformed Services University of the Health Sciences, and Chief, Child and Adolescent Psychiatry Service, Walter Reed Army Medical Center, Washington, D.C.

MEYER SONIS is Professor of Child Psychiatry, University of Pittsburgh School of Medicine.

ARTHUR D. SOROSKY is Assistant Clinical Professor of Child Psychiatry, University of California at Los Angeles.

MAX SUGAR is Clinical Professor of Psychiatry, Louisiana State University School of Medicine. He is Past President, American Society for Adolescent Psychiatry.

JAIME TRUJILLO is Chief of Inpatient Services, Adolescent Program, Illinois State Psychiatric Institute, Chicago.

THEODORE VAN PUTTEN is Associate Professor of Psychiatry, University of California at Los Angeles.

NOAH WEINSTEIN is a Juvenile Court Judge, St. Louis, Missouri.

SIDNEY L. WERKMAN is Professor of Psychiatry, University of Colorado School of Medicine.

LYNN WHISNANT is Assistant Professor of Clinical Psychiatry and Associate Director of Undergraduate Education in Psychiatry, Yale University School of Medicine.

LEONARD ZEGANS is Professor of Psychiatry and Director of Education, University of California School of Medicine at San Francisco.

CONTENTS OF VOLUMES I–VI

NAME INDEX

559

SUBJECT INDEX